Three-Dimensional
Biomedical Imaging

Three-Dimensional Biomedical Imaging

Principles and Practice

Richard A. Robb

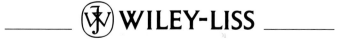

A JOHN WILEY & SONS, INC., PUBLICATION
New York • Chichester • Weinheim • Brisbane • Singapore • Toronto

Copyright © 1998 by John Wiley & Sons, Inc. All rights reserved.

Published simultaneously in Canada.

Library of Congress Cataloging-in-Publication Data:

Robb, Richard A.
   Three-dimensional biomedical imaging : principles and practice /
Richard A. Robb.
      p.   cm.
   "A Wiley-Liss Publication."
   Includes bibliographical references and index.
   ISBN 0-471-25238-7 (pbk. : alk. paper)
   1. Three-dimensional imaging systems in medicine.   2. Three
-dimensional imaging systems in biology.   I. Title.
   [R857.T47R63   1998]
   616.07'54--dc21   97-40459
                                               CIP

Printed in the United States of America.

10 9 8 7 6 5 4 3 2 1

Preface

"I want to reach a point of condensation of sensations to make a picture."

Henri Matisse

As an artist, Matisse intuitively sensed the potency of images for synthesis and expression of information. Human vision provides an extraordinarily powerful and effective means for acquiring information. Much of what we know about ourselves and our environment has been derived from images—images produced by various instruments, ranging from microscopes to telescopes, which extend the range of human vision into realms beyond that which is naturally accessible. In addition to art and aesthetics, images have profound scientific significance and value. More than "pretty" pictures, science needs "useful" pictures. Recent development of advanced quantitative methods to fully analyze the intrinsic information contained in images has begun to unearth the rich treasures they contain and to exploit their full scientific, educational, and biomedical value.

Imaging science involves the study of imaging processes and products (i.e., the images themselves). The challenge of imaging science is to define and facilitate development of advanced capabilities for acquisition, processing, visualization, and quantitative analysis of images in order to significantly increase the faithful extraction of the scientific, educational, and clinical information which they contain. This is a formidable task, one which consistently suggests that continued advances are required to address it effectively. The need for new approaches to image analysis has become increasingly important and pressing as advances in imaging technology enable more complex objects and processes to be imaged and simulated.

The traditional disciplines of biological and medical science are significantly grounded in the observation of living structures and in the measurement of various properties of these structures (e.g., their functions). These observations and measurements are often recorded as images. Ever since the invention of the microscope and the discovery of X-rays, physicians, surgeons, and life scientists have been using images to diagnose and treat disease and to better understand basic physiology and biology. The value of biomedical images depends upon the context in which they are obtained and the scientific or medical interests and goals that motivate their production and use. The importance of mensuration in biomedical visualization cannot be overstated. Measurable pictures are useful pictures!

Medical imaging has its roots in the discovery of the X-ray by Röntgen in 1895. However, it wasn't until 75 years later that a major innovation in medical imaging had revolutionary impact on the use of imaging in diagnosis and treatment. The advent of X-ray computed tomographic (CT) scanning in the early 1970s provided the capability for seeing into the body in a way not possible before, with accuracy and precision not delivered by conventional X-ray techniques. The ensuing two decades saw 3-D imaging develop slowly as a useful technology in medicine and clinical practice. However, with the current availability of advanced computers and associated software programs, and the ever-improving fidelity and increased resolution of medical imaging systems, the initial promise of 3-D imaging for significant improvements in diagnosis and treatment of disease is now beginning to be realized. 3-D imaging is becoming routinely used in such clinical applications as surgery simulation, radiotherapy planning, and quantification of tissue pathology.

The imaging modalities used in biology and medicine are based on a variety of energy sources, including light, electrons, lasers, X-rays, radionuclides, ultrasound, and nuclear magnetic resonance. The images produced span orders of magnitude in scale, ranging from molecules and cells to organ systems and the full body. The advantages and limitations of each modality are primarily governed by the basic physical and biological principles that influence the way each energy form interacts with tissues, and by the specific engineering implementation for a particular medical or biological application. The variety of disease processes and abnormalities affecting all regions of the human body are so numerous and different that each imaging modality possesses attributes that make it uniquely helpful in providing the desired understanding and/or discrimination of the disease or abnormality, and therefore no single method has prevailed to the complete exclusion of others. In general, the methodologies are complementary, together providing a powerful armamentarium of clinical diagnostic, therapeutic, and biomedical research capabilities which has potential to significantly advance the practice of medicine and the frontiers of biological understanding.

The complementary nature of many of the 3-D imaging modalities has given rise to the era of *multimodality imaging* and provides a new emphasis in imaging science. This emphasis might be referred to as the *calculus of imaging,* namely, differentiation and integration of 3-D images. Arguably the most important challenges, and the most profound promises, of 3-D imaging in biology and medicine are automatic segmentation and classification (i.e., differentiation) of tissues and tissue properties, and conversely the registration and "fusion" (i.e., integration) of the complementary information provided by different imaging modalities into a single multivalued image (i.e., a vector image). Significantly, the synthesis of multimodal, multidimensional images into registered vector images provides enhanced opportunities for accurate selective segmentation, and accurate segmentation provides improved capabilities for truly synergistic and more precise measurements of local features and properties (i.e., analogous to piecewise differentiation in the integral calculus).

Imaging science and biomedical visualization have benefited by the significant advances in the microelectronics industry during the last three decades. The capabilities of the supercomputers of yesterday are now available in desktop workstations for a fraction of the cost. These powerful computational capabilities made available at modest cost have virtually "liberated" programmers and software developers to be more creative—to be able to develop and test algorithms without spending significant periods of time and effort in optimizing code or compromising functionality to achieve acceptable performance. Concomitantly, the quality of the images produced by medical and biological imaging systems has increased dramatically in the last decade, providing faithful high-resolution recordings of 3-D objects. The combination of high-quality 3-D images and high-performance low-cost computing provides an ideal opportunity for the development of powerful yet practical software for *useful* biomedical image visualization, manipulation, and measurement.

The algorithms and processes required for useful display and analysis of multidimensional, multimodal biomedical images have been synthesized into several types of available 3-D software packages. These software programs feature integrated, comprehensive tools for fully interactive 3-D display, manipulation, and measurement of biomedical image data. Such 3-D software incorporates many functions for solving the calculus of imaging, and for exploring, developing, testing and applying solutions to real problems. The software systems have proven readily extensible, so that new approaches and paradigms can be tested, evaluated and documented. The rapid improvement and deployment of 3-D software has been facilitated and nurtured by concomitant improvements in computer performance, software development aids, and network environment support tools.

This book features one such 3-D software system—ANALYZE™—developed at the Mayo Clinic and currently in use in hundreds of universities, hospitals, and other institutions around the world. ANALYZE™ has been applied to data from many different imaging modalities. It runs efficiently on standard workstation computers without the need for special-purpose hardware.

The 3-D packages like ANALYZE℠ are successful when they are comprehensive, integrated, and provide functionality that addresses a broad range of medical and biological problems. They must feature solutions to the most important challenges in biomedical imaging, including segmentation, classification, registration, and display. Current packages are largely generic; they can be applied to any imaging modality or image forms. In medicine they can be used productively on magnetic resonance (MR) images, CT images, position emission tomographic (PET) or single photon emission tomographic (SPECT) images, and ultrasound images. In basic science they can be used on images from conventional light microscopy, electron microscopy, or confocal microscopy. They can be used in education to teach anatomy and function to medical students and clinical trainees. They can be used in nonmedical applications, such as industrial inspection, geology, meteorology and astronomy.

Biomedical imaging software has provided a strong bridge between science and practice, spanning the gap from basic research to clinical usefulness. ANALYZE℠, for example, is being used in a large number of multidisciplinary research and clinical projects. Thousands of scientists, engineers, physicians, and surgeons use it on hundreds of computer workstations. Its applications are broad in scope, wide in scale, and penetrating in impact. It can be used on microscopic or telescopic images to study molecules or galaxies; it can be used to study functions of cells or to plan surgical operations; it can be used to display and measure properties of organelles, organs, or organ systems; indeed, it can be used to analyze the structure–function relationships within cell bodies, human bodies, or heavenly bodies. It has significantly contributed to the establishment of 3-D imaging as a powerful new technology in basic research and clinical medicine.

Although the ANALYZE℠ software system is used to illustrate many concepts and processes throughout this book, the work is not strictly about ANALYZE℠. ANALYZE℠ is much more than a software system: it is a philosophy, a paradigm for scientific investigation, an efficient environment to support biological imaging research and medical imaging practice. This book is about that philosophy, about that paradigm, about that environment.

The book provides an overview of 3-D biomedical imaging, from science to practice. It begins with first principles, progresses from simple to sophisticated technology and methods, and concludes with examples of current applications and implications for future advances. Within this spectrum are included eight chapters which respectively describe: 1) historical perspectives, fundamental principles and definitions, contemporary issues, and current approaches in 3-D biomedical imaging; 2) multimodality systems for acquisition and representation of 3-D biomedical image data; 3) computational systems for 3-D image display and analysis; 4) processing and visualization methods for enhancing and rendering 3-D biomedical image data; 5) methods for segmenting, registering, and integrating multimodality 3-D biomedical images; 6) mensuration of 3-D biomedical image features and properties, and the meaning of such measurements; 7) examples of practical applications of 3-D biomedical imaging in basic biology, clinical diagnosis, and medical treatment; and 8) summary and prognostications for future advances in multidimensional, multimodality biomedical imaging.

These themes comprise a publication that should serve as a useful and enduring reference for those interested and engaged in the field of 3-D biomedical imaging.

Richard A. Robb
Rochester, MN
September, 1994

Preface to the Paperback Edition

I am pleased that Wiley has determined to provide a paperback edition of *Three-Dimensional Biomedical Imaging: Principles and Practice,* and hope this will facilitate access to the book by a broader segment of the imaging sciences community, particularly students and educators. The "principles and practice" described and illustrated in this book are enduring, and provide the reader with a comprehensive basic introduction to three-dimensional biomedical imaging science and applications. Consequently, I feel it would be an ideal text for an initial academic course in the discipline. In addition, familiarity with the fundamental theories, systems, and methods presented in *Three-Dimensional Biomedical Imaging,* along with some of their practical applications, will be useful preparation for understanding a sequel to this book, entitled *Biomedical Imaging, Visualization, and Analysis,* which I am currently preparing with Wiley. This second book will expose the reader to new ideas and paradigms, advanced methodologies, and extensive applications of imaging in medicine and biology.

Richard A. Robb
September, 1997

Acknowledgments

The author is grateful for the important contributions to this work by the staff of the Biomedical Imaging Resource (BIR) and their collaborators at the Mayo Foundation. In particular, Jon Camp, Dennis Hanson, Ron Karwoski, and Mahlon Stacy assisted in developing several of the chapters. Special appreciation is expressed to Gina Croatt for preparation of the manuscript and to Margret Ryan and Eileen McMahon for editorial assistance. The combined dedication, talents, and experience of the BIR staff have helped define and realize the field of 3-D biomedical imaging and expand it from theory and principles to practice and applications.

Contents

Chapter 3 The Image Computer 73

Chapter 4 Image Processing and Visualization   117

Figure Credits

Figure 2.1 (From Robb, R. A., *Three-Dimensional Biomedical Imaging*, 1, 7, 1985, Chapter 2, Nudelman, S. and Roehrig, H. Photoelectronic-Digital Imaging for Diagnostic Radiology. Reprinted by permission of CRC Press, Boca Raton, Florida). **Figures 2.2, 2.3a, 2.4a, 2.5a, 2.6a, 2.7a** (From Drew Consultants, Inc., Carlisle, MA. With permission). **Figure 2.8** (From Instrumentarium Corporation, Helsinki, Finland. With permission). **Figure 2.10** (From Robb, R. A., *Critical Reviews in Biomedical Engineering*, 7, 4, 271, 1982. Reprinted by permission of CRC Press, Boca Raton, Florida). **Figure 2.11** (From Robb, R. A., *Critical Reviews in Biomedical Engineering*, 7, 4, 272, 1982. Reprinted by permission of CRC Press, Boca Raton, Florida). **Figure 2.12** (From Robb, R. A., *Critical Reviews in Biomedical Engineering*, 7, 4, 274, 1982. Reprinted by permission of CRC Press, Boca Raton, Florida). **Figure 2.13** (From Robb, R. A., *Critical Reviews in Biomedical Engineering*, 7, 4, 276, 1982. Reprinted by permission of CRC Press, Boca Raton, Florida). **Figure 2.14** (From Robb, R. A., *Critical Reviews in Biomedical Engineering*, 7, 4, 277, 1982. Reprinted by permission of CRC Press, Boca Raton, Florida). **Figure 2.15** (From Robb, R. A., *Critical Reviews in Biomedical Engineering*, 7, 4, 279, 1982. Reprinted by permission of CRC Press, Boca Raton, Florida). **Figure 2.16** (From Robb, R. A., *Critical Reviews in Biomedical Engineering*, 7, 4, 280, 1982. Reprinted by permission of CRC Press, Boca Raton, Florida). **Figure 2.18** (From Robb, R. A., *Critical Reviews in Biomedical Engineering*, 7, 4, 285, 1982. Reprinted by permission of CRC Press, Boca Raton, Florida). **Figure 2.19** (From Robb, R. A., *Critical Reviews in Biomedical Engineering*, 7, 4, 291, 1982. Reprinted by permission of CRC Press, Boca Raton, Florida). **Figure 2.20** (From Robb, R. A., *Critical Reviews in Biomedical Engineering*, 7, 4, 292, 1982. Reprinted by permission of CRC Press, Boca Raton, Florida). **Figure 2.21** (From Robb, R. A., *Critical Reviews in Biomedical Engineering*, 7, 4, 293, 1982. Reprinted by permission of CRC Press, Boca Raton, Florida). **Figure 2.22** (From Robb, R. A., *Critical Reviews in Biomedical Engineering*, 7, 4, 294, 1982. Reprinted by permission of CRC Press, Boca Raton, Florida). **Figure 2.23** (From Robb, R. A., *Critical Reviews in Biomedical Engineering*, 7, 4, 304, 1982. Reprinted by permission of CRC Press, Boca Raton, Florida). **Figure 2.24** (From Harris, L. D., Ritman, E. L., and Robb, R. A., Computer generated 3-D display of x-ray computed tomographic volume image data, *Proceedings of the 1st European Conference on Cineradiography with Photons or Particles*, SPIE 312, 177, 1981. With permission). **Figure 4.18** (From Heffernan, P. B. and Robb, R. A., A new method for shaded surface display of biological and medical images, *IEEE Transactions on Medical Imaging*, MI-4(1)28 (March) 1985. © 1985 IEEE). **Figures 4.20, 4.21** (From Robb, R. A. and Barillot, C., Interactive display and analysis of 3-D medical images, *IEEE Transactions on Medical Imaging*, 8(3)222, September, 1989. © 1989 IEEE). **Figures 4.22, 4.23, 4.24** (From Robb, R. A. and Barillot, C., Interactive display and analysis of 3-D medical images, *IEEE Transactions on Medical Imaging*, 8(3)223, September, 1989. © 1989 IEEE). **Figure 5.32** (From Jiang, H., Robb, R. A., and Holton, K. S., A new approach to 3-D registration of multimodality medical images by surface matching, *Proceedings of Visualization in Biomedical Computing 1992*, SPIE 1808, 209, 1992. With permission). **Figure 5.34** (From Jiang, H., Robb, R. A., and Holton, K. S., A new approach to 3-D registration of multimodality medical images by surface matching, *Proceedings of Visualization in Biomedical Computing 1992*, SPIE 1808, 210, 1992. With permission). **Figure 5.37** (From Jiang, H., Robb, R. A., and Holton, K. S., A new approach to 3-D registration of multimodality medical images by surface matching, *Proceedings of Visualization in Biomedical Computing 1992*, SPIE 1808, 212, 1992. With permission).

1

First Principles

Seeing. We might say that the whole of life lies in that verb.
Pierre Teilhard de Chardin, *The Phenomenon of Man*

1.1 Introduction

To be able to "see" into the body has always been and remains a primary capability desired and necessary to study and elucidate the basic processes of life, and to diagnose and treat the disease conditions that perturb and endanger the normal function of biological processes. This capability can be achieved by surgically cutting into the body to look directly at the structures and functions of interest. However, because of the life-threatening risk and pain involved, this approach should be restricted to treatment of disease and not used for diagnosis.

The viability of organisms, including humans, is critically dependent on the virtually continuous movements of fluids that supply nutrition to and carry waste from all tissues.[1] In humans, the life-sustaining movements of these vital fluids are actuated and controlled by voluntary and involuntary musculature. Consequently, physiological function is, to a major degree, based on the functions of the muscle cells that generate the forces which result in and control these movements. The function of these cells is determined by their atomic composition, biochemical nature, metabolic characteristics, and geometric arrangement and by the changes in these properties within the 3-D configuration and dimensions of the anatomic structures in which they are imbedded. Improved understanding of both the normal and the pathophysiological processes of life in humans depends on the development of methods to *directly* and *accurately* visualize and measure these anatomic domains and functional variables.

Because the function and interaction of bodily organs and tissues are readily affected by physical interventions into their working environment, and since these interventions may result in alterations of the anatomic and/or functional status being studied, it is desirable to devise direct measurement techniques that involve the minimum possible degree of morphological and physiological disturbance. The transmission of radiant energy (e.g., X-rays, gamma rays, radio waves, or ultrasound waves) through the body produces images without subjective sensations and does not directly affect the function of bodily tissues at the dose levels required to produce useful images. A beam of radiation passing through the body is absorbed and scattered by structures in the beam path to varying degrees, depending on the composition of these structures and on the energy level of the beam.[2] It is this differential absorption and scatter pattern by tissues within the body which is carried in the transmitted beam and recorded by a detector to produce an image of the tissues. Since a variety of sources of radiant energy are available that can be administered at levels selected and/or controlled to readily penetrate and be absorbed to some degree by all bodily tissues, radiographic images can be produced of every body organ, ranging in density from bone to lung. The images produced from radiant emanations passing through parts of the body provide a direct recording of internal, unseen structures.

1.2 Historical Perspectives

In 1895, Wilhelm Conrad Röntgen, a German physicist working in his laboratory at the University of Würzburg, made the "great discovery of the invisible ray" as he was making observations of fluorescence using cathode ray tubes[3] (see Figure 1.1). The initial discovery was followed quickly by a number of carefully contrived experiments to elucidate the properties of this marvelous new ray. The potential applications of "Röntgen's ray" (subsequently nicknamed X-rays) in medicine and biology were quickly recognized, as many scientists repeated, improved, and expanded Röntgen's experiments[3-5] (see Figure 1.2). In a remarkably short time, scientists and physicians began exploiting this exciting new capability to at long last "see into the body" in a painless, nondestructive way. Röntgen was hailed by scientific and medical peers as a messiah, ushering in a new century with his revolutionary discovery.

The discovery of X-rays heralded a new era in the practice of medicine that permitted visualization into the body without painful and often dangerous surgery. The discovery was almost immediately recognized and accepted for its potential as a new medical diagnostic technique. X-ray imaging is esssentially noninvasive. Modest risks are incurred due to the ionizing effect of the X-rays,[3] but these risks are usually acceptable because of the diagnostic advantages provided by direct visualization of intracorporeal

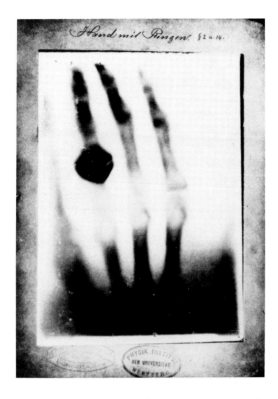

Figure 1.1.   First radiograph of hand made by W. C. Röntgen on December 22, 1895. Historical notes[3,4] suggest it is the hand of Röntgen's wife. Note the ring on the third finger. Original plate is in the Deutsche Museum, Munich, Germany. (From Glasser, O., *Wilhelm Conrad Röntgen and the Early History of the Röntgen Rays*, Charles C. Thomas, Springfield, IL, 1934.)

structures when such examination is indicated by illness and associated symptoms. The intervening years since the discovery of X-rays have been characterized by a succession of evolutionary improvements in radiographic instrumentation and photographic procedures. One notable development was the introduction of fluoroscopic imaging with an image intensifier in the late 1940s.[6] This technology was coupled with that of television to provide dynamic X-ray imaging systems. Nuclear medicine tomographic imaging[7] and ultrasonography were important developments of the 1950s and 1960s. However, not until the 1970s did the field again witness an "epoch-making" development of similar magnitude to that of Röntgen's discovery. The basic radiographic process used by Röntgen to photograph the internal structures of the body had not changed for more than 75 years. A film or screen containing a radiation-sensitive material is exposed to the X-rays transmitted through a region of the body. The developed film or excited phosphorus

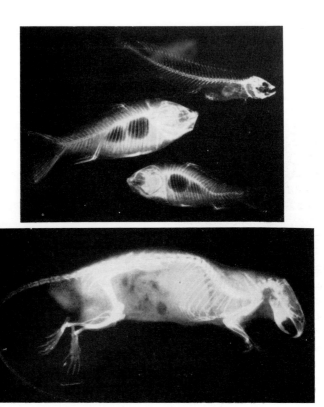

Figure 1.2. X-radiographs of goldfish and a rat made in February 1896, by J. A. Eder and E. Valentin.[4] These are negative plates, which is the same format used today in most conventional radiographic methods. The anatomic detail is remarkably excellent, considering that the X-ray had been discovered only two months prior to recording of these radiographs. (From Glasser, O., *Wilhelm Conrad Röntgen and the Early History of the Röntgen Rays,* Charles C. Thomas, Springfield, IL, 1934.)

screen exhibits a geometric pattern produced by the structures in the beam path.

The ongoing development of radiologic imaging instrumentation[2] and techniques perhaps has accomplished more to benefit man in the detection and delineation of disease than any other medical diagnostic procedure. The techniques provide clear photographs of internal structures. Rapid imaging systems can provide dynamic recordings of internal moving organs. Contrast angiography, which involves injection of radiopaque substances into the bloodstream, enables visualization of the circulation to, from, and within almost any organ of the body.

However, conventional X-ray imaging techniques have several important limitations. Small characteristic differences (1% to 2%) in X-ray atatenuation by various body tissues are not detectable in recordings on X-ray film or fluoroscopic screens. A large percentage of the radiation detected is scattered from the body, thus reducing the true signal-to-noise ratio of the recorded information. And much detail is lost in the radiographic process due to superposition of 3-D structural information onto a 2-D detector.

The development of X-ray computed tomography (CT) in the early 1970s[8,9] was based on a classic treatise by Radon in 1915 which described a mathematically rigorous inversion formula for reconstruction of an object from its projections.[10] CT had a revolutionary impact on diagnostic imaging with X-rays because it eliminated or greatly minimized these problems. Transaxial scanning, with a highly collimated rotating X-ray source, coupled with computer-based image reconstruction techniques, provides unambiguous images of the cross-sectional dimensions of the body with excellent discrimination of soft tissue differences.

During the decade of the 1970s, the development of X-ray CT advanced rapidly. Although the method is based upon a complementary synthesis of several basic and applied science principles,[11] its success is due primarily to the power and speed of the computer. In only a few years, the X-ray CT technique had a meteoric rise from its inception in the laboratory to widespread, routine clinical utilization. It has literally revolutionized medical imaging, particularly in the field of radiology. This achievement was recognized with the awarding of the Nobel Prize in 1979.[12] The co-recipients were Allan Macleod Cormack and Godfrey Newbold Hounsfield for their independent and unique contributions to the invention of X-ray computer-assisted tomography (CAT), also known as computed tomography (CT). It is notable that the award was made in physiology and medicine because, although the CT method is based upon a complementary synthesis of basic and applied science principles, its most prolific and profound application has been in clinical medicine,[9,11] enabling physicians, without surgery, to examine internal structures of the body with a sensitivity and specificity never available to them before.

In the mid 1950s, Bracewell[13] published one of the earliest works on the problem of reconstructing an object from its projections. In the late 1950s, Cormack became interested in the determination of the distribution of attenuation coefficients in tissues of the body in order to improve radiation treatment planning. He recognized that perhaps if enough X-ray views were taken at different angles, sufficient information would be available to uniquely determine the internal structure of the body, and diagnostically useful images could be reconstructed from these determinations. His early studies[14] led to a mathematically accurate way of quantitatively reconstructing cross-sectional images from X-ray projections (radiographs).

In the late 1960s, the British scientist Godfrey Hounsfield was independently developing his ideas that mathematical techniques could be used to reconstruct the internal structure of the body from a number of X-ray measurements. He developed an intuitive mathematical approach to the image reconstruction problem and carried out significant theoretical calculations to conclude that the quantitative tomographic technique could produce up to 100 times more accurate measurements of the absolute value of X-ray attenuation coefficients within the body than conventional radiographic methods.[15] This realization motivated the construction and testing of several prototype scanners in the Central Research Laboratories of Elector-Musical Instruments, Ltd. (EMI), progressing from bench-top gamma-ray sources to X-ray sources, with computers coupled to the scintillation detectors in order to complete a scan and process the data in a practical period of time.

These efforts eventually resulted in construction of the first clinical X-ray CT scanner for the head, called simply the EMI brain scanner, which was installed at Atkinson Morleys Hospital, Wimbledon, England, in 1971. After more than a year of collection of experimental and clinical data, the results from the EMI brain scanner were presented in 1972, followed by the now classic publications in 1973,[8,9] which heralded the revolutionary era of diagnostic X-ray CT. Hounsfield accomplished a remarkable synthesis by 1) recognizing the diagnostic need, 2) developing a numerically implementable mathematical solution to the image reconstruction problem, and 3) organizing electromechanical and X-ray technology into a precisely engineered instrument that resulted in a successful clinical machine.

With the successful introduction of the EMI brain scanner into the clinical arena, an explosive development and marketing of CT scanners by a variety of manufacturers followed. By 1976, more than 20 companies were producing one or more models of X-ray CT scanners for commercial purposes. By 1980, this number had decreased significantly, as smaller companies realized they could not compete with major radiographic equipment manufacturers. The beginning of the 1980s saw CT scanners in many medical institutions throughout the world,[15] with an ever-increasing accumulation of published data[16] and experience with these systems relating to a wide variety of clinical applications.[17] Perhaps more importantly, both the disadvantages of X-ray CT (e.g., use of ionizing radiation) and its promise (high-resolution 3-D imaging) gave birth to 3-D *multimodality* CT using other imaging forms.

The potential utilization of 3-D imaging in biomedical research is just beginning to be explored. The realization that this tool may be useful in basic biological investigations has been precipitated by the continually improving capability of 3-D imaging for quantitative tissue characterization[18,19] and by the promise of dynamic scanning for measurement of functional parameters.[20–24] 3-D imaging provides excellent visualization of anatomic detail, but its potential for elucidating several important biological questions requires continuing improvement of capabilities for measurement of tissue composition and organ function, as well as anatomic structure. 3-D imaging, using energy sources other than X-ray, such as radioisotopes and radiopharmaceuticals,[25,26] nuclear magnetic resonance,[27,28] and ultrasound,[29,30] can provide certain information about tissue functions and properties not obtainable with radiographic 3-D imaging. This information is clinically significant and also has prospects for use in biomedical investigations.

Improved specificity in 3-D imaging may be accomplished by development of near-simultaneous multienergy scanning methods,[31-33] wherein 3-D image scanning is performed using two or more different radiant energies, either at the same time, in quick succession, or in an "interleaved" scan mode. These capabilities, sometimes called "tomochemistry" or "tomodensitometry," show definite promise but are in the infancy of development, progress being slow because of the physical constraints in building 3-D imaging systems that can scan efficiently with multiple energy sources. Techniques for simultaneous multienergy scanning would be greatly expedited by the development of efficient and economical energy-selective detectors and/or monoenergetic sources.

Over the years there have been numerous improvements in the basic tomographic methodology. These advances have been spurred by the development of more sophisticated and powerful instruments and techniques using a variety of energy forms that have broadened and refined the uses of medical imaging. The physician is now provided with significant capabilities for noninvasive examination of internal structures of the body with an accuracy and specificity never before available. The ability to extract objective and quantitatively accurate information from either conventional or tomographic radiographic images has developed slowly since the discovery of X-rays. But modern computers have made possible the development of several new imaging modalities that use different sources of radiant energy to elucidate different properties of body tissues. These methods have significant potential for providing greater specificity and sensitivity (i.e., precise objective discrimination and accurate quantitative measurement of body tissue characteristics and function) in clinical diagnostic and basic investigative imaging procedures than ever before possible. The momentous role of the computer and associated software advances in making these capabilities possible cannot be overemphasized.

Imaging science and biomedical visualization have benefited by the significant advances in the microelectronics industry during the last three decades. The capabilities of the supercomputers of yesterday are now available in desktop workstations for a fraction of the cost. These capabilities have virtually liberated programmers and software developers to develop and test algorithms without spending significant time and effort in optimizing code or compromising functionality to achieve acceptable performance. Concomitantly, the improvements in the quality of images produced by medical and biological imaging systems have increased dramatically in the last decade, providing faithful high-resolution recordings of 3-D objects. The combination of high-quality 3-D images and high-performance, low-cost computing has provided an ideal opportunity for the development of powerful yet practical software for *useful* biomedical image visualization, measurement, and manipulation. As suggested in Figure 1.3 (see color figure 1), these computational and 3-D biomedical visualization capabilities have been applied to a wide variety of organs, tissues, and cells. Almost a century later, Röntgen's

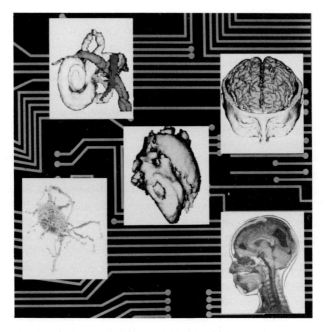

Figure 1.3. Depiction of 3-D biomedical images of structure and function of organs, tissues, and cells, made possibly by modern electronic computing methods. See color figure 1.

discovery of seeing into the body continues to take on remarkable new dimensions.

1.3 Fundamental Issues and Definitions

Although the various modern imaging modalities differ somewhat in the energy forms, equipment, and computational approaches used in the image formation process, they all have in common a unique and powerful capability—to produce, by noninvasive means, accurate numerical representations of the distributions of various structures and functional processes within the body.[34] In many of the modalities, this capability provides an unambiguous view of the "third dimension," often presented as images of cross-sectional slices through the body region of interest. The general principles of physics and mathematics upon which these different imaging modalities are based are fundamentally similar.[2,35] Some form of energy is measured after its passage through a region of the body, and from these measurements, mathematical estimates are computed and images produced of the 2-D or 3-D distribution of interactions between the energy and the body tissues (e.g., absorption, attenuation, or nuclear mechanical disturbances). However, the specific details of applying these principles, the engineering and instrumentation developed to reduce them to practice, and, most significantly, the information content and quality of the final images are quite different. This is primarily due to the different energy–tissue interactions that are measured and to the varying biological, physical, and technological constraints imposed in obtaining these measurements in a practical way.[2]

The imaging modalities used in biology and medicine are based on a variety of energy sources, including light, electrons, lasers, X-rays, radionuclides, ultrasound, and nuclear magnetic resonance. The images produced span orders of magnitude in scale, ranging from molecules and cells to organ systems and the full body. The advantages and limitations of each imaging modality are primarily governed by the basic physical and biological principles that influence the way each energy form interacts with tissues, and by the specific engineering implementation for a particular medical or biological application. The variety of disease processes and abnormalities affecting all regions of the human body are so numerous and different that each imaging modality possesses attributes that make it uniquely helpful in providing the desired understanding and discrimination of the disease or abnormality, and therefore no single method has prevailed to the complete exclusion of others. Even though significant disparity in scale and characteristic features separate the imaging realms, striking parallels and common approaches exist relative to visualization and analysis of these images. In general, the methodologies are complementary, together providing a powerful and synergistic armamentarium of clinical diagnostic, therapeutic, and biomedical research capabilities which has potential to significantly advance the practice of medicine and the frontiers of biological understanding.

The process of forming an image involves *mapping* an object or some property of an object into or onto "image space." This space is used to visualize the object and its properties, and may be used to quantitatively characterize its structure or function. *Imaging science* may be defined as the study of these mappings and the development of ways to understand them, improve them, and use them productively. Generally, the steps involved in imaging procedures include image-data acquisition, image display and analysis, and image interpretation (i.e., perception, cognition, and understanding). Most modern imaging devices are digital computer-based and produce images in the form of arrays of 2-D picture elements (pixels) or 3-D volume elements (voxels). The numbers associated with these pixels and voxels represent the mappings of object properties that can be detected and localized spatially and/or functionally and which quantitatively characterize the object properties. The agenda for the field of imaging science is to develop a comprehensive understanding of all of the steps involved in the biomedical imaging process and the complex ways in which they are interdependent, so that parameters pertaining to each step can be optimized to improve the basic scientific, diagnostic, and therapeutic value of biomedical images.

Closely associated with imaging science is scientific visualization. Visualization is more than simply observing images. It involves 1) realistic and faithful display of objects captured or synthesized as images, 2) effective manipulation and editing of images, and 3) precise and accurate measurement of image (object) properties. Visualization supports imaging science as its principal *modus operandi.*

Four postulates fundamentally important in imaging science and scientific visualization derive from these definitions. 1) Image mappings, varied as they are, provide direct measurements of form or function. 2) The "gestalt" or whole of a digital or computer image is significant: the contextual "glue" that holds discrete images together contains important information. 3) The individual pixel is also important, since it contains subtle details fundamental to understanding the mapping of the real object and its properties into image space. 4) There are many ways, mostly arbitrary, to display, manipulate, and measure digital images; a rational basis for their selection and use is important to both the scientist and physician.

The particular challenge of biomedical computing in visualization is to define and formulate such a rational basis and to develop the associated capabilities for acquisition, processing, display, and quantitative analysis that will significantly increase the faithful extraction of both scientific and clinical information contained in biomedical images. This is a formidable task, one which consistently suggests that continued advances are required to address it effectively. The need for new approaches to image visualization and analysis will become increasingly important and pressing as improvements in imaging technology enable more complex objects and processes to be imaged and simulated.

The complementary nature of many of the 3-D imaging modalities has given rise to several new approaches in imaging science, particularly medical imaging.[34,36] A common emphasis in these approaches might be referred to as the "calculus of imaging," namely, differentiation and integration of 3-D images. Arguably the most important challenges and the most profound promises, of 3-D imaging in biology and medicine are automatic segmentation and classification (i.e., differentiation) of tissues and tissue properties and conversely the registration and "fusion" (i.e., integration) of the complementary information provided by different imaging modalities into a single multivalued image. The synthesis of multimodal, multidimensional images into an integrated multispectral image would provide capabilities for truly synergistic measurements and advanced analyses of the life processes and their perturbations (e.g., disease).

1.4 Current Approaches

Although imaging science and biomedical visualization include significant components of theoretical research, they are primarily applied sciences.

They are largely devoted to solving real problems. This is particularly true in biomedical imaging, where the goal of imaging science is to apply the principles of imaging to diagnosing and treating disease and to gaining basic insights into the processes of life. The development of such capabilities in the research laboratory is a time-honored tradition. However, rarely do research methods developed primarily to solve one problem emerge to provide a viable solution to other problems for which they were not initially designed. Even less often are they sufficiently robust to result in advancing the entire field for good. Among the exceptions are certain advanced 3-D software packages. This book will be liberally illustrated with results from one such package, ANALYZE™, developed entirely at an academic biomedical institution, the Mayo Clinic.[37–39] Although not intended as the subject of this work, an "analysis of ANALYZE™" with regard to first principles is instructive.

The algorithms and programs developed for many research projects over several years were synthesized by the research staff at Mayo's Biomedical Imaging Resource into a comprehensive software system called ANALYZE™, now proven useful in a variety of multimodality, multidimensional biomedical imaging and scientific visualization applications. It is written entirely in the C programming language and contains approximately 500,000 lines of source code. It utilizes several features of the workstation operating system to facilitate and complement its modular architecture. The system is composed of over 50 individual programs or modules, each representing a specific function or class of functions, all of which are built on a base of a dozen libraries providing common I/O, graphics and other basic operations. Table 1.1 illustrates the organization of these ANALYZE™ modules into integrated, logical groups for file management, display, processing, measurement, ancillary utilities, and interactive tools. Table 1.2 provides a list of the modules with a brief description of each one.

ANALYZE™ features integrated, complementary tools for fully interactive display, manipulation, and measurement of multidimensional image data. It has been applied to data from many different imaging modalities. The software runs efficiently on many standard workstations without the need for special-purpose hardware.

Five complementary attributes of ANALYZE™ make it a uniquely powerful visualization package:

1. It is *comprehensive* and generic, containing a large number of intelligently and synergistically *integrated tools* for display, manipulation, and measurement of *multimodality* images;
2. It has several original algorithms that deal *directly* and *accurately* with *multidimensional* image data;
3. It is highly *operator-interactive;* most operations are performed in fractions of a second while preserving accuracy and image quality;
4. It is *intuitive and easy to use;* surgeons, physicians, and basic scientists can use it productively with little knowledge of computers;

Table 1.1. ANALYZE™ Module Groupings

Files	Display	Process	Measure
Load Images	**Section**	**Transform**	Line Profile
Save Images	Multiplanar	Image Albegra	Region of Interest
Header Edit	Oblique	Matrix Ops	Stereology
File Manager	Curved	Wavelet	Volume Estimator
Tape Read	Cube	**Filter**	Tree Trace
Convert Images	**Render**	Spatial	Plot
	Volume	Designer	
	Surface	3D FFT/Deconv	
	Other	**Histogram**	**Other**
	Contours	Global	Configure
	Intensity Grid	Adaptive	Screen Edit
	Movie	**Segment**	
		Image Edit	Macro Record
		2D Morphology	Macro Play
		3D Morphology	
		Connect	ERASE SCREEN
		Extract Contours	
		Classify	
		Multi-Spectral	
		Fusion	
		Surface Matching	

Tool Table		
HELP	Image Viewer	New Session
Magnifying Glass	Hardcopy	Toggle Session
Interactive Color	Text Editor	Disk Usage
Snap Shot	Calculator	Session Log
Caliper	UNIX Shell	

5. It is *extensible and transportable;* its modular design facilitates expedient enhancements, additions, and workstation implementations.

ANALYZE™ was not originally conceived as an exportable or marketable product. It was not even initially intended for clinical applications. It was based on first principles of imaging science and visualization and developed in a basic research environment to address important research questions involving biomedical images. It was "born" in 1985 as a streamlined, optimized synthesis of several proven approaches to relevant, important questions in biomedical imaging science. After only approximately two years of testing and use, the Mayo Clinic began to specifically explore the possibilities of transferring the software to the outside world. Because of the state-of-the-art capabilities of the software, the experience and expertise of the development team, their extensive international collaborations, and their understanding of the practical problems in the biomedical community, ANALYZE™ soon achieved wide-scale acceptance.

The ANALYZE™ software is successful because it incorporates many functions for solving the calculus of imaging and for exploring, developing, testing, and applying solutions to real problems. It is readily extensible so that new approaches and paradigms can be tested, evaluated, and documented. Indeed, ANALYZE™ functions and features have approximately doubled every year over its lifetime. This significant growth has been facilitated and nurtured by concomitant improvements in workstation performance, software development aids, and network environment support tools. Even though many of the new functions in evolving versions have incorporated more and more sophisticated algorithms and compute-intensive procedures, the performance of ANALYZE™ has still increased and improved. This is primarily attributable to the steady increases in performance provided by workstation manufacturers. But the first, uncompromised principle of developing the software entirely in a high-level language, independent of any customized hardware, firmware, or other software, permits the software to readily take immediate advantage of improvements in workstation performance.

ANALYZE™ has also been successful because it is readily portable, comprehensive, and integrated, providing functionality that addresses a broad range of problems and provides solutions to some of the most important challenges in contemporary biomedical imaging. These include segmentation, classification, registration, and display of 3-D biomedical images. Additionally, it has been designed and carefully programmed to be highly efficient and user-interactive, performing powerful 3-D image processing and display operations in near real-time or fractions of a second. As stated, ANALYZE™ is also generic; it has been and can be applied to any imaging modality and to any image data. In medicine it can be used productively on magnetic resonance (MR) images, CT images, positron emission tomographic (PET) or single photon emission tomographic (SPECT) images, and ultrasound images. In basic science it can be used on images from conventional light microscopy, electron microscopy, confocal microscopy, or tunneling microscopy. It can be used in education to teach anatomy and function to medical students and clinical trainees. It can even be used in nonmedical applications, such as industrial inspection, geology, and meteorology.

There is a growing market for useful 3-D imaging software. However, the software must meet the following criteria: 1) it must be comprehensive, 2) it must be directed toward relevant problems, and 3) it must be highly operator-responsive (interactive). The software system should be really *useful*, not (only) glamorous! It should manifest the visual metaphor that defines usefulness in 3-D image analysis, that is, it must produce realistic displays, generate precise and accurate quantitative measurements, and allow useful

Table 1.2. ANALYZE™ Module Description

Analyze	Coordinates all of the programs in the ANALYZE™ package.
Adaptive Histo	Performs Adaptive Histogram Equalization on images in the shared memory.
Calculator	Displays a calculator on your screen which performs quick on line calculations (*Tool Table*).
Caliper	Performs geometric measurements on the screen (*Tool Table*).
Configure	Enables the ANALYZE™ run time and workstation environment to be configured to specific preferences.
Connect	Segments a binary volume image using region growing from a selected seed pixel.
Contours	Enables the display of contours extracted from surface descriptions.
Convert Images	Converts images from one file format to another.
Cube Sections	Enables interactive generation and display of orthogonal sections in a 3-D cubic viewing environment.
Curved Sections	Extracts and displays curved planar section images.
Disk Usage	Displays the disk usage of the mounted directories (*Tool Table*).
Extract Contours	Extracts a surface contour from a binary volume.
File Manager	Provides file management facilities.
Filter Designer	Performs 2-D and 3-D convolution and deconvolution in the frequency domain using the *Fast Fourier Transform* (*FFT*).
3D FFT/Deconv	Performs 2-D and 3-D forward and inverse FFTs, convolutions, and deconvolutions on images.
Global Operations	Performs general-purpose histogram operations on images.
Header Edit	Enables editing and creation of image database header files.
Help	Displays the on-line manual pages (*Tool Table*).
Image Algebra	Facilitates formula-based algebraic image manipulation.
Image Edit	Enables the editing and changing of images in the shared memory segment.
Image Viewer	Enables the display of slices from ANALYZE™ database files (*Tool Table*).
Intensity Grid	Generates wiregrid displays of images.
Interactive Color	Enables manipulation of the display lookup table (*Tool Table*).
Line Profile	Enables interactive sampling and plotting of image intensities from profiles, lines, and curvilinear traces.
Load Images	Enables the selection of image files from disk to be loaded into the shared memory segment.
Macro Play	Plays back a recorded ANALYZE™ session.
Macro Record	Records an ANALYZE™ session.
Magnifying Glass	Magnifies regions of the screen, displays histograms of the regions, or enables viewing of the underlying screen pixel values (*Tool Table*).
Matrix Ops	Performs arbitrary geometric transformations on volume images.

(Continued)

Table 1.2.   (*Continued*)

2D Morphology	Performs 2-D binary math morphology on images.
3D Morphology	Performs 3-D binary and grayscale math morphology on images.
Movie	Enables rapid display of images from memory producing an animation effect.
Multi-Spectral	Provides a set of tools for exploring and classifying multispectral images.
Multiplanar Sections	Enables the generation and display of orthogonal images.
New Session	Starts a completely new ANALYZE™ session (*Tool Table*).
Oblique Sections	Extracts arbitrarily oriented image planes from the volume image.
Plot	Plots information sampled from the measurement programs in ANALYZE™.
Preserve Histo	Performs data range reduction by histogram equalization on images.
Region of Interest	Enables interactive defining and sampling of regions of interest (ROI).
Save Images	Enables the saving of images in memory to a named disk file.
Screen Edit	Provides the ability to prepare presentation slides with ANALYZE™ screens.
Session Log	Displays the file *session.txt* (ANALYZE™ redirects *stderr* to this file) (*Tool Table*).
Snapshot	Provides the capability to capture an ANALYZE™ screen and store it as an image, raster, tiff, or screen file.
Stereology	Measures volume of an object using a stereological method.
Surface Matching	Determines geometric transformation parameters which can be used to spatially register two volume images.
Surface Render	Enables generation and display of shaded surface images.
Tape Read	Enables reading in images from magnetic tape.
Text Editor	Provides a full screen text editor (*Tool Table*).
Toggle Session	Toggles between multiple ANALYZE™ sessions (*Tool Table*).
Tree Trace	Provides a method of tracing 3-D structures.
UNIX Shell	Activates a UNIX system command shell (*Tool Table*).
Volume Estimator	Measures and estimates the volume of an arbitrary three-dimensional object using a probabilistic model.
Volume Render	Provides multipurpose 3-D volume viewing, volume editing, and volume measurement.
Wavelet	Performs 1-D, 2-D, and 3-D wavelet transforms and image compression based on these transforms on images.

editing and manipulation of the objects being imaged. The cost and performance of the software should be in line with the cost and performance of the workstation. The software may cost more than the hardware, but the overall cost/benefit ratio should remain clear and favorable.

   The most important element in developing a successful 3-D software system like ANALYZE™ is the people. The second most important element is effective tools. A combination of people with different skills is required—those who have overall vision, those who can transform vision into working protocols, those who have implementation talents, and those who can test, evaluate, and maintain. ANALYZE™ was developed by a gifted staff of imaging scientists, systems analysts, computer engineers, and programmers, all of whom worked synergistically together to produce a robust image visualization and analysis system. Fast, friendly computers and reliable server-client networks were important tools, well-matched to the talent of the team.

Another critical factor, of course, is financial support. It might be argued that the critical factors needed to produce a comprehensive system like ANALYZE™ could only exist in a well-endowed laboratory and that success depended on just the right combination of gifted, dedicated people, availability of modern computing equipment, access to state-of-the-art imaging devices, an environment of relevant and definable problems, and support of a 'benevolent" governing institution. Critical to the success of ANALYZE™ was internal empowerment to pursue research without a specific product in mind. Had there been an attempt from the outset to design ANALYZE™ as a commercial product whose functions and performance were defined by the needs of the marketplace, it clearly would never have evolved in the way that it did; it would have been inadequate, incomplete, and obsolete when it was finished. Rather, ANALYZE™ has always looked ahead and addressed tomorrow's problems; it is living software, changing and growing to respond to both current and future needs. There has also been an element of serendipity in the success of ANALYZE™: its timing was fortunate, coinciding with other technological advances and user readiness to try new solutions. The best-laid plans may not have resulted in success, but in retrospect, it is not difficult to recognize why ANALYZE™ is useful and successful. ANALYZE™ involves the user in exploring and analyzing data in such a way that new insights and understanding are achieved. The combination of addressing the relevant problems in imaging science and integrating methods to permit interactive exploration, visualization, and quantitative analysis of multidimensional biomedical images provided the elements for success.

Systems like ANALYZE™ will continue to be extended and expanded to include an ever-increasing array of functions and capabilities for visualization and analysis of biomedical images. Specific clinical applications, such as surgery simulation and radiation therapy planning, will be developed, refined, and advanced. These developments will be facilitated and greatly aided by continuing improvements in performance and adaptability of workstations produced by computer manufacturers. One of the elements that has directly contributed to the success of ANALYZE™ is its implementation on general-purpose computers; no special-purpose hardware is required. Additional increases in speed of central processing units, memory size and performance, and data transfer rates, both internally (e.g., display) and externally (storage), will continue to be an important factor in the acceptability and usefulness of 3-D software packages.

Computer system manufacturers will assist significantly by building bridges between the user and the developer. They should recognize and understand end-user problems, and can help match these to basic science developments in the laboratories, that is, provide the bridge. Ongoing education by technology vendors in the capabilities and promises of new advances and environments, and how these might apply to the problems in the user community, are important. For the basic scientist and the practitioner of medicine, such efforts go a long way to fostering the evolution[40,41] of 3-D biomedical imaging and visualization from principles to practice.

1.5 References

1. Schmidt, R. F., Thews, G. (Eds.) *Human Physiology*. Springer-Verlag, 1983.

2. Sprawls, P. *Physical Principles of Medical Imaging*. Aspen Publications, Gaithersburg, MA, 1987.

3. Etter, L. E. "Some historical data relating to the discovery of the röntgen rays." *Am. J. Röntgenol.*, 56, 220, 1946.

4. Glasser, O. *Wilhelm Conrad Röntgen and the Early History of the Röntgen Rays*. Charles C. Thomas, Springfield, IL, 1934.

5. Dessauer, F. *Die Offenbarung einer Nacht. Leben und Werk von W. C. Röntgen*. 4th ed., Joseph Knecht, Frankfurt-am-Main, 1958.

6. Sturm, R. E., Morgan, R. H. "Screen intensification systems and their limitations." *Am. J. Röntgenol. Rad. Ther.*, 62, 617, 1949.

7. Kuhl, D. E., Edwards, R. Q. "Image separation radioisotope scanning." *Radiology*, 80, 653, 1963.

8. Hounsfield, G. N. "Computerized transverse axial scanning (tomography). I. Description of system." *Brit. J. Radiol.*, 46, 1016, 1973.

9. Ambrose, J. "Computerized transverse axial scanning (tomography). II. Clinical application." *Brit. J. Radiol.*, 46, 1034, 1973.

10. Radon, J. Über die Bestimmung von Funktionen durch ihre Integralwerte längs gewisser Mannigfaltigkeiten. *Bu. Succhss. Akad. Wiss. Leipzig, Math. Phys. K.*, 69, 262, 1917.

11. Robb, R. A. *Critical Reviews in Biomedical Engineering*. CRC Press, Boca Raton, FL, Vol. 7, Iss. 4, 1982.

12. DiChiro, G., Brooks, R. A. "The 1979 Nobel Prize in Physiology and Medicine." *J. Comput. Assist. Tomogr.*, 4, 241, 1980.

13. Bracewell, R. N. "Strip integration in radioastronomy." *Aust. J. Phys.*, 9, 198, 1956.

14. Cormack, A. M. "Representation of a function by its line integrals, with some radiological applications." *J. Appl. Phys.*, 35, 2908, 1964.

15. Hounsfield, G. N. "Computed medical imaging." Nobel Lecture, December 8, 1979. *J. Comput. Assist. Tomogr.*, 4, 665, 1980.

16. Dwyer, S. J., III, Brenner, D. J., Takasugi, S., Goldberg, H. "Annotated Bibliography of Computed Tomography." Special Publication Series UMC-HCTC/E-001, University of Missouri-Columbia, 1979.

17. Ring, B. A. "An overview: computed axial tomography." *Appl. Radiol.*, November-December, 1979.

18. Fullerton, G. D. "Fundamentals of CT tissue characterization." In: *Medical Phsyics of CT and Ultrasound Tissue Imaging and Characterization, AAPM, Med. Phys. Monogr.*, 6, 125, 1980.

19. Pullan, B. R., Fawcett, R. H., Isherwood, I. "Tissue characterization by an analysis of the distribution of attenuation values in computed tomography scans." *J. Comput. Assist. Tomogr.*, 2, 49, 1978.

20. Taber, P., Chang, L. W. M., Campion, G. M. "Left brachiocephalic vein simulating aortic dissection on computed tomography." *Radiology,* 133, 562, 1979.

21. Lipton, M. J., Brundage, B. H., Doherty, P. W., Herfkens, R., Berninger, W. H., Redington, R. W., Chatterjee, K., Carlsson, E. "Contrast medium-enhanced computed tomography for evaluating ischemic heart disease." *J. Comput. Assist. Tomogr.*, 4, 571, 1980.

22. Gur, D., Drayer, B. P., Borovetz, H. S., Griffith, B. P., Hardesty, R. L., Wolfson, S. K. "Dynamic computed tomography of the lung: regional ventilation measurements." *J. Comput. Assist. Tomogr.*, 3, 749, 1979.

23. Heinz, E. R., Dubois, P. J., Drayer, B. P., Hill, R. A. "A preliminary investigation of the role of dynamic computed tomography in renovascular hypertension." *J. Comput. Assist. Tomogr.*, 4, 63, 1980.

24. Young, S. W., Noon, M. A., Nassi, M., Castellino, R. A. "Dynamic computed tomography body scanning." *J. Comput. Assist. Tomogr.*, 4, 168, 1980.

25. Kuhl, D. E., Phelps, M. E., Kowell, A. P., Metter, E. J., Selin, C., Winter, J. "Effects of stroke on local cerebral metabolism and perfusion: mapping by emission computed tomography of ^{18}FDG and ^{13}NH$_3$." *Ann. Neurol.*, 8, 47, 1980.

26. Ter-Pogossian, M. M., Klein, M. S., Markham, J., Roberts, R., Sobel, B. E. "Regional assessment of myocardial metabolic integrity *in vivo* by postiron/emission tomography with "C/labelled palmitate." *Circulation*, 61, 742, 1980.

27. Lauterbur, P. C. "Medical imaging by nuclear magnetic resonance zeugmatography." *IEEE Trans. Biomed. Eng.*, 26, 2808, 1979.

28. Hawkes, R. C., Holland, G. N., Moore, W. S., Worthington, B. S. "Nuclear magnetic resonance (NMR) tomography of the brain: preliminary clinical assessment with demonstration of pathology." *J. Comput. Assist. Tomogr.*, 4, 577, 1980.

29. Greenleaf, J. F., Bahn, R. C. "Clinical imaging with transmissive ultrasonic computerized tomography." *IEEE Trans. Biomed. Eng.*, BME-27(12), 1980.

30. Carson, P. L., Oughton, T. V., Hendee, W. R., Ahuja, A. S. "Imaging soft tissue through bone with ultrasound transmission tomography by reconstruction." *Med. Phys.*, 4, 302, 1979.

31. Smith, V., Parker, D. L., Stanley, J. H., Phillips, T. L., Boyd, D. P., Kan, P. T. "Development of a computed tomographic scanner for radiation therapy treatment planning." *Radiology,* 136, 489, 1980.

32. Marshalla, W. H., Jr., Enster, W., Zatz, L. M. "Analysis of the dense lesion at computed tomography with dual kVp scans." *Radiology,* 124, 87, 1977.

33. Alvarez, R. E., Macovski, D. "Energy-selective reconstruction x-ray computed tomography." *Phys. Med. Biol.,* 21, 733, 1976.

34. Robb, R. A. *Three-Dimensional Biomedical Imaging. Vol. I & II.* CRC Press, Boca Raton, FL, 1985.

35. Udupa, J. K., Herman, G. T. *3D Imaging in Medicine.* CRC Press, Boca Raton, FL, 1991.

36. Höhne, K. H., Fuchs, H., Pizer, S. M. *3D Imaging in Medicine, Algorithms, Systems, Applications.* NATO ASI Series, Series F: Computer and Systems Sciences, Vol. 60, Springer-Verlag, Berlin, Heidelberg, 1990.

37. Robb, R. A., Hanson, D. P., Karwoski, R. A., Larson, A. G., Workman, E. L., Stacy, M. C. "ANALYZE™: A comprehensive, operator-interactive software package for multidimensional medical image display and analysis." *Comput. Med. Imag. Graph.,* 13:433–454, 1989.

38. Robb, R. A. "A software system for interactive and quantitative analysis of biomedical images." In: Höhne, K. H., Fuchs, H., Pizer, S. M. (Eds.), *3D Imaging in Medicine.* NATO ASI Series, 1990, Vol. F 60:333–361.

39. Robb, R. A., Hanson, D. P. "The ANALYZE™ software system for visualization and analysis in surgery simulation." In: Lavallee, S., Taylor, R., Burdea, G., Mosges, R. (Eds.), *Computer Integrated Surgery.* MIT Press, Cambridge, MA, 1994.

40. *Proceedings of Visualization in Biomedical Computing 1990.* Atlanta, GA, May 22–25, 1990.

41. Robb, R. A. (Ed.) *Proceedings of Visualization in Biomedical Computing 1992.* SPIE, Vol. 1808, Chapel Hill, NC, October 13–16, 1992.

CHAPTER

2

Multimodality Imaging

There are two ways of acquiring knowledge: namely by argumentation and by experience . . . But argumentation does not banish doubt so effectively that the mind rests in intuition of the truth until it is discovered by way of experience.

Roger Bacon, *Opus Magnus*

2.1 Introduction

Technological advances in biomedical imaging systems have provided routine capabilities for 3-D image acquisition and, in a few cases, 4-D image acquisition (fast scanning in 3-D).[1] The first step in biomedical image formation occurs when some form of energy is measured after its passage through and interaction with a region of the body. Mathematical estimates are computed and images produced of the 2-D and 3-D distribution of interactions of the energy with body tissue (absorption, attenuation, nuclear magnetic disturbances, etc.). Various types of instrumentation may be used to measure the energy–tissue interactions, but the *representation* of the resulting image space is similar among all imaging systems. This chapter will discuss some of the characteristics of the systems that acquire the raw data for 3-D biomedical images, the basic physical, mathematical, and computational principles used in reconstructing the 3-D images, and common forms for representing them for display and analysis on computers.

2.2 Some Biomedical Imaging Systems

Common characteristics of imaging systems that form a basis for comparison between them include spatial resolution, contrast resolution, and temporal resolution. Most imaging systems can also be characterized as those which produce images of structure and those which produce images of function, although several modalities can be used for either.[2]

In discrete digital images, each pixel or voxel has specific dimensions in the measurement space of the object. These dimensions are determined by the "space-resolving" power of the image acquisition system and image formation mechanism, and are referred to collectively as the spatial resolution of the imaging system. The resolution and dimensions may differ for each orthogonal direction represented in the image (anisotropic) or they may be equal (isotropic). The limits to spatial resolution in the final image are the smallest dimensions of the object differentiable by the total imaging system.

The ability of the imaging system to detect differences in signal intensity (e.g., electron density, proton density) between two structures is called the contrast resolution and is dependent on the image acquisition system and the energy form being measured. Contrast resolution is usually specified as a percentage of the largest signal difference that can be detected and quantified by the imaging system. The temporal resolution of an imaging system has two definitions: the "aperture time" and the "frame (or repetition) rate." The aperture time is the amount of time it takes to capture a single image. The frame rate is defined by the smallest interval of time required to produce successive images.

2.2.1 Digital Radiography

Conventional X-ray projection images are now, in many cases, being stored digitally rather than on standard radiographic film. Although digital radiography is not inherently a 3-D biomedical imaging modality many image processing and analysis techniques created for 3-D imagery can be applied to these 2-D digital radiographs. Laser scanning of standard films and direct laser readout from new digital electrostatic cartridges can be used to create digital radiographs. Digital radiography techniques are also often used in real-time X-ray imaging systems, called cine systems, in applications like digital subtraction angiography (DSA) and bi-plane cardiac function imaging. Figure 2.1 compares a typical film-based X-ray system and an electronic/digital X-ray system.[3]

Most digital radiography is used for structural imaging, with real-time techniques like DSA providing functional information.[4] Since the energy source is X-ray, the recorded parameter is absorption (based on X-ray attenuation due to variances in electron density of structures in the beam path). The dimensionality of these images is strictly 2-D (in fact, a projection of a 3-D structure onto 2-D). The spatial resolution is characteristically very high, in the range of 0.1 to 0.5 mm^2. This results in very large discrete images, anywhere from 2000 $\times$ 2000 to 4000 $\times$ 4000 digital values. The contrast resolution is on the order of 1% of full range, with the temporal resolution equal to the time of exposure of the X-ray (i.e., 10 msec). These digital

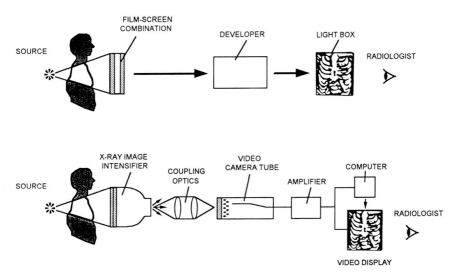

Figure 2.1. Diagram comparing conventional (top) and digital (bottom) radiography systems.

images are characteristically represented in a 12-bit dynamic range, with values from 0 to 4096 (16-bit representation in a computer system).

2.2.2 X-Ray CT and Fast CT

X-ray computed tomography (CT) involves the determination of the 2-D or 3-D distribution of X-ray densities (tissue attenuation coefficients) within the structure being imaged by mathematically reconstructing the X-ray transmission measurements from many angles of view.[5] Conventional X-ray CT scanners utilize a single X-ray tube which rotates through a full 360° rotation while recording projections at fine angular increments during this rotation (every 0.5° to 1°). These projection images are processed and an image is formed through mathematical reconstruction techniques, including filtered back projection or Fourier reconstruction. The X-ray beam originates as a point source and is collimated to a single slice, forming a flat fan-beam geometry. The detectors are usually solid-state detectors (xenon-filled chambers). Figure 2.2 is an illustration of a rotating source X-ray CT system.

Conventional CT imaging systems are used for structural imaging and, in selective cases, for functional imaging associated with dye distribution.[6] The energy source again is X-rays. The measured parameter is the variation in transmission of the X-rays based on attenuation due to the electron density of structures. The dimensionality of a single image is 2-D, but each 2-D image does have a defined thickness and thus can be thought of as a 3-D image composed of voxels. 3-D volume images are constructed of sequential

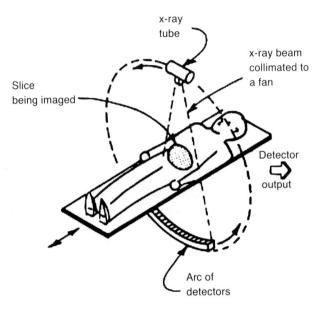

Figure 2.2.   Diagram of X-ray CT system with rotating source and detector.

adjacent CT sections, each separately acquired by changing the position of the structure being imaged. The spatial resolution[7] of voxels in CT data ranges from 0.1 to 1 mm^2 in the plane of acquisition, with the slice thickness ranging from 1 to 10 mm. The number of images sequentially acquired depends on the 3-D extent of the structure of interest, usually ranging from a few sections to over 100. Often, 3-D scans are done with varying slice thickness through the extent of the structure, with thicker sections used outside the immediate area of interest and thinner, higher-resolution sections within the area of interest, reducing overall X-ray exposure while capturing a fuller 3-D extent of the structure being imaged.

Images are usually reconstructed in a 512×512 matrix, resulting in volume images that range anywhere from $512 \times 512 \times 1$ to $512 \times 512 \times 100$. Contrast resolution[7] is in the range of 0.5% of full signal differences. Temporal resolution for conventional CT systems is approximately 1–2 sec, the time necessary to rotate the X-ray system a full 360°. Most CT data are represented in a calibrated range called the Hounsfield scale, ranging in discrete value from -1000 to 1000. Often these values are represented in a positive integer range (0–2048), stored as a 16-bit computer value.

Fast "cine-CT" X-ray CT imaging systems are finding increased use in functional CT imaging, primarily for cardiac imaging and functional assessment. These scanners use a single, curved anode (180 degrees of curvature) with multiple targets, and the beam is rapidly swept across these multiple targets to produce the multiple angles of view necessary to reconstruct an image. The beam is usually collimated to produce four to eight sections. Images can be acquired approximately every 50 msec, giving these scanners very high temporal resolution. The dimensionality of image data produced is either 2-D (single-slice), 3-D when multiple adjacent sections are acquired (although the four- to eight-section limitation compromises the use of these data for most 3-D visualization operations), 3-D when a single section is imaged through time, and 4-D when multiple adjacent sections are acquired at each time point through the time course of the scan (the most common scan type). Often, time-varying scans are acquired with cardiac gating, allowing more adjacent sections to be acquired through time. The spatial resolution is on the order of 0.5 mm^2 in plane, with a slice thickness of 10 mm, which again compromises the ability for these volume images to be used with 3-D visualization functions. Reconstructions are characteristically done in a 512×512 matrix, with 1 to 40 sections in the volume image. Contrast resolution is approximately 1% of full difference in signal, with dynamic range the same as for conventional CT. Figure 2.3 illustrates a fast CT system.

2.2.3 MRI

Magnetic resonance imaging (MRI) technology[8] can produce images with a wide range of characteristics. MRI systems provide mechanisms for intricate control of the signal being measured through modulation of the magnetic field and radio-frequency (RF) pulse sequences used to alter the spins of protons in the structure being imaged. Since MRI selectively images the distribution of protons, it is an excellent soft tissue imaging modality, providing highly detailed structural images. Techniques are being rapidly developed for doing fast MRI to capture functional characteristics such as flow or evoked neurofunctional responses.[9] MRI can further be used to study the biochemical constituency of tissues, using a technique called magnetic resonance spectroscopy (MRS).[10] Figure 2.4 shows an MRI system.

The energy source in MRI is electromagnetic energy emitted from protons that have been knocked out of alignment with a magnetic field and that resonate as they precess back to alignment. This produces an RF signal at a characteristic frequency (Larmor frequency) which can be measured. Relaxation times for the signal as these protons return to equilibrium are measured for both longitudinal (T1) and transverse (T2) orientations. These proton densities and relaxation times are the values reconstructed in the image, with variances in the values due to differing densities and response times of protons in different tissues. Given different scanning protocols, the dimensionality of the data acquired can range from 2-D to 5-D. 2-D images are single-slice reconstructions from a single section of the structure (although there is a thickness, as with CT). 3-D volume images can be acquired using either 2-D multiple adjacent slice techniques or true 3-D volume acquisitions.[9] Most MR images are reconstructed into a 256×256 matrix (inter-

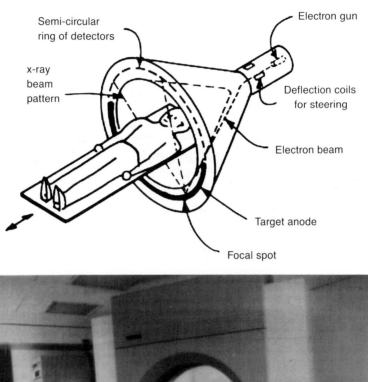

Semi-circular
ring of detectors

x-ray
beam
pattern

Electron gun

Deflection coils
for steering

Electron beam

Target anode

Focal spot

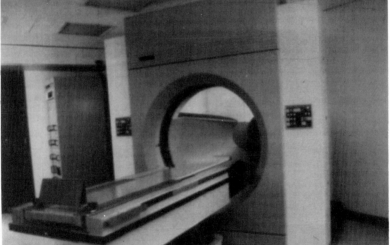

Figure 2.3. Diagram (top) and photograph (bottom) of X-ray CT system for high speed 3-D imaging.

polated from frequency and phase encodings ranging from 128 to 256) with 1 to 128 sections in a given volume image. The spatial resolution in plane ranges from 0.5 to 1 mm, with the slice thickness from 1 to 10 mm. The 3-D spoiled gradient recalled echo (SPGR)[11] sequences used to acquire volume images can sample each voxel isotropically with a resolution of approximately 1 mm^3. MRI contrast is greatest in soft tissue, detecting 5% differences in signal, and can be enhanced with the use of contrast materials like GdDTPA (gadolinium base) or newer superparamagnetic contrast agents.

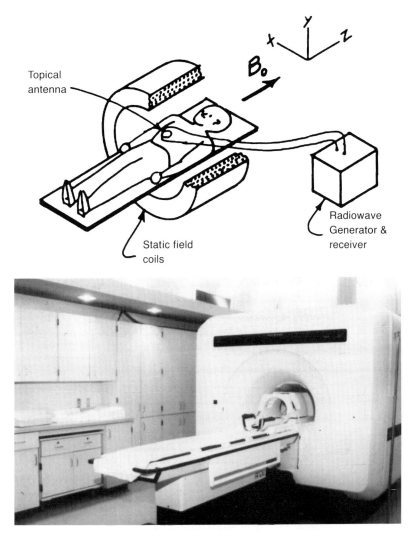

Figure 2.4. Diagram (top) and photograph (bottom) of MRI system.

MRI acquisition times range from seconds to minutes, depending on the pulse sequence, the number of repetitions, and the number of slices acquired. Recent fast MRI sequences allow subsecond acquisition using techniques like echo planar imaging (EPI).[11] MRI data are acquired in the frequency domain (called k-space) and reconstructed using inverse Fourier transforms. Once reconstructed, the data are characteristically represented in a 10- to 12-bit data range, although most MR images do not contain more than 8 bits of dynamic range in discrete value.

2.2.4 Nuclear Medicine Imaging

Nuclear medicine imaging systems image the distribution of radioisotopes distributed within the body, preferably to a specific organ or structure of interest. Several different radioisotopes are used, with the particular element or tag selected based on the physiological function to be measured. The images acquired from these systems provide a direct representation of metabolism or function in the organ or structure being imaged. Currently, there are two main types of nuclear medicine scanning technologies: Single photon emission computed tomography (SPECT) and positron emission tomography (PET).

2.2.4.1 SPECT

SPECT systems image the distribution of radiopharmaceuticals that emit photons upon decay. These photons are imaged using gamma cameras, and several designs exist for SPECT imaging systems based on the number and placement of the gamma cameras. Many SPECT systems simply rotate the gamma camera around the structure being imaged, similar to X-ray CT in principle, with projections acquired at many angles of view. Other SPECT systems use multiple gamma cameras to acquire more angles of view rapidly, providing better spatial resolution and faster scan times.[12]

Image reconstruction processes for all types of medical computed transaxial tomographic imaging are remarkably similar. As in other modalities, the primary purposes of producing SPECT images are to remove superposition of complex structural information and to provide a quantitative image of a body section or sections. SPECT images represent the distribution of small amounts of injected or inhaled physiological radioisotopic tracers which provide functional information that is generally very difficult or nearly impossible to obtain by other imaging methods. It is important to consider that the principal strength of nuclear medicine imaging is its ability to provide functional information through the use of radiopharmaceuticals such as labeled substrates, analogs, drugs, and other compounds which are indicators of in vivo biochemical or hemodynamic functions. Figure 2.5 illustrates a SPECT system.

Although the most rapid advances in clinical applications of CT have occurred in X-ray CT and MRI, research utilizing single-photon emitters actually preceded Hounsfield's work.[13] Although the earliest clinical applications of any form of CT were SPECT imaging of the head, the growth of SPECT as a clinical entity pales in comparison to X-ray CT. Still, advances have steadily occurred, as has been observed by both clinical and technical experts in this field. The principal strength of SPECT is its potential to provide quantitative measurements of the 3-D distribution of radiopharmaceuticals. Concurrently, SPECT provides an advantage over conventional scintigraphy for imaging of low-contrast distributions. However, these ca-

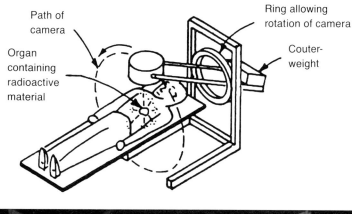

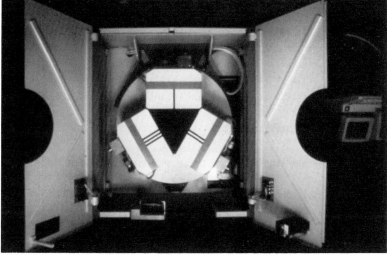

Figure 2.5. Diagram (top) and photograph (bottom) of SPECT system with three heads (gamma cameras).

pabilities are achieved, as with any complex imaging system, only when each part of the image-forming system performs correctly. There is a predominance of gamma camera-based SPECT systems which use gantry rotation to provide 360° angular range.

2.2.4.2 PET

PET is a nuclear medicine imaging modality that yields transverse tomographic images of the distribution of positron-emitting radionuclides systemically administered to the subject.[14] In PET the image-forming variable is the distribution of the radionuclide administered, and the data required for the generatiaon of the image are supplied by the detection of the annihilation radiation emitted as a result of the annihilation of positrons in matter.

The utilization of positron-emitting radionuclides in nuclear medicine imaging is not obviously attractive. The number of radionuclides decaying by positron emission is small in comparison to those decaying by the emission of gamma rays. The high energy (approximately 511 keV) of the annihilation photons renders their "conventional" collimation by means of "heavy" absorbers such as lead or tungsten difficult and inefficient. Their detection requires the use of much more massive detectors than normally used in nuclear medicine imaging of radionuclides emitting lower-energy gamma-ray photons. Finally, the most widely used cameras for conventional nuclear medicine imaging are not well suited for the imaging of annihilation photons. Probably because of such considerations, in its early development positron-emitting radionuclide imaging attracted relatively little attention in the scientific community except in a limited number of centers.

Despite early discouraging perceptions of positron imaging, PET has matured into an imaging modality which is recognized as a highly useful research tool with clinical potential.[15] This has occurred mostly because of a reevaluation of the above factors, which led to a more attractive perspective of PET. Figure 2.6 shows a PET system.

The most compelling factor in the development of PET has been the recognition that a small number of radionuclides, specifically carbon-11, nitrogen-13, oxygen-15, and, to a lesser degree, fluorine-18, possess chemical characteristics which render them particularly useful in the study of biochemical processes of fundamental importance in biology and medicine. In spite of the short half-lives of these radionuclides (^{11}C = 20 min; ^{13}N = 10 min; ^{15}O = 2 min; ^{18}F = 110 min), they have now been incorporated into a very large number of radiopharmaceuticals of great importance in the study of chemical processes of living organisms.[14,15]

As mentioned above, the collimation of the annihilation radiation by conventional means is inefficient because of the large amount of the collimating material required to absorb the high-energy annihilation photons. However, because of the fact that the annihilation radiation, in most instances, consists of two photons traveling nearly colinearly in opposite directions, the collimation of this radiation can be achieved very efficiently electronically. Electronic collimation of the annihilation photons also permits the localization of the annihilation event by the so-called photon time-of-flight method.[14] The latter approach further improves the signal-to-noise ratio that can be achieved in the imaging of positron-emitting radionuclides as compared to radionuclides decaying by the emission of single photons. Last, but not least, the detection of the annihilation photons through their coincidence detection is particularly propitious for the tomographic reconstruction of images from projections, as it is utilized in PET. The spatial resolution achievable in such reconstructions is on the order of 0.5 cm.

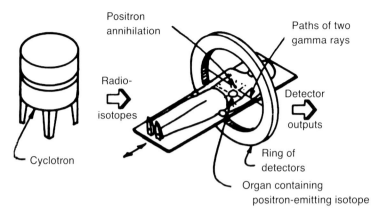

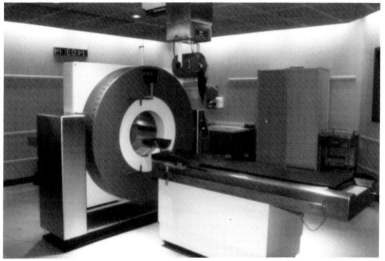

Figure 2.6.   Diagram (top) and photograph (bottom) of PET system.

Thus, the usefulness of PET relies essentially on three factors: 1) the desirable chemical characteristics of some radionuclides which happen to decay through the emission of positrons; 2) the efficient collimation of the annihilation radiation which can be achieved electronically; and 3) the desirable characteristics of electronic collimation and tomographic reconstruction.

2.2.5 Ultrasound

As well as revolutionizing diagnostic radiology, X-ray CT made the concept of high-technology imaging acceptable to clinicians and the general public alike and stimulated research into diagnostic imaging using other forms of energy. Of these other forms, ultrasound is the only imaging modality that does not directly or indirectly involve electromagnetic radiation.[16]

Ultrasound is any type of acoustical energy that contains frequencies higher than the upper audible limit. However, when the term ultrasound is used in a diagnostic imaging context, longitudinal waves with frequencies between 0.5 and 15 MHz are generally implied. Acoustical energy is the dynamic disturbance from equilibrium of the extrinsic properties (e.g., pressure, temperature, and particle position) of some medium. This chapter is specifically concerned with media consisting of biological tissues. It is convenient to regard the disturbance as propagating through the tissue in the form of a wave. Any one of the extrinsic properties can be taken as a descriptor of the wave motion, although it is usual to consider pressure variations. As well as "supporting" wave motion, the tissue intimately affects the behavior of the wave. There is a strong and complicated interaction between the intrinsic or physical properties (e.g., the density and compressibility) of the tissue and wave propagation. The basis of ultrasonic imaging is to determine information about intrinsic tissue properties from observations of the way in which probing waves are perturbed or "scattered" by the tissues. The presentation of such information is typically in visual form, i.e., as image displays. Figure 2.7 shows a clinical ultrasound imaging system.

Because of the strong and complicated dependence of the wave motion on the intrinsic tissue properties, probing a body with ultrasound and recording the scattered waves provides the investigator with a wealth of information. The great difficulty and challenge of ultrasonic imaging is to "unravel" the information in the form of a useful image. B-scan imaging, which is inherently tomographic, has the advantage of relatively simple and inexpensive implementation. In principle, a computer is not required to reconstruct images from the raw echo data, although very often a computer is incorporated into the scanner for versatility of control and image manipulation.

Many ultrasonic imaging techniques[16] have been developed recently in an effort to produce images that are either quantitative or at least better than those obtainable by B-scanning. A common feature of all these techniques, which distinguishes them from B-scan, is that a computer is necessary to reconstruct images from the raw or measured data.

2.2.6 Biomagnetic Imaging

Biomagnetic imaging utilizes relatively new scanning technology for imaging of the electrical activity of the brain. The technology is based on the use of superconducting quantum interference devices (SQUID) to detect the very weak magnetic fields caused by flux of the electrical signals in the brain and other organs such as the heart.[17] The field strength from the heart (magne-

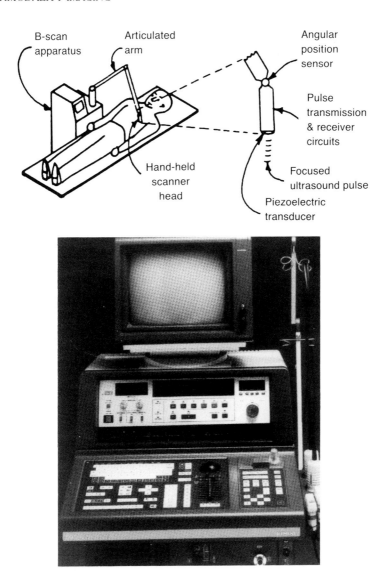

Figure 2.7. Diagram (top) and photograph (bottom) of ultrasound imaging sytem used for diagnostic echocardiography.

tocardiogram) is approximately 10^{-10} T (tesla) and for evoked responses in the brain is about 10^{-13} T.[18] Given the earth's magnetic field at 10^{-4} T, with fluctuations in this field of 10^{-7} T, it is quite remarkable that technology exists to capture the magnetic fields induced by electrical activity in the human body.

SQUID devices are highly sensitive detectors based on the effect of superconductivity. Given a current in a loop of superconducting wire, which will continue as long as the wire is in a superconductive state, the magnetic flux through this loop is constant. If an external source changes the magnetic field, the current in the superconducting loop changes so that the flux remains the same. The detector in biomagnetic imaging systems utilizes this principle to detect small magnetic flux changes in the body. These detectors, called gradiometers, were initially based on rf-SQUID technology (1983), and evolved to dc-SQUID technology based on detection coils which contain a Josephson junction (nonsuperconducting area). The phase of the wave function of the moving electrons in the two branches of the coils differs by an amount relative to the magnetic flux. Gradiometer coils are built with multiple loops, either as first-order gradiometers or second-order gradiometers, in order to transport the change in magnetic flux from a location near the structure being imaged to the superconduction loop which is contained in a superconducting Dewar containment vessel. Current biomagnetic imaging systems contain many gradiometers arranged to be evenly distributed over the whole head. These multiple detector devices allow the identification and imaging of multiple current dipoles generating the magnetic flux measured by the system within the structure being imaged. Each detector measures the magnetic field contributions from the current density. Reconstruction of the location of these current dipoles has no unique solution for multiple dipoles. A single equivalent current dipole representing the center of electrical activity can be computed, or a spatial arrangement of the dipoles can be assumed (usually a grid) with linear estimation techniques used to compute the current density at each location, resulting in a map of current density distribution.

Biomagnetic or magnetoencephalography (MEG) techniques can be used to measure current density changes resulting from spontaneous activity or from transient activity as a result of evoked response studies.[19] These changes can be measured in acquisition times on a millisecond scale, permitting fast functional imaging of the brain and other organs. The location of the current dipoles can be localized within a few millimeters, depending on the location of the dipole in relation to the detecting device. Given the localized signal and the poor spatial resolution of the imaging system, MEG studies need to be correlated to other imaging modalities which present the structural detail of the organ being studied. This is most often done using a coordinate system for the MEG data within which specific markers attached to the patient are localized (or using anatomic landmarks), followed by CT or MRI scanning in which these same markers can be identified for coregistration with the MEG data.[19] Applications of this technology include neurofunctional imaging in normal people, where evoked response studies would reveal information about the function of the normal brain, and in patients with defined neurologic abnormalities, such as epileptic foci. Figure 2.8 illustrates a biomagnetic imaging apparatus.

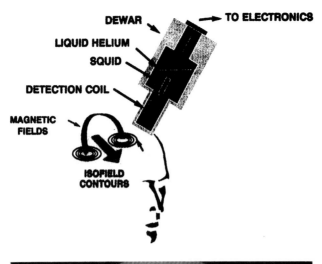

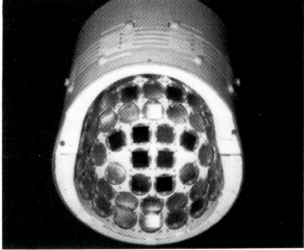

Figure 2.8. Diagram (top) and photograph (bottom) of biomagnetic imaging system for imaging magnetic signals from the brain.

2.2.7 Microscopy Imaging

The microscope was the first powerful tool available to cell biologists, and it remains one of the most useful. Several different microscope technologies have developed since the advent of the first light microscope, including the electron microscope, the scanning electron microscopy, and the even newer technologies of digital fluorescence microscopy and confocal microscopy.[20] Changes in microscope technology have allowed the imaging of increasingly smaller structures through improvements in resolution, and have permitted the imaging of functional aspects of structures as well. From the standpoint of 3-D biomedical visualization, each microscopy technology provides a different set of features and constraints.

The most common form of microscopy is light microscopy. Structures are examined using the transmission of light through the structure of interest and optically magnifying this image for viewing. The resolution of the light microscope is directly related to the optics in the system, within which the wavelength of the illuminating radiation, the refractive index of the lens, and the optical aperture are the controlling characteristics. The aperture is fixed in most microscopes, so resolution enhancement is achieved by using different wavelengths of light, such as ultraviolet rather than visible light, or by changing the refractive index by using film (oil) substances to fill the space between the specimen and the lens.

For 3-D imaging, the thickness of the structure observed through the microscope also influences the axial resolution in the volume image. This may be fixed at the time of sectioning, if serial sections are created of the structure and individually placed on slides, requiring each section to be viewed, digitized, and registered in order to capture the full 3-D volume. Or, the thickness of the section may be determined by incrementally adjusting the plane of focus to image specific planes through an intact specimen. This provides a stack of images with the out-of-focus structures blurred into each image throughout the volume. If the in-focus structure of interest is imaged with sufficient clarity in each image, this 3-D volume may be used directly, but frequently the out-of-focus structures need to be removed, generally by the use of deconvolution techniques. Digital images are often acquired using a video camera, video digitizing hardware, and software integrated with a computer system and the microscope, and with a stepping motor to control the z-axis position of the focal plane. These images can be digitized at different resolutions, but 512×512 is typical. Anywhere from a few to several hundred sections comprising the entire volume may be digitized, resulting in relatively large volume images. Resolutions range down to the 0.1-μm range, with slice thicknesses of approximately 10 μm (an axial disparity of 100 to 1). The data usually contain more than 8 bits of dynamic signal range, so often 10- or 12-bit digitizers are used to capture the full dynamic range of the signal. Tissues are often selectively dyed with color dyes to enhance the visualization of particular structures for color digitizing systems which capture the image in full Red-Green-Blue (RGB) color resolution. Such colored data are amenable to multispectral feature space classification for automated segmentation of the different structures in the specimen. Polarized light, dark-field microscopy, and phase-contrast microscopy are other techniques used to more clearly image specific structures.

The transmission and scanning electron microscopes use electron interactions with the cells and tissues of the specimen and the subsequent release of energy to form images of the structures. Electrons at high voltage have very short wavelengths. For example, at 50,000 V an electron has a wavelength of about 0.05 Å. This small wavelength provides for the high-resolution imaging ability of electron microscopes, permitting imaging with 1- to 5-Å resolution. The scanning electron microscope moves a thin beam of electrons back and forth across the specimen. As the electrons strike the specimen, they are scattered as secondary electrons are knocked from the sample, which are detected and used to form the image. Scanning electron microscopes provide only surface details of the specimen, requiring a priori sectioning of the surface to be scanned for a full 3-D volume. Transmission electron microscopy can be focused like light microscopy, permitting the acquisition of adjacent multiplanar images by changing the depth of focus. Images from these sources are digitized like those for light microscopy, and the number and size of images are approximately the same (i.e., large data sets). However, the resolution is now at the angstrom level, providing much higher resolution for the data.

The advent of confocal microscopy has led to an increasing utilization of 3-D visualization techniques in microscopic applications.[20] The key feature of a confocal microscope is that illumination and detection are confined to the same spot in the specimen at any one time. Only what is "in focus" is detected, with out-of-focus regions of the sample appearing as voids (or black in the image). The confocal microscope needs to scan the point probe over the field of view, as a complete optical image is not captured directly. There are many possible types of confocal microscopes, but the most common is the epi-illumination type, which uses the same lens as both the condenser and the objective. Light from an aperture is reflected into the rear of the objective lens and is focused on the specimen, while light returning from the specimen as a result of either reflection or fluorescence passes back through the lens and is focused on a second aperture, which allows a portion of the beam to pass to a detector. Most confocal systems are based on laser scanning, using lasers as the light source to provide the highest resolution and sensitivity. Most laser light confocal systems use fluorescence of selected dyes to acquire the images, with some allowing the acquisition of two different epifluorescent images in conjunction with a confocal reflectance image and a nonconfocal transmission image.[21] Many different fluorochromes are available, including dyes like Texas Red and Lucifer Yellow. 3-D volume image acquisition is achieved by using focus depth control driven by a z-axis stepping motor for accurate optical sectioning. The images are directly digitized from the microscope at similar dimensions to other microscope systems (512 × 512), with several hundred sections common throughout a particular structure of interest, resulting again in large 3-D volume image data sets. The pixel resolution is in the 0.1-μm range, with slice thicknesses of about 0.5 μm, providing a better-sampled data set in the axial dimension (5 to 1 disparity) than with other microscopy techniques. The images can be acquired in near real time, with computer-controlled triggering of the acquisition possible, which is useful for imaging physiologic events at the cellular level. For example, confocal imaging has been used[21] to image the efflux of calcium from the sarcoplasmic reticulum in an oocyte stimulated by the activation of various receptors in the cell wall (e.g., muscarinic receptors). Figure 2.9 is a photograph of a 3-D confocal microscopy system.

2.3 Image Reconstruction

A diversion into the semantics associated with the term "computed tomography" (CT) is made here. Such a tangent is important, since the underlying mathematical and physical principles of computed tomography form the basis for most approaches to 3-D biomedical imaging, namely, that multiple slices or planes are computed as "graphical cuts" (the definition of tomography) through a 3-D object, and its 3-D form is then modeled as a "stack" of these slices or planes. Tomography literally means the representation of a slice, and implies the formation of 2-D cross-sectional images free of blurring from structures not in the planes of interest. Such images are correctly called tomograms. Popular usage of X-ray CT systems has resulted in the term "computed tomography" acquiring the restricted meaning of the formation of tomograms of X-ray absorption coefficient by the method of re-

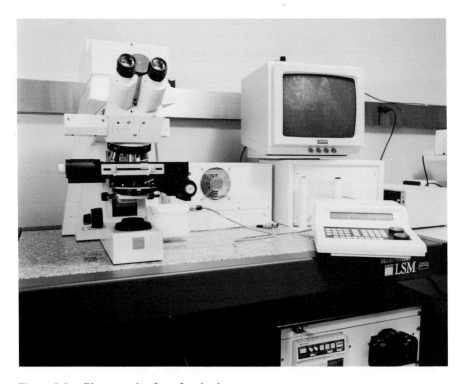

Figure 2.9. Photograph of confocal microscope system.

construction from recorded projections.[22] However, in general, the term is applicable to any technique that requires computation in order to reconstruct an image with nonambiguous resolution in three dimensions.

Generally, all biomedical imaging systems that produce 3-D volume images use a form of reconstruction called computed tomography. This now well-established technique is a computer implementation of an appropriate inversion formula to mathematically reconstruct adjacent cross sections of an object from measured fluctuations of some energy traversing (transmitted through and/or reflected by) the object from several different directions.[5]

To better understand a review of the basic physical and mathematical principles upon which CT is based, an intuitive appreciation must be gained of the problems encountered with conventional radiographic imaging, and the approach to these problems represented by transverse section scanning. X-ray CT will be used to demonstrate the principles.

2.3.1 Conventional Radiography

A beam of X-rays passing through the body is differentially absorbed and scattered by structures in the beam path. The amount of absorption depends on the physical density and atomic composition of these structures and on the energy of the X-ray beam. For equivalent X-ray energy, a more dense structure will attenuate the beam more than a less dense structure. It is this differential absorption pattern by tissues within the body which is carried in the transmitted X-ray beam and recorded by the X-ray detector, usually film.[4]

Even though two spatially separated X-ray beams of equal energy may be recorded by the detector as having nearly equal total attenuation, they may have passed through entirely different materials. This is because attenuation is dependent on path length through an object as well as on its physical density and atomic composition. In such cases, it is impossible to "see" or determine from the detector (film) the different materials which the beam passed through. The attenuations at different points along the beam path "add up" and are superimposed onto the same points on the detector, as illustrated diagrammatically at the top of Figure 2.10.

This superposition problem is clearly demonstrated in a conventional chest X-ray, like that shown at the bottom of Figure 2.10, where structures within the chest are superimposed on top of one another at each point in the film. Since exposure to X-rays blackens film, the image is dark where many X-rays are detected by the film due to low absorption (e.g., through the lungs), and the image is light where fewer X-rays are detected due to greater absorption and scatter of the beam (e.g., through the heart, ribs, and spine). The result is that only in those regions where high density differences exist between adjacent structures can details be clearly discerned in the film, as in the case of the ribs (bone) against the lungs (air). Structures of relatively low density (for example, the tracheal passage) which are in the same beam

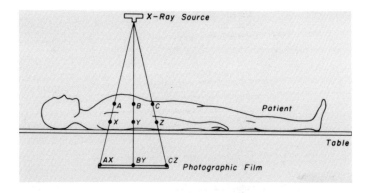

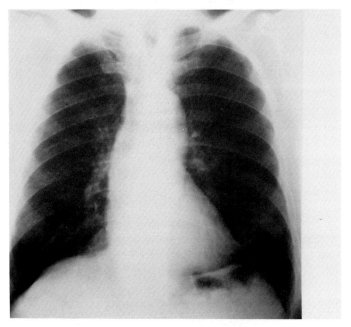

Figure 2.10. Diagram (top) and photograph (bottom) of conventional projection X-radiography technique.

path as high-density structures (for example, the spine) cannot be seen due to the superposition problem.

2.3.2 Conventional Axial Tomography

Conventional axial tomography was developed in an attempt to overcome the superposition problem.[23–25] Figure 2.11 illustrates this technique. The X-ray source and photographic detector (film) are moved in opposite directions parallel to the plane of the body desired to be imaged. By appropriately

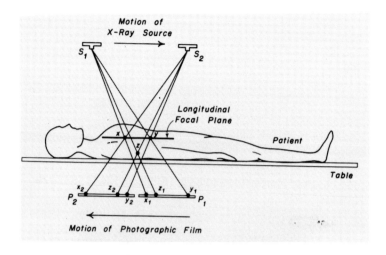

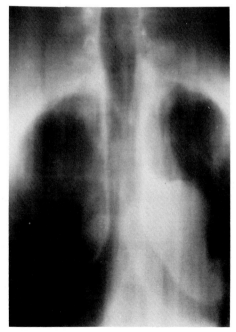

Figure 2.11. Diagram (top) and photograph (bottom) of conventional axial tomography technique.

adjusting the speed of the X-ray source relative to the speed of the photographic plate, all points in the focal plane will always project onto the same points on the photographic plate, while points outside of this plane will project onto different points on the plate. The result is that the distribution of densities within the focal plane will be sharply recorded on the film, and densities outside of the focal plane will be blurred. In the conventional to-mogram of a patient shown at the bottom of Figure 2.11, the plane of focus was selected to be the trachea. The tracheal anatomy can be quite clearly visualized, an impossible result in a conventional chest X-ray. However, the problem of superposition is not eliminated. Image quality is significantly de-graded due to the presence of variable-density objects outside the focal plane. The blurred structures of the spinal vertebrae are superimposed on the focused structures of the trachea and appear as if within the trachea.

Such superposition often causes problems in accurate interpretation of anatomic boundaries. Small density differences are very difficult to detect or estimate in conventional tomograms, for much the same reasons as in the conventional radiograph. Due to superposition and scattering, even under favorable conditions of small field size and low X-ray energy, differences in X-ray transmission of less than 5% to 10% generally are not detectable with these conventional radiographic techniques.

2.3.3 Computed Transaxial Tomography

In computed transaxial tomography,[5] scatter is minimized by collimating the beam, and superposition is eliminated by scanning around a transaxial plane, as shown in Figure 2.12. The X-ray transmitted through the plane or slice is measured with detectors that can record intensity differences less than 0.1%, and the individual attenuation coefficients of structures in the beam path then can be determined to within 0.5% accuracy from these measurements by techniques that are described in the following sections.

A cross section of a patient's chest determined from measurements with a current generation CT scanner is shown at the bottom of Figure 2.12. The location, size, and density of all structures within the chest are accurately visualized for this particular transaxial slice through the mid-thorax. Such sets of cross sections produced by X-ray CT solve the superposition prob-lem. A full 3-D representation of the chest could be obtained by reconstruct-ing similar cross sections over the entire anatomic extent of the thorax and "stacking" these sections like a roll of coins.

2.3.4 Some Principles of Radiation Physics

X-rays interact with objects by reasonably well-known mechanisms. In gen-eral, these can be described as photoelectric and Comptom effects,[4,26] but the principal manifestation of these for consideration in X-ray CT is absorp-tion and its variations, including beam hardening and scatter. Enumeration of the incremental attenuation of X-rays by bodily tissues has been stan-dardized using calibration scales for clinical X-ray dose levels.

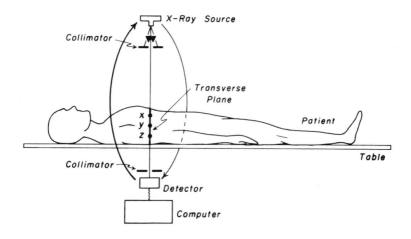

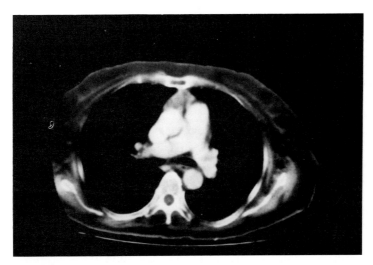

Figure 2.12. Diagram (top) and photograph (bottom) of computed transaxial tomography technique.

2.3.4.1 Absorption Law

It is a well-known law of radiation physics (Lambert-Beer's law)[27]

$$I_t = I_o e^{-\mu \ell} \tag{2.1}$$

that when a monoenergetic X-ray beam (i.e., a beam with a single X-ray wavelength) passes through an object of uniform density, it is attenuated according to the exponential relationship where I_o is the incident intensity, I_t is the transmitted intensity, ℓ is the length of the path of the beam through the object, and μ is the absorption coefficient (often called the linear attenuation coefficient in CT) for the object, which is determined by the physical density and atomic composition of the object, and is dependent on the energy (voltage or wavelength) of the X-ray beam.[28,29]

In the usual case, the density of the object along the path of the X-ray beam is not uniform. If the attenuation coefficients and path lengths of varying density structures within an object are known, the total attenuation is cumulative, which may be expressed by

$$I_t = I_o e^{-\Sigma_L \mu_i \ell_i} \qquad (2.2)$$

where L is the total path length through all structures.

In the practical case, the path segment lengths, ℓ_i, are made small enough to assume that the attenuation coefficients, μ_i, are uniform in each small segment. If the ℓ_i are made equal, say to ℓ, then the equation may be written as

$$\sum_L \mu_i = \frac{1}{\ell} \ln \frac{I_o}{I_t} \qquad (2.3)$$

Thus, if I_o, I_t, and ℓ are known, the sum of the attenuation coefficients along the beam path can be calculated. In CT, I_o and I_t are measured from many different angles of view by X-ray detectors, and ℓ is mathematically defined to be arbitrarily small in order to assume uniform density segments throughout an object. These measurements give multiple equations in the same unknowns, the individual μ_i, which then can be solved by various mathematical approaches that are discussed in the next section. The result is a map of attenuation coefficients within the object that can be displayed as an image by assigning brightness values (gray levels) proportional to the attenuation coefficients at each point throughout the object.

This principle is idealized relative to the practical situation, since monoenergetic X-ray sources of sufficient intensity to irradiate the body are not available, and tissues within the body, particularly bone, may alter beam direction resulting in the detection of "scattered" as well as linearly transmitted x-rays. The latter problem is reduced significantly in CT by appropriate collimation of the X-ray beam at the source and at the detector. However, problems due to X-ray spectral changes during irradiation of an object with a polyenergetic X-ray source are not resolved so simply.

2.3.4.2 *"Beam Hardening"*

A conventional X-ray tube emits a beam which is a distribution of different X-ray energies (or wavelengths) across a certain range. (For most CT scanners, the average energy is between 40 and 60 keV before entry into the subject.) Different energies of X-ray are attenuated by different amounts when passed through an object of uniform density. The lower energies (longer wavelengths) are absorbed more readily than the higher energies (shorter wavelengths), so that the spectral distribution of energies within the beam shifts toward the higher energies as the beam passes through the object. (The average energy in the beam of most CT scanners after transmission through the subject is approximately 70 to 75 keV.) This effect is sometimes called "beam hardening," and it causes the attenuation values within a particular irradiated volume to be position dependent, since each point along the beam's path is exposed to a slightly different energy spectrum.

This problem is illustrated in Figure 2.13. Ideally, the beam attenuation is directly proportional to the thickness of the body traversed by the beam. However, since the X-ray beam is polyenergetic (i.,e., possessing a distribution of energies), lower-energy X-rays are preferentially absorbed as the beam passes through the object, and the continuing X-ray beams are more

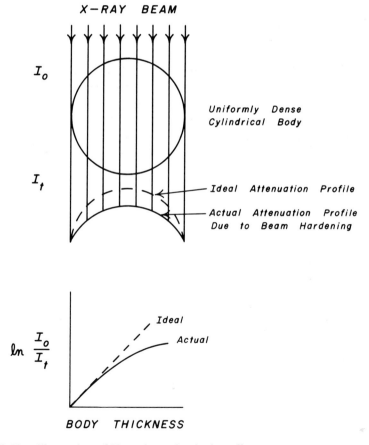

Figure 2.13. Illustration of X-ray beam hardening effect.

penetrating because of their increasing average energy, causing the object to appear less dense than if a monoenergetic beam equivalent to the average incident energy of the polyenergetic beam was used. Relative to the average energy in the incident beam, the average energy of the transmitted beam is increased more for longer pathways through the body than for shorter pathways, and thus their relationship to body thickness departs from linearity.

This problem has been well described in X-ray CT,[28-30] with several approaches proposed and implemented to correct it.[31-34] The initial approach used in the first CT scanner[35] was to use a water bag around the head to serve as a "compensating" filter.[28] The water bag made all beam path lengths similar, so that beam hardening was "linearized." This same linear correction can be obtained by mathematical processing[31,32] of the measured transmission data within the computer, thus eliminating the need for the water bag. However, more sophisticated mathematical approaches[33,34] are required to adequately correct the decidedly nonlinear beam hardening caused by dense material within the body, such as compact bones, X-ray contrast agents, or prosthetic implants.

Generally, these more exact methods for correction of beam hardening involve an iterative approach to first approximate the distribution and amount of dense material (e.g., bone) in the scan region, and then correct the absorption measurements relative to the known (assumed or measured) X-ray energy spectrum before making the final reconstruction. Therefore, these procedures increase the computational time required to reconstruct a CT image, but this is generally an acceptable trade-off for obtaining improved image quality.

Several investigators have performed actual tissue attenuation studies,[36-40] both in vitro and in vivo, and with both monoenergetic photons generated by isotope sources and polyenergetic X-ray beams in CT systems. Current X-ray CT methods that include beam-hardening corrections provide excellent accuracy in measurement of tissue attenuation coefficients compared to other radiographic techniques (10 to 100 times better).[41] Typical standard deviations in measurement of absorption coefficients of tissue are about $\frac{1}{2}\%$ relative to water, that is, an accuracy of $\pm\frac{1}{4}\%$.

2.3.4.3 CT Numbers

Figure 2.14 shows a typical scale of CT numbers used to represent the computed values of attenuation coefficients of human body tissues and organs,[36-40] and illustrates the precision with which they can be obtained with current X-ray CT scanners. The range of the soft tissue values includes statistical deviations due to measurement errors[38] and actual attenuation differences between the same types of tissue in different specimens. For example, the CT numbers for whole blood are significantly affected[37] by hematocrit (ratio of red blood cells to plasma). The CT numbers for fat change with water content; those for lungs change with blood and/or water content.

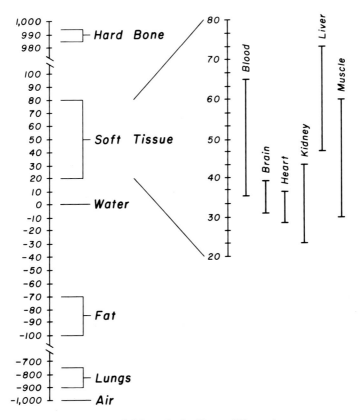

Figure 2.14. Standard (Hounsfield) scale for X-ray CT numbers.

The CT number produced by X-ray CT scanner systems is an expression of the relationship of the linear attenuation of X-rays by a given material (tissue) to that by water for the same X-ray energy.[28] This relationship is:

$$\text{CT number} = k \cdot (\mu - \mu_w)/\mu_w \tag{2.4}$$

where μ is the attenuation coefficient of the material and μ_w is the attenuation coefficient of water. The constant, k, is a "magnifying value" chosen to produce a numerical resolution scale sufficient to represent the precision of the scanner measurements. For most current scanners, the value of k is either 500 or 1000, with most recent scanners employing the -1000 to $+1000$ scale.

On this scale (see Figure 2.14), often called the Hounsfield scale in honor of the inventor of the first clinical X-ray CT scanner, the CT number, often called a Hounsfield unit (H), is given by:

$$H = 1000 \cdot \left(\frac{\mu}{\mu_w} - 1 \right) \tag{2.5}$$

or to obtain the value of the attenuation coefficient relative to water

$$\frac{\mu}{\mu_w} = 1 + H/1000 \tag{2.6}$$

This is the ideal formulation for the CT number, H, on the Hounsfield scale. Conversion of the CT number measured on any given scanner (H_s) to this scale can be obtained by measuring the CT numbers for air (H_a) and water (H_w) and using these as calibration values[41] in the formula, so that

$$H = 1000 \cdot (H_s - H_w)/(H_w - H_a) \tag{2.7}$$

However, due to variations in X-ray beam energies, detector efficiency, electronic noise, etc., normalized values of CT numbers and their relationship to actual tissue densities may vary significantly between different scanners.

2.3.5 Mathematical and Computational Principles

The mathematical and computational principles of image reconstruction form the predominant concept in X-ray CT, and therefore they will be described in some detail from a historical perspective. Image reconstruction algorithms are formulations of these mathematical principles into procedures which can be numerically implemented on a computer to estimate, in the general case, the 3-D distribution of X-ray attenuation coefficients throughout an object from a finite number of its 2-D projections. In the special case of transverse section scanning, the problem reduces to estimation of a 2-D distribution of X-ray attenuation coefficients in a plane (or "slice") from a number of 1-D projections.

2.3.5.1 *Projection and Reconstruction Space Geometry*

Figure 2.15 diagrammatically illustrates the concept of generating projections of a slice of an object by scanning an X-ray beam and detector across and about the object. Several different schemes and geometries for scanning have been implemented, with various advantages for speed and calibration, as will be discussed in the next section. Two of these are known as parallel-beam geometry and fan-beam geometry. For intuitive simplicity, the parallel scanning geometry scheme, as illustrated in Figure 2.15, will be used to describe the basic mathematical approach to reconstruction. Either fan-beam geometry can be reduced to parallel-beam geometry,[42] or appropriate geometric calculations can be used to do fan-beam reconstruction directly.[43,44]

All conventional image reconstruction algorithms require that during CT scanning, the X-ray source and detector lie in the same plane as the slice to be reconstructed. The projection data are samples of the detector readings at discrete positions of the X-ray source and detector as they rotate 180° (up

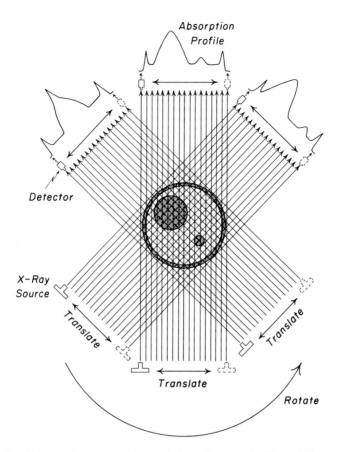

Figure 2.15.   Scheme for generating multiple projections in X-ray CT.

to 360° for fan-beam geometry) around the body. The set of projection data collected at each angular setting of the X-ray source and detector is often called a "profile," or "view" (the terms "projection," "profile," and "view" are used interchangeably). It is composed of the values of detector readings as a function of source-detector position. The value of the profile at each position is proportional to the intensity of the X-ray transmitted along the path between the X-ray source and detector. The intensity readings are converted to attenuation values by computing the natural logarithms of the ratios of incident X-ray intensities, as measured with no attenuating material in the beam, to transmitted X-ray intensities. According to Equation 2.3, each profile sample represents the sum of all attenuation coefficients of structures within the plane which intersect the line between the X-ray source and detector at each sample position. These profile samples are often called "line integral values" or "ray sums" (the terms "profile sample," "line integral value," and "ray sum" are used interchangeably), and when collected from many angles of view, are the values used to mathematically reconstruct the distribution and magnitude of attenuation coefficients throughout the plane.

In order to discuss types of algorithms used for reconstructing cross-sections of X-ray attenuation coefficients, it is useful to consider the reconstruction space and how it is discretely represented in digital computers. Figure 2.16 is a diagram illustrating such a representation. A reconstruction algorithm implemented on a computer generally specifies a finite planar region in the space irradiated which contains all structures of interest to be reconstructed, with attenuation of the beam outside this region assumed to be zero. This planar region is usually bounded by a square or a circle, and is always partitioned into a matrix (grid) of nonoverlapping smaller regions (usually square) called pixels (for picture elements), each of which is assumed to have a uniform X-ray attenuation coefficient (or X-ray density). The number and size of pixels selected are somewhat arbitrary but should be based on the resolution in the projection data, the spatial resolution desired in the picture, and the spatial resolution which is practically achievable.[45–48] In general, if d is the linear dimension (side) of a resolution element (pixel), D is the linear dimension (diameter) of the region to be reconstructed, M is the number of projection views recorded around 180°, and

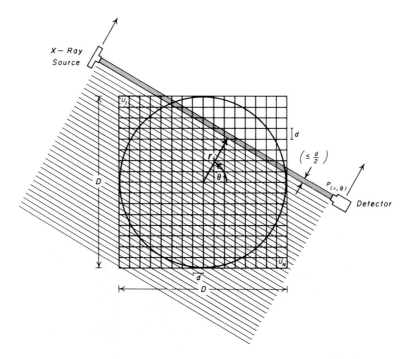

Figure 2.16. Representation of discrete, finite planar region used for image reconstruction from projections.

each view is sampled (ray sums) at intervals of $d/2$ or smaller in each view, then the maximum theoretically[49] achievable resolution is given by:

$$d = \pi D/2M \tag{2.8}$$

However, the actual resolution achievable in a reconstruction is highly dependent on the asymmetry of the object being reconstructed, the frequency and distribution of projection data samples, the noise in the sampled projection data, and the reconstruction algorithm used.[47-49] The task of the reconstruction algorithm is to geometrically determine the paths of the X-ray beams passing through the pixels of the reconstruction matrix and to mathematically relate the measurements of total attenuation (ray sums) for many such intersecting paths obtained from different views in such a way as to solve for the fractional attenuation by each pixel. When this is done, the computer can display the matrix of attenuation values as a grid of brightness levels in order to visualize an image of the structures in the reconstruction region, as illustrated in Figure 2.17.

2.3.5.2 Image Reconstruction Algorithms

The reconstruction problem may be described in equation form for the infinite continuous case as:

$$P(r, \theta) = \int_{-\infty}^{\infty} U(x, y) d\ell \tag{2.9}$$

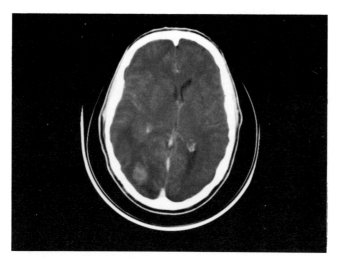

Figure 2.17. Example of image reconstructed from multiple X-ray projections. Image is a cross-sectional slice through head scanned in X-ray CT system.

where the projection ray sums $P(r, \theta)$ are expressed in polar coordinates as a function of distance r from the origin and angle θ relative to the x-axis of the cartesian coordinate reconstruction plane, $U(x, y)$ is a function of position within the reconstruction plane whose magnitude evaluated at any point (x, y) is the linear attenuation coefficient at that point, and ℓ is the differential path length along any ray. This equation forms the basis for all approaches to image reconstruction and may be called the general "projection formula." The problem is to invert Equation 2.9 to solve for $U(x, y)$.

The Austrian mathematician Radon proved[50] the existence of a valid inversion formula for Equation 2.9, assuming ideal conditions of continuity and compact support of the function, U, and infinite, noiseless projections, P. One form[47] of the Radon transform expressed in polar coordinates is

$$U(t, \theta) = \frac{1}{2\pi^2} \int_0^\pi \int_{-\infty}^\infty \frac{\partial P(r, \phi)}{\partial r} \frac{1}{t\cos(\phi - \theta) - r} \, dr d\phi \qquad (2.10)$$

Before reviewing methods that have been derived to solve Equation 2.9, or that have been developed to evaluate Radon's transform, Equation 2.10, a discrete form of the projection formula should be considered, since infinite and perfect (noiseless) projection data are not available in the real world. Since the true function $U(x, y)$ is not known, the goal is to obtain an approximation by assigning an estimate of its value to each partition element or pixel in a bounded, discretized region of space. Note in Figure 2.16 that the pencil X-ray beam has finite width and does not equally intersect every pixel. This means that some pixels contribute more and some less to the total absorption along any given ray path. With these considerations, for a reconstruction matrix with N total pixels, and for M total measured ray sums, Equation 2.9 may be written in discrete form as:

$$P_j \simeq \sum_{i=1}^N W_{ij} \cdot U(i) \qquad j = [1, M] \qquad (2.11)$$

where each of the measured projections or ray sums, P_j, is approximately equal to a weighted sum of the pixel attenuation values $U(i)$, where i indexes all x, y points. However, the weighting array, W_{ij}, is very sparse, being nonzero only where ray j intersects with pixel i. Several different ray paths may intersect with the same pixel. Conversely, each ray sum may contain information about several pixels. The relationship of ray sums to pixel attenuation along linear ray paths forms a set of simultaneous linear equations, as suggested by Equation 2.11. The minimum number of ray sums required for unique solution of the attenuation coefficients is equal to the total number of pixels, but since the measurements are contaminated with noise (photon, electronic, discretization) and may in fact not all be simultaneously linear and/or independent (for example, due to motion during the scan), often many more measurements than unknowns are required to obtain the best reconstructions.[45-49]

It is generally not practical to solve the set of Equation 2.11 by direct matrix inversion. In typical applications, N may be on the order of 10^4 to 10^5, and M on the order of 10^5 to 10^6, so that matrix W_{ij} can be on the order of 10^9 by 10^{11} in size! Therefore, a wide variety of mathematical approaches to the reconstruction problem have been developed. Most approaches can be classified[51] into one or more of the following four categories:

1. Summation methods (e.g., simple back projection);
2. Series expansion methods (e.g., iterative estimate-correct);
3. Transform methods (e.g., Fourier transform);
4. Direct analytic methods (e.g., convolution or filtered back projection).

The method most universally used at present is called either the Fourier transform method or the convolution or filtered back projection (FBP) method. The convolution method has fundamental components in categories 1, 3, and 4 but is primarily considered a direct analytic solution in closed form to the integral equations derived from the basic projection formula. However, before describing this now routine approach to image reconstruction, a brief description and simple illustrations will give a broader understanding of the variety of approaches available and the computational processes involved in image reconstruction.

The most elementary approach to image reconstruction is to estimate the densities for each pixel in the reconstruction matrix by adding together all the ray sums of rays that pass through each point. This algorithm is called the summation method or simple back projection.

An intuitive understanding of the image formation process and consequent errors in the summation method can be achieved with a simple graphical example, as shown in Figure 2.18. The summation method has been shown[51] to be equivalent to the simple back projection method. For a finite total number M of projections, P_j, the discrete values of the back projection image, $U(i)$, at each pixel i can be described mathematically by the formula:

$$U(i) = \sum_{j=1}^{M} P_j \cdot K_{[ij]} \qquad i = 1, N \qquad (2.12)$$

where K_{ij} is a special unit function:

$$K_{ij} = \begin{cases} 1, & \text{if ray } j \text{ intersects pixel } i \\ 0, & \text{if ray } j \text{ does not intersect pixel } i \end{cases} \qquad (2.13)$$

The starlike object reconstructed by simple back projection of the single circular point, as shown in the example of Figure 2.18, is essentially repeated for every point in an image reconstructed by this method. The number of spikes on the star depends on the number and direction of the projections.

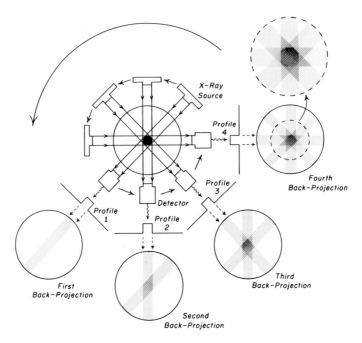

Figure 2.18. Graphical example of summation method for image reconstruction—simple back projection.

The density of the star is greatest at the center, where all projections overlap. This star-pattern density distribution is the point spread function of the summation method. Since the spikes of each reconstructed point spread into adjacent reconstructed points in the image plane, the reconstructed image is blurred.

Since the superposition of a continuous set of straight lines around a point is equivalent to rotation of a line about a point over a circumference of $2\pi r$, as the number of back-projected rays through a point is increased, the density distribution becomes proportional to $1/r$, where r is the distance from the point. The back projection image can thus be shown[52,53] to be a convolution of the true image with this $1/r$ blurring function. Several ways to partially correct the back projection image have been suggested.[52–54] One is to make the average density of the reconstructed object identical with the estimated average density of the original object (computed from the ray sums) by subtracting from each pixel a constant which is the product of the estimated mean density and the number of projections minus one. Such corrections, however, do not achieve the spatial resolution and sharpness that can be obtained by other reconstruction methods.

Even though algebraic reconstruction techniques (ART) and other iterative algorithms[51,55,56] were among the first practical methods for image reconstruction, they have given way to more efficient and accurate direct analytic approaches, and virtually no current commercial CT scanner uses an iterative algorithm.

As previously mentioned, the reconstruction method most widely used is the FBP algorithm. As the name suggests, it is related to the simple back projection method already discussed, but with a significant important difference: it corrects the blurring problem by appropriate prefiltering of the projection data before the back projection (summation) process. This prefiltering step involves a direct convolution of the projection data with a weighting function selected to compensate for the smoothing introduced by the $1/r$ point spread function of the back projection process.

However, another approach to applying such a weighting function is based on the Fourier inversion formula, and although both approaches lead to relatively equivalent algorithms (the relationship between convolution in the spatial domain and Fourier filtering in the frequency domain is well known in filter theory),[57] the Fourier approach is classified as a different type of algorithm than the direct convolution method because it involves different computational considerations. Before describing the direct convolution approach to the FBP method, it is instructive to first briefly develop the Fourier transform method, because, in fact, it comprises the fundamental theory underlying the convolution approach.

The Fourier transform method involves three steps:

1. Transforming the projections of an object into Fourier space, where they yield values on a central section defining part of the Fourier transform of the object (i.e., they are lines intersecting the origin at an angle corresponding to the direction of the projection in real space);
2. Interpolating from the values on the central sections to fill the Fourier transform space;
3. Performing an inverse Fourier transform to provide an estimate of the object.

Mathematically, this can be expressed by considering again the integral equations of the projection formula, Equation 2.9, and taking the Fourier transform of both sides:

$$\rho(\omega, \theta) = \int_{-\infty}^{\infty} P(r, \theta)e^{-i\omega r}dr$$

$$= \int_{-\infty}^{\infty} \int_{-\infty}^{\infty} U(x, y)e^{-i\omega(x\cos\theta + y\sin\theta)}dxdy \quad (2.14)$$

where $\omega = 2\pi k$, with k being the wave number, or spatial frequency along the r-axis, and where the substitution $r = (x \cos\theta + y \sin\theta)$ has been made on the right side. Equation 2.14 has been called[47] the Fourier Theorem of

Image Reconstruction, and can be used directly, with some difficulty, for reconstruction.[58] However, the resolution limits and computational difficulties are significant, primarily because of the required interpolation in the Fourier plane. Therefore, several approaches to making the method practical have been developed,[41,43,44,59] generally involving an explicit inverse Fourier transform of Equation 2.18. With a transformation of coordinates, this time from cartesian to polar and integrating over the angle variable θ from $0°$ to $180°$, the inversion may be expressed as:

$$U(x, y) = \frac{1}{4\pi^2} \int_{0}^{\pi} \int_{\infty}^{-\infty} \rho(\omega, \theta)e^{i\omega(x\cos\theta + y\sin\theta)}|\omega|d\omega d\theta \qquad (2.15)$$

where $|\omega|$ comes from the Jacobian of the transformation.[60] The validity of this inversion process was first proven, in a somewhat different form (see Equation 2.10), by Radon[50] in 1917 for the ideal case of infinite, perfect projection data [i.e., $P(r, \theta)$ noiseless and available for all θ]. It has been shown that Radon's inversion formula can be evaluated using Fourier integrals.[61]

Equation 2.15 can be considered in two parts: first, the projection data are "filtered" in the inner integral ($|\omega|$ is the filter function), and second, the filtered projection data are summed up, or "back-projected," by the outer integral over all points (x, y). Hence, Equation 2.15 represents the analytic derivation by Fourier transforms of the filtered back projection reconstruction algorithm. It is, perhaps, the most elegant and mathematically rigorous algorithm used in image reconstruction.

However, computational difficulties can arise in numerically implementing Equation 2.15 because projection data of the inner integral filtered in frequency space are not spatially bound ($|\omega|$ is a continuous ramp function), and therefore cannot be represented by a finite discrete Fourier series.[62] Although the choice of filter function may be varied conveniently to produce a desirable high-frequency bound or roll-off, the most common approach used in current X-ray CT scanner systems is to do the filtering directly in the spatial domain as a convolution integral.[63]

The convolution approach has proven to be both accurate and computationally efficient and is a direct solution to the inverse integral equations derived from the projection formula. Several methods[52,53,59,63,64] either were developed to evaluate Radon's formula directly or were derived from it. The approach again is simply to filter the projection data with a function selected to negate the blurring ($1/r$) effect of the back projection process, and then to back project the filtered projections. The spatial domain filtering step may be expressed as the convolution:

$$P^*(r, \theta) = \int_{-\infty}^{\infty} P(r', \theta) \cdot h(r - r')dr' \qquad (2.16)$$

where P^* denotes "convolved projection" and $H(r)$ is called the convolution kernel. The second step is to integrate (back project) the filtered projections over all projection angles (0° to 180°):

$$U(x, y) = \int_0^\pi P^*(x \cos \theta + y \sin \theta, \theta)d\theta \qquad (2.17)$$

Under appropriate conditions,[47,65] Equations 2.16 and 2.17 may be numerically implemented by replacing the integrals with sums, where the convolution sum is performed over the number of projection samples in each view, and the back projection sum is performed over the number of views available. The resultant discrete equations comprise the FBP algorithm and are computationally efficient, being amenable to very rapid parallel processing,[66] since projections can be filtered and back projected independently of each other. The number of multiplications and additions involved is approximately $4M(m^2 + N)$, where M is the number of view, m is the number of ray sums, and N is the number of pixels to be reconstructed.[65] The accuracy of the method is excellent if sufficient samples are available (i.e., if Nyquist frequency sampling is used and the number of views approaches the criterion of Equation 2.8) and an appropriate filter function is used.[65] Interpolation of the projection data may be performed to increase the number of ray sums required for back projection.

From consideration of Equation 2.15, the Fourier transform of the convolution kernel, h, in Equation 2.16 should be the ramp function, so that

$$h(r) = \int_{-\infty}^{\infty} |\omega|e^{i\omega r}d\omega \qquad (2.18)$$

To insure convergence of Equation 16, the filter function is generally defined to be a ramp for frequencies up to a specified limit, and zero beyond that limit. However, to avoid artifacts due to the sharp cut-off and to save extra computation time required to smooth the final image, a modified filter, which is the product of a ramp and roll-off filter, is commonly used. Idealized ramp, roll-off, and combination filters are depicted in Figure 2.19. An upper frequency bound, ω_m, is selected such that h is zero for $|\omega| > \omega_m$ and therefore

$$h(r) = \int_{-\omega_m}^{\omega_m} |\omega|e^{i\omega r}d\omega \qquad (2.19)$$

Figure 2.20 shows two examples of current, commonly used convolution filter functions.[60,63] The purpose of the "negative side lobes" in each filter is to compensate for the positive side lobes or spokes of the $1/r$ point spread distribution introduced by back projection. If the filter is carefully chosen,

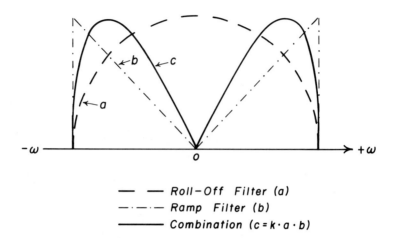

Figure 2.19. Example of idealized convolution filters.

these negative and positive side lobes cancel each other out when the filtered projections are summed, resulting in an unblurred image of the original object. This result, in effect, is a "deconvolution" of the point spread function and the blurred picture obtained by simple back projection and is, under appropriate sampling conditions, equivalent to convolution of the inverse point spread function with the simple back-projected image.

The FBP algorithm may be graphically illustrated in a way similar to the simple back projection method depicted in Figure 2.18. Figure 2.21 is a dia-

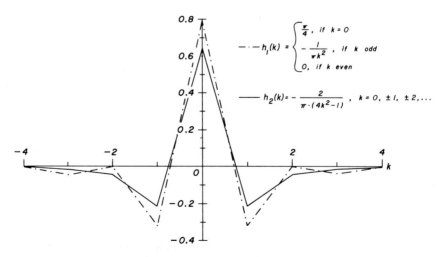

Figure 2.20. Examples of two practical convolution filters used for image reconstruction by filtered back projection.

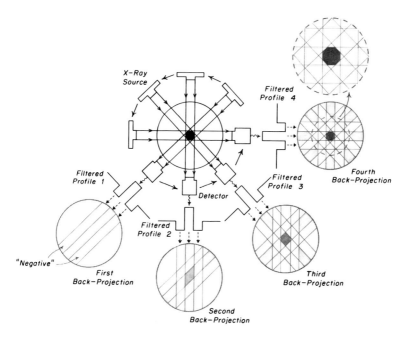

Figure 2.21.   Graphical example of filtered back projection method.

grammatic example of the FBP method using a simplified convolution kernel to show the compensating effect of the filter function on the density distributions of the back projection.

2.3.5.3 Fan Beam vs. Parallel Beam

The previous discussion of projection formulas, inversion formulas, and algorithms to numerically evaluate these formulas has been based on what is known as parallel-mode geometry (refer to Figures 2.15 and 2.16), in which the ray sum profile is produced by the projection of beams along many parallel paths at each of many equally spaced angles. In order to reduce the time for scanning, most of the newer X-ray CT scanners employ a different mode of scanning, namely fan-beam geometry, wherein each ray sum profile consists of many projection paths fanning out from a single focal point. The basic geometry is depicted in Figure 2.22. The focal point lies on a circle, concentric with but external to the reconstruction plane, which is the focus of X-ray source positions during rotation about 360°. The fan angle subtends the diameter of the reconstruction space, and the transmitted diverging rays are recorded by an array of detectors. The parallel mode geometry may be considered a special case of the fan-beam mode geometry, where, in the limit, the radius of the focal point circle approaches infinity.

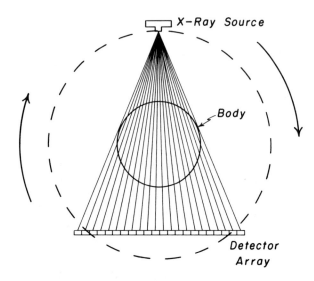

Figure 2.22.   Geometry for fan beam generation of projections for image reconstruction.

Two approaches are used in the reconstruction of fan-beam data. The first is to reorganize the fan data into parallel data (called "re-binning"), using interpolation if necessary, for use with a "parallel-mode" algorithm. The second, and more common, approach is to reconstruct the fan-beam data directly. Fan-beam versions of the FBP algorithm have been developed which were derived both from the Fourier inversion formula[67] and from the Radon inversion formula.[68] In each case a change of variables is made to adapt parallel-mode formulas and their approximations to the fan-beam data. These modifications include:

1. Multiplying each fan-beam ray sum by the cosine of the fan angle relative to the center ray of the fan;
2. Incorporating a fan angle term in the convolution kernel;
3. Providing a fan distance correction in the back projection formula.

These factors can be readily introduced into the FBP Equations 2.16 and 2.17, with only a slight increase in the computation time required to evaluate them, and with accuracy equivalent to the parallel-mode algorithms. They have been successfully applied for image reconstruction of all parts of the body.[22,59,65,69]

2.4 3-D Volume Image Representation

3-D biomedical images are generally modeled in the "stack of slices" representation described in the previous section. This model is effectively represented in the computer as a 3-D array. The organization of the tomographic data, the reference coordinate system used to uniquely address its values in 3-space, transformations to obtain desired isotropicity and orientation, and, finally, useful display of the data in either "raw" or processed format are important considerations in approaching effective utilization of 3-D imaging in real applications.

2.4.1 Data Organization

Multidimensional biomedical images reconstructed from tomographic imaging systems are characteristically represented as sets of 2-D images. A biomedical image is a real or virtual spatial representation of an organic object or objects. Digital representations of images are made up of discrete values, often called picture elements, or pixels for short. A pixel contains a value that represents and is related to some local property of the object. A pixel has a defined spatial position in 2-D (x, y) relative to some coordinate system imposed on the imaged region of interest, and each pixel has a size dictated by the discretization process used. Even though a 2-D image may be considered a basic building block for higher dimensionality, a 2-D biomedical image is really a 3-D image, as each such image has a thickness dimension associated with the imaging aperture. Characteristically, the shape of a pixel is dimensionally square in the plane of the image (e.g., 0.5 mm $\times$ 0.5 mm), but the thickness of the pixel is often significantly greater in dimension (e.g., 3 mm). Figure 2.23 illustrates the concept of pixels in an image and their thickness, suggesting the term "voxel" for volume picture element or volume pixel.[44]

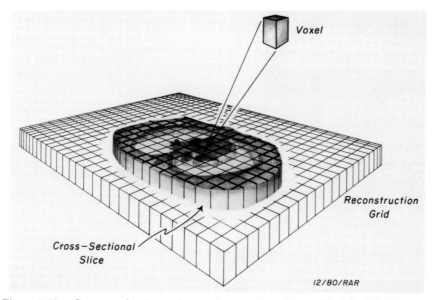

Figure 2.23. Concept of volume picture elements (voxels) used in 2-D digital images.

3-D biomedical images are often organized as collections of 2-D images, where the third dimension may be another spatial dimension, time, or the same object imaged by different modalities. Most often, 3-D images represent the object as adjacent planes through the structure. This results in a stack of 2-D images spanning the extent of the 3-D structure of interest. This may be called a volume image. Each element of the volume image is called a voxel. A voxel contains a value that is a representation of some local property of the structure being imaged. Each voxel has a defined spatial position and dimension in 3-space. Since most 3-D data sets are composed of stacks of 2-D images in which the "thickness" of each 2-D image is often greater than the size of the pixels, a 3-D volume image most often contains voxels that are not cubic, i.e., the volume image is anisotropic. One common step in processing 3-D biomedical image data prior to visualization and analysis is to create an isotropic volume image from the anisotropic data, using various spatial interpolation methods. This volume can then be displayed a variety of ways, which are described in Chapter 4. Figure 2.24 indicates a representation of a volume image with isotropic voxels used for projection imaging onto a screen.

Another possible representation for 3-D biomedical images includes a collection of 2-D images that vary through time. Many imaging systems can acquire 2-D images repetitively through the course of time, primarily to study function of structures. In this context, the collection of 2-D images into a 3-D time-varying data set can be thought of as having two spatial dimensions (the pixel) and one time dimension, although any 2-D image still has a thickness dimension.

Finally, another 3-D representation may consist of spatially correlated 2-D images from different scanning modalities, or different scan types within a modality, often called a multispectral image set. For example, a single 2-D image may have been created for the same structure of interest on a structural imaging system (MRI), as well as a functional imaging system

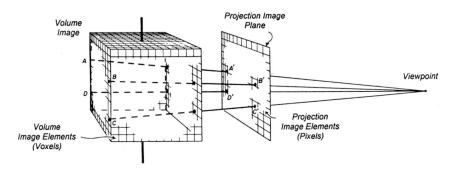

Figure 2.24. Concept of volume elements (voxels) used in 3-D digital images. Voxels are often projected into pixels for viewing 3-D volume on a 2-D screen.

(PET), in order to correlate function with structure. The number of different modalities or scan types defines the number of spectra (i.e., the "z" dimension) in the 3-D image set.

4-D biomedical images are organized as collections of 3-D image sets. For example, a 4-D image set may consist of 3-D volume images that are time varying, a common format for imaging systems that can acquire 3-D spatial volume images rapidly through time.[1,69] Another 4-D organization consists of 3-D multispectral volume image sets, where each volume image represents a different modality or type of acquisition. This concept extends beyond 4-D image sets to 5-D and more, where each new dimension is added to prior dimensions (e.g., a 5-D data set may consist of 4-D time-varying 3-D volume images for different modalities).

2.4.2 Coordinate Systems and Object Orientation

Typically, volume images are represented as a 3-D discrete regular grid of voxels within a defined coordinate system. The orientation of the structure being imaged is often specified in order to standardize the location and orientation of the object in a regular grid, permitting spatial correlation and comparison between volume images.

There are at least two consistent ways of conceptualizing the arrangement of multiple 2-D images as a coherent 3-D volume image. One system, called *origin-order consistency,* is mathematically rigorous but not always intuitively obvious. Another system, called *view-order consistency,* is a more natural and intuitive way of conceptualizing 3-D volume images, but it is not mathematically consistent.

In the *origin-order system,* the coordinate system maintains an unambiguous, single 3-D origin in the volume image, with the order of all voxels in a single line of a plane, the order of all lines in a plane, and the order of all planes in the volume proceeding from the same origin. With this coordinate consistancy applied to a left-handed coordinate system, the projection of the origin is always displayed at the lower left of the screen and the order of the images is always from the origin outward, as shown in Figure 2.25. Volume images in this system can be correctly reformatted, as demonstrated by the orthogonal sections in Figure 2.26, and structures in the volume image will be correctly rendered using volume image visualization techniques. Flipping images about one or three of the axes corrupts the integrity of the image and results in a volume image which is mirror-reversed and can no longer be self consistent. Reformatted and/or rendered displays of such data will generate mirror images.

Structure orientation within this left-handed, origin-order coordinate system is also critical to the consistent comparison or direct utilization of multiple volume images. Most medical imaging devices acquire transaxially oriented 2-D images as the default image set, with multiple adjacent transaxial images comprising the 3-D volume image. In this coordinate system, these

Volume

- Transverse slices are in the XY plane.
- Sagittal slices are in the ZY plane.
- Coronal slices are in the ZX plane.

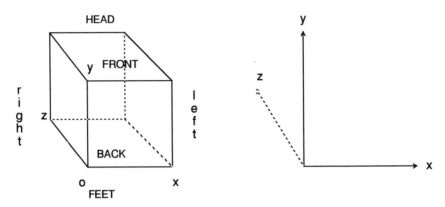

Figure 2.25. Origin-order based, left-handed coordinate system representation for 3-D volume images.

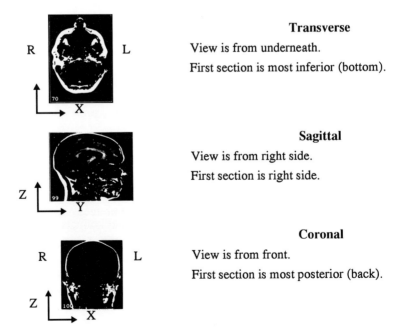

Transverse

View is from underneath.

First section is most inferior (bottom).

Sagittal

View is from right side.

First section is right side.

Coronal

View is from front.

First section is most posterior (back).

Figure 2.26. Correct orientation for mutually orthogonal sections in origin-order, left-handed coordinate system.

images are placed in the *x-y* plane, with the *x-z* plane sectioned coronally and the *y-z* plane sectioned sagittally.

View-order consistency is not concerned with the maintenance of a single unambiguous 3-D origin. It simply posits a relationship that should hold between the orientation of the sectional images and their order in the data file. A view-order-based system accepts sectional images in any of six orientations, and assigns the axes to the row, column, and image directions of the image data regardless of the physical section orientation. The main advantage of the view-order system is that it is highly intuitive and is completely insensitive to orientation. Its major drawback is that the location of the origin and orientations of the axes will vary depending upon the section orientation.

2.4.3 Value Representation

As each pixel or voxel in a discrete image is represented by a value that is measured and/or computed by the image acquisition system, the range of representation must encompass the entire range of possible measured and/or computed values and must be of sufficient accuracy to preserve precision in the measured values. This range of representation is called the dynamic range of the data. This range is defined both by the imaging system, which determines the inherent range of values required to capture the entire signal, and by the numeric scale used to represent the images, which is usually related to the discrete representation by the computer system. Often, the discrete representation of value in the computer system cannot capture the entire dynamic range of the acquired signal from the imaging system. Figure 2.14 shows a typical range used for representing X-ray CT values.

2.4.4 Interpolation and Transformation

As previously mentioned, most 3-D biomedical volume images are sampled anisotropically, with the slice thickness often significantly greater than the in-plane pixel size. Either prior to display and measurement or during these operations, the volume image must be transformed in order to accommodate for this anisotropy. This is often required for proper visualization, as the 3-D data must be isotropic in order to produce the correct aspect ratio along each dimension when displayed. Similarly for resectioning functions, sections created through nonisotropic voxels will exhibit aliasing artifacts due to the difference in sampling frequency along the orthogonal axes if anisotropy is not corrected. Actual voxel interpolation to produce an isotropic volume is often not required when the goal is simply to look at acquisition planes or make in-plane measurements. But in most cases, 3-D biomedical volume images will need to be interpolated to isotropic dimensions and potentially transformed in orientation in order to achieve the desired visualization or quantitative analysis tasks.

The most commonly used interpolation scheme for 3-D volume images is first-order linear interpolation of the gray level values in the volume image. In this scheme, values of "new pixels" are simply interpolated linearly between the values of the existing pixels. In 3-D, this operation becomes trilinear interpolation, where the value of any given voxel is interpolated among voxels in the surrounding 3-D region. Given that this operation is linear, the interpolation in each of the dimensions is completely separable, permitting the computation to be done in the three orthogonal directions sequentially. Trilinear interpolation works well for most biomedical images, but when the ratio in size between any of the voxel dimensions in 3-D becomes greater than approximately 5:1, linear interpolation should probably not be used for measurement or display of the gray level information between the sampled voxels. This is commonly the case with biomedical imagery, and particularly with X-ray CT and MRI where the in-plane x-y dimension of the pixels may be less than 1 mm, while the slice thickness and/ or separation is commonly greater than 5 mm. In these instances, trilinear interpolation will provide poor approximations between voxels, particularly in the slice acquisition direction (e.g., z-axis), and often a jagged staircase artifact is produced, which is very visible in renderings of these volumes. To compensate for this problem, either in-plane resolution needs to be reduced to decrease the ratio between the slice thickness and the pixel size, requiring less interpolation in the z-direction and hence less artifact, or other interpolation mechanisms must be utilized. Higher-order interpolants such as cubic spline interpolation[70] may be used in such cases, with an increase in computation time. These algorithms use more than the immediately adjacent voxels and use a cubic polynomial to estimate intermediate values. If a particular structure of interest can be defined and segmented from the volume image, shape-based interpolation methods[71] can be used to estimate the intermediate voxels that would (or would not) be contained in the structure based on shape criteria. These methods often use distance transforms, which compute the closest distance to the desired edge of the structure (both inside and outside) for every voxel in the volume image and interpolate these distance values to estimate the location of the structure.[72] Shape-based interpolation works well when a particular surface is desired, and the visualizations of the 3-D surface are without the staircase artifact, but the a priori requirement of specific structure identification limits the usefulness of this interpolation technique.

2.4.5 Display

Does multidimensional biomedical imaging, defined as the process of generating digital volume image data by any one of several techniques, imply the need for multidimensional display? The answer is yes, if the nature of the insights, understanding, or measurements to be derived from the image data requires an appreciation of 3-D shapes and/or spatial relationships. The term 3-D display includes, in a broad sense, those methods which attempt to display information of three dimensions utilizing all or a subset of possible depth cues. Computer display and visualization methods can assist the observer to process, manipulate, and measure useful information in 3-D biomedical images.[73]

The need for 3-D display is emphasized by gaining an appreciation of the fundamental dilemma of studying 3-D irregularly shaped objects like the organs of the body, using tomographic images. Tomography provides clear, unambiguous views of 2-D sections through the body utilizing images that, by definition, contain no 3-D information. Often it is very difficult to interpret (understand) isolated tomographic images, especially if the image is of an organ system that has an abnormal shape or the orientation of the scanning plane is not "standard." The most common method used to resolve this difficulty is to scan and display a "stack" of parallel tomographic images, side-by-side on multiformat film or on a television screen. If, however, the objective in collecting the volume image requires cognition (appreciation or understanding) of the 3-D shapes or spatial relationships of an organ or image region, then 3-D displays avoid the necessity of mentally reconstructing a representation of the structure of interest. Mental reconstruction is often both difficult and highly subjective; that is, different observers mentally reconstruct or "see" different shapes.

Multidimensional display techniques for 3-D tomographic image analysis can be classified into two basic display types based on what is shown to the observer.[74] The first type, referred to as direct display, extends the concept of the 2-D frame buffer display of tomographic images into three dimensions by presenting the volume image 3-D array of voxels as a 3-D distribution of brightness. Frame buffers generate 2-D images on a TV monitor which are visible representations of 2-D arrays of image elements (pixels). Generally, the brightness of each displayed pixel is proportional to the magnitude of the pixel, although pixel brightness transformations such as gray level windowing are often employed before display to enhance the visibility of selected gray levels. By representing the volume image as a 3-D distribution of brightnesses, direct display enables the direct visualization of the unprocessed image data. The second type of multidimensional display, utilized in conjunction with 3-D biomedical images, is called surface display. The rationale for the use of surface displays is that visualization of the surfaces which exist within the volume is useful. The surface is first identified either manually or in an automated fashion by computer algorithm. The identified surface is then represented either as a set of contours or as a surface locus within a volume which reflects light from an imaginary light source. The output of this latter process is made visible with a 2-D frame buffer relying mainly on the monocular depth cues of shading and/or motion parallax (rotation) to convey depth and shape. In contrast to direct display, surface displays present information (surfaces) derived from the image data. The information is presented as a 3-D distribution of light reflectors, i.e., each pixel in the output image represents the magnitude of light reflected off the surface. This fundamental difference of display methods to show either light emitters or light reflectors forms the basis for virtually all computer workstation display types. More direct 3-D displays using augmenting equipment, including stereo holograms, stereo viewers, head mounted display, etc., still use one or the other of these types of displays in the image formation process.[75]

Because these two display types differ fundamentally, they are useful for different and somewhat complementary image analysis procedures. Direct display enables the direct visualization of the unprocessed image data, which, in turn, facilitates procedures such as editing, e.g., searching for a desired region within the volume image to make a measurement. Conversely, surface displays facilitate the analysis of cognition of shapes and spatial relationships.[76]

2.5 References

1. Robb, R. A., Hoffman, E. A., Sinak, L. J., Harris, L. D., Ritman, E. L. "High-speed three-dimensional x-ray computed tomography: The Dynamic Spatial Reconstructor." *Proc. IEEE*, 71, 308–319, 1983.

2. Robb, R. A. *Three-Dimensional Biomedical Imaging. Vol. I & II*. CRC Press, Boca Raton, FL, 1985.

3. Nudelman, S., Roehrig, H., Capp, M. P. "A study of photoelectronic-digital radiology. III. Image acquisition components and system design." *Proc. IEEE*, 70, 715, 1982.

4. Curry, T. S., Dowdey, J. E., Murry, R. C. *Christensen's Physics of Diagnostic Radiology*. 4th Ed. Lea & Febiger, Malvern, PA, 1990.

5. Robb, R. A. "X-ray computed tomography: An engineering synthesis of multiscientific principles." *CRC Crit. Rev. Biomed. Eng.*, 7, 265–334, 1982.

6. Ring, B. A. "An overview: computed axial tomography." *Appl. Radiol.*, November 1979.

7. McCullough, E. C. "Specifying and evaluating the performance of computed tomography (CT) scanners." *Med. Phys.*, 7, 291, 1980.

8. Lauterbur, P. C. "Image formation by induced local interactions: examples employing nuclear magnetic resonance." *Nature (London)*, 242, 190, 1973.

9. Jack, C. R., Thompson, R. M., Butts, R. K., et al. "Sensory motor cortex: correlation or presurgical mapping with functional MR imaging and invasive cortical mapping." *Radiology,* 190, 85–92, 1994.

10. Sprawls, P., Bronskill, M. (Eds.) *The Physics of MRI*. American Association of Physicists in Medicine, Monograph 21, Woodbury, NY, 1992.

11. Wehrli, F. W. *Fast-Scan Magnetic Resonance, Principles and Applications*. Raven Press, New York, 1991.

12. Gustafson, D. E. "Single Photon Emission-Computed Tomography." In: Robb, R. A. (Ed.) *Three-Dimensional Biomedical Imaging. Vol. II.* Chapter 1. CRC Press, Boca Raton, FL, 1985.

13. Oldendorf, W. H. "Isolated flying spot detection of radiodensity discontinuities: displaying the internal structural pattern of a complex object." *IRE Trans. Bio-Med. Electron.*, 8, 68, 1961.

14. Ter-Pogossian, M. M. "Positron Emission Tomography (PET)." In: Robb, R. A. (Ed.) *Three-Dimensional Biomedical Imaging. Vol. II.* Chapter 2. CRC Press, Boca Raton, FL, 1985.

15. Spinks, T. J., Jones, T., Bailey, D. L., et al. "Physical performance of a new commercial positron tomograph with retractable septa." *IEEE Med. Imaging Conf. Rec.*, 1991, pp. 1313–1317.

16. Greenleaf, J. F. *Tissue Characterization with Ultrasound. Vol. I & II.* CRC Press, Boca Raton, FL, 1986.

17. Black, W. C. "Biomagnetism—Magnetic Imaging." Reprint published by Medical Electronics, October 1991.

18. Hobbie, R. K. *Intermediate Physics for Medicine and Biology.* 2nd Ed. John Wiley & Sons, New York, 1988.

19. Fuchs, M., Wischmann, H.-A., Dössel, O. "Overlay of neuromagnetic current density images and morphological MR images." In: Robb, R. A. (Ed.) *Proceedings of Visualization in Biomedical Computing 1992.* SPIE, Vol. 1808, Chapel Hill, NC, October 13–16, 1992.

20. Kriete, A. *Visualization in Biomedical Microscopies, 3-D Imaging and Computer Applications.* VCH Publishers, Germany, 1992.

21. Lechleiter, J., Girard, S., Peralta, E., Clapham, D. "Spiral calcium wave propagation and annihilation in *Xenopus laevis* oocytes." *Science*, 252, 123–126, 1991.

22. Herman, G. T. (Ed.) *Image Reconstruction from Projections: Implementation and Applications. Top. Appl. Phys., Vol. 32,* Springer-Verlag, Berlin, Heidelberg, New York, 1979.

23. Vallebona, F. "Radiography with great enlargement (microradiography) and a technical method for radiographic dissociation of the shadow." *Radiology*, 17, 340, 1931.

24. Ziedes des Plantes, G. B. "Eine neue Methode zür Differenzierung in der Röntgenographie." *Acta Radiol.*, 13, 182, 1932.

25. Edholm, P. "The tomogram—its formation and content." *Acta Radiol. Suppl.*, 193, 1, 1960.

26. Rossman, K., Moseley, R. D. "Measurement of the input to radiographic imaging systems." *Radiology*, 92, 265, 1969.

27. Bürsch, J., Johs, R., Heintzen, P. H. "Validity of Lambert-Beer's Law in roentgendensitometry of contrast material using continuous radiation." In: *Roentgen-, Cine-, and Videodensitometry,* Georg Thieme Verlag, Stuttgart, 1971, 81.

28. McCullough, E. C., Baker, H. L., Houser, O. W., Reese, D. F. "An evaluation of the quantitative and radiation features of a scanning x-ray transverse axial tomograph: the EMI scanner." *Radiology*, 111, 709, 1974.

29. Zatz, L. M., Alvarez, R. G. "An inaccuracy in computed tomography: the energy dependence of CT values." *Radiology*, 124, 91, 1977.

30. Brooks, R. A., DiChiro, G. "Beam hardening in x-ray computed tomography." *Phys. Med. Biol.*, 21, 390, 1976.

31. McDavid, W. D., Waggener, R. G., Payne, W. H., Dennis, M. J. "Correction for spectral artifacts in cross-sectional reconstructions from x-rays." *Med. Phys.*, 4, 54, 1977.

32. Herman, G. T., Simmons, R. Illustrations of a beam hardening correction method in computerized tomography. *Appl. Opt. Instrumen. Med.*, III, SPIE, 173, 264, 1979.

33. Ruegsegger, P., Hangartner, T., Keller, H. U., Hinderling, T. "Standardization of computed tomographic images by means of a material-selective beam hardening correction." *J. Comput. Assist. Tomogr.*, 2, 184, 1978.

34. Joseph, P. M., Spital, R. A. "A method for correcting bone induced artifacts in computed tomography scanners." *J. Comput. Assist. Tomogr.*, 2, 100, 1978.

35. Hounsfield, G. N. "Computerized transverse axial scanning (tomography). I. Description of system." *Brit. J. Radiol.*, 46, 1016, 1973.

36. Phelps, M. E., Hoffmann, G. J., Ter-Pogossian, M. M. "Attenuation coefficients of various body tissues, fluids, and lesions at photon energies of 18 to 136 KeV." *Radiology*, 117, 573, 1975.

37. New, P. E. J., Aronow, S. "Attenuation measurements of whole blood and blood fractions in computed tomography." *Radiology*, 121, 635, 1976.

38. Fullerton, G. D. "Fundamentals of CT tissue characterization in medical physics of CT and ultrasound tissue imaging and characterization." *AAPM, Med. Phys. Monogr.*, 6, 125, 1980.

39. Pullan, B. R., Fawcett, R. H., Isherwood, I. "Tissue characterization by an analysis of the distribution of attenuation values in computed tomography scans." *J. Comput. Assist. Tomogr.*, 2, 49, 1978.

40. Mategsano, V. C., Petasnick, J., Clark, J., Chung Bin, A., Weinstein, R. "Attenuation values in computed tomography of the abdomen." *Radiology*, 125, 135, 1977.

41. Hounsfield, G. N. "Computed medical imaging." Nobel Lecture, December 8, 1979, *J. Comput. Assist. Tomogr.*, 4, 665, 1980.

42. Drieke, P., Boyd, D. "Convolution reconstruction of fan beam projections." *Comput. Graphics Image Proc.*, 5, 459, 1976.

43. Herman, G. T., Lakshminarayanan, A. V., Naparstek, A. "Convolution reconstruction techniques for divergent beams." *Comput. Biol. Med.*, 6, 259, 1976.

44. Robb, R. A., Greenleaf, J. F., Ritman, E. L., Johnson, S. A., Sjostrand, J. D., Herman, G. T., Wood, E. H. "Three-dimensional visualization of the intact thorax and contents: a technique for cross-sectional reconstruction from multiplanar x-ray views." *Comp. Biomed. Res.*, 7, 395, 1974.

45. Glover, G. H., Eisner, R. L. "Theoretical resolution of computed tomography systems." *J. Comput. Assist. Tomogr.*, 3, 85, 1979.

46. Huesman, R. H. "The effects of a finite number of projection angles and finite lateral sampling of projections on the propagation of statistical errors in transverse section reconstruction." *Phys. Med. Biol.*, 22, 511, 1977.

47. Brooks, R. A. "Computational principles of transmission CT." In: *Medical Physics of CT and Ultrasound and Tissue Imaging and Characteristics*, AAPM, *Med. Phys. Monogr.*, 6, 37, 1980.

48. Frieder, G., Herman, G. T. "Resolution in reconstructing objects from electron micrographics." *J. Theor. Biol.*, 33, 189, 1971.

49. Crowther, R. A., DeRosier, D. J., Klug, A. "The reconstruction of a three-dimensional structure from projections and its application to electron microscopy." *Proc. R. Soc. London Ser. A*, 317, 319, 1970.

50. Radon, J. "Über die Bestimmung von Funktionen durch ihre integralwerte längs gewisser Mannigfaltigkeiten." *Bu. Succhss. Akad. Wiss. Leipzig, Math. Phys. K.*, 69, 262, 1917.

51. Gordon, R., Herman, G. T. "Three-dimensional reconstruction from projections: a review of algorithms." *Int. Rev. Cytol.*, 38, 111, 1974.

52. Vainshtein, B. K. "Finding the structure of objects from projections." *Kristallografiya*, 15, 894, 1970.

53. Gilbert, P. F. C. "The reconstruction of a three-dimensional structure from projections and its application to electron microscopy. II. Direct methods." *Proc. R. Soc. London Ser. B*, 182, 89, 1972.

54. Budinger, T. F., Gullberg, G. T. "Three-dimensional reconstruction in nuclear medicine imaging." *IEEE Trans. Nucl. Sci.*, 21(3), 2, 1974.

55. Goitein, M. "Three-dimensional density reconstruction from a series of two-dimensional projections." *Nucl. Instrum. Methods*, 101, 509, 1917.

56. Gilbert, P. F. C. "Iterative methods for the reconstruction of three-dimensional objects from projections." *J. Theor. Biol.*, 36, 105, 1972.

57. Bracewell, R. N. *The Fourier Transform and Its Applications*. 2nd Ed. McGraw-Hill, New York, 1978.

58. DeRosier, D. J., Klug, A. "Reconstruction of three-dimensional images from electron micrographs." *Nature (London)*, 217, 130, 1968.

59. Ledley, R. S., DiChiro, G., Luessenhop, A. J., Twigg, H. L. "Computerized transaxial x-ray tomography of the human body." *Science*, 186, 207, 1974.

60. Shepp, L. A., Logan, E. C. "The Fourier reconstruction of a head section." *IEEE Trans. Nucl. Sci.*, 21(3), 21, 1974.

61. Bracewell, R. W., Riddle, A. C. "Inversion of fan-beam scans in radioastronomy." *Astrophys. J.*, 150, 427, 1967.

62. Marr, R. B. "On the reconstruction of a function on a circular domain from a sampling of its line integrals." *J. Math. Anal. Appl.*, 357, 1974.

63. Ramachandaran, G. N., Lakshminarayanan, A. V. "Three-dimensional reconstruction from radiographs and electron micrographs: application of convolutions instead of Fourier transforms." *Proc. Natl. Acad. Sci. U.S.A.*, 68, 2236, 1971.

64. Cho, Z. H., Ahn, I., Bohm, C. Huth, G. "Computerized image reconstruction methods with multiple photon/x-ray transmission scanning." *Phys. Med. Biol.*, 19, 511, 1974.

65. Shepp, L. A., Kruskal, J. B. "Computerized tomography: the new medical x-ray technology." *Am. Math. Mo.*, 85, 420, 1978.

66. Gilbert, B. K., Harris, L. D., Beistad, R. D., Robb, R. A., Atkins, D. E. "Implementation of computational-intensive reconstruction algorithms for x-ray computed tomography." *IEEE Proc. Comp. Soc. Conf. Pattern Recog. Proc.*, CH1428-2C, 256, 1979.

67. Lakshminarayanan, A. V. *Reconstruction from Divergent Ray Data.* Department of Computer Science, SUNY/Buffalo Technical Report 92, 1975.

68. Herman, G. T., Naparstek, A. "Fast image reconstruction based on Radon inversion formula appropriate for rapidly collected data." *SIAM J. Appl. Radiol.,* 4, 81, 1976.

69. Robb, R. A., Sinak, L. J., Hoffman, E. A., Kinsey, J. H., Harris, L. D., Ritman, E. L. "Dynamic volume imaging of moving organs." *J. Med. Syst.,* 6, 539–554, 1982.

70. Foley, J. D., Van Dam, A., Feiner, S., Hughs, J. *Computer Graphics: Principles and Practice.* 2nd Ed. Addison-Wesley Publishing Co., Reading, MA, 1990.

71. Raya, S., Udupa, J. "Shape-based interpolation of multidimensional objects." *IEEE Trans. Med. Imaging,* 9(1), 564–567, March 1990.

72. Herman, G. T., Zheng, J., Bucholtz, C. A. "Shape-based interpolation." *IEEE Comput. Graph. Appl.,* 12(3), 69–79, May 1992.

73. Harris, L. D. "Display of multidimensional biomedical image information." In: Robb, R. A. (Ed.) *Three-Dimensional Biomedical Imaging. Vol. II.* Chapter 5. CRC Press, Boca Raton, FL, 1985.

74. Robb, R. A. (Ed.) *Proceedings of Visualization in Biomedical Computing 1992.* SPIE, Vol. 1808, Chapel Hill, NC, October 13–16, 1992.

75. Camp, J. J., Stacy, M. C., Robb, R. A. "A system for interactive volume analysis (SIVA) of 4-D biomedical images." *J. Med. Syst.,* 2, 287–310, 1987.

76. Uttal, W. R. *Visual Form Detection in 3-Dimensional Space.* Lawrence Erlbaum Associates, Hillsdale, NJ, 1983.

CHAPTER

3

The Image Computer

Scientist Russell A. Kirsch and his colleagues, working at the National Bureau of Standards in the mid 1950's, constructed a mechanical drum scanner and traced the intensities of a photograph. They converted the photomultiplier signals into arrays of 176 by 176 binary digits, and fed them into a SEAC 1500 word memory computer. They then programmed the computer to extract line drawings, count objects, recognize characters, and produce oscilloscope displays of images.

William Mitchell, *The Reconfigured Eye*[1]

3.1 Introduction

The evolution of electronic imaging has paralleled the evolution of computers. Since Kirsch published his paper on electronic imaging, many efforts have been made to capture, compute, and display images with computers. Like some early predictions regarding the impact computers would have on society,[2] some promises for computer imaging remain unfulfilled. This is partly because the complexities of real image data have grown, and implementation of computer technology has lagged somewhat behind the most advanced concepts of imaging science. However, the tremendous advances in the microelectronics industry between 1960 and 1990 have facilitated concomitant advances in image processing, display, and analysis (understanding), particularly in biomedical imaging and scientific visualization.

3.2 A Brief History of Computers

As written language accelerated the ability of humans to communicate, learn, and understand, computing devices have enhanced our ability to calculate and do arithmetic. Early math was performed on fingers and toes. The Babylonians extended this capability with the abacus, and in the 1780s, the Jacquard loom was invented to speed up the process of creating patterns in cloth. The loom is credited with being the first primitive stored program computer.[3] In a sense, the loom was also an image reproduction device, as it stored the pattern for the final "image" of the cloth in coded, punched cards.

Later developments in computers were generally driven by the need to solve complex mathematical equations. Charles Babbage developed a mechanical calculating machine that provided a basis for computer units.[3] Computers built from relays at MIT in the 1930s performed simple arithmetic. In the 1940s, IBM developed the first large-scale computer, called Mark I, at Harvard, followed by ENIAC, a computer based on 18,000 vacuum tubes. The development of the transistor at Bell Labs allowed smaller, faster, and more reliable computers, such as the IBM 360 in 1964. In the late 1960s, the integrated circuit enabled companies like Cray Research and Digital Equipment to build supercomputers and commercially successful minicomputers. The early 1980s saw the Personal Computer "revolution," officially started when IBM began selling the "PC." Figure 3.1 illustrates the time course in evolution of some important computer landmarks.

As the electronics and hardware for computers developed, software for computers also evolved to provide the tools that made the computers much more powerful. Operating systems, programming languages, software libraries, subroutines, and standardized recipes for computing were devised and shared. For the abacus, the operating system is the design of the instrument. Its programming language is the technique used to operate the machine. Neither can be changed. But the electronic computer allows for considerable change in its operating principles. This is accomplished through computer programs, or "software."

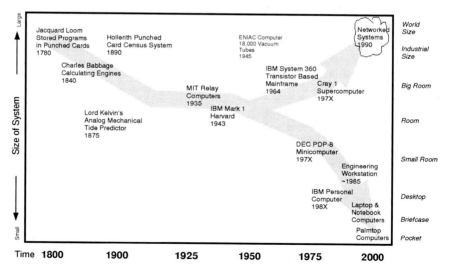

Figure 3.1. Timeline for evolution of important computers and their relative physical sizes.

The early computers were programmed from wired plug boards, a time-consuming process. As the size of computer memories grew, from the 72 cells of the Mark I in 1944 to the 20,000 digits of the IBM 701 processors in the early 1950s[4] to the 16 gigabytes (16×10^9) available in systems today, operating systems grew to accommodate the many new features of computers. For example, the "device driver," a module in modern operating systems, was used in the Atlas operating system in the 1950s[5] and provided a convenient method to attach new input and output devices to the computer.

As the operating system developed, programming languages also evolved, and programming techniques were standardized and collected in programming libraries. Initially all programming was done in the "language" of the machine, but as the memories and storage devices became larger, programmers had to move away from "machine" languages into "assembly" language, a kind of shorthand for machine language, but with one significant difference: numbers used in the program were referred to symbolically, not by their real addresses. This allowed the programmer to concentrate more on the purpose of the code and less on the mechanics of it.

Over time many so-called programming languages have developed, each filling some specific purpose. In the sciences, FORTRAN (for FORmula TRANslator) was developed in 1954[4] and is still widely used today. In the early 1970s, the C programming language was developed by Dennis Ritchie on a DEC PDP-11 computer, in conjunction with the development of the UNIX operating system.[6] In the mid 1980s, Bjarne Stroustrup extended C, and called it C++, adding important constructs to assist with managing objects.

3.3 Capturing and Displaying Images with Computers

Computers are machines that function largely by analogy. For example, a computer that is programmed to compute the trajectory of a rocket does not actually fly rockets until the right answer appears. Instead, the mathematics of rocket flight are translated into a suitable analogy for rocket flights, and the results are returned by exercising the analogy. Rocket flights are simple mathematical constructs, and computers can solve them easily because the mathematics convert easily and the number of variables is small. By comparison, computer programs for predicting weather are immense and not well defined, and the number of variables is extensive. Since weather prediction is a time-crucial activity (getting yesterday's "forecast" today is not particularly useful), attempts to solve this problem with computers had to wait until suitable computer power was available.

Electronic imaging on computers had to wait for suitable hardware before significant progress could be made. On early computers, image processing was crude, at best. For example, creative programmers found ways to generate rough images of the Mona Lisa by using appropriate characters on line printers and teletypes to form proportional halftone intensities. These techniques were mostly for fun.

The digital image might be considered to be a form of visual display, like photographs without chemicals, or paintings without paint. But the distinction between digital imagery and photography is more profound than that. Whereas a photograph is a continuous or analog image, the digital image is made up of discrete elements, each of which has one or more values associated with it. Copies of photographs can be made by photographing the photograph, but duplication by this method will never render a copy with all of the same information contained in the original. Successive copies will degrade further, as more information is lost or replaced by noise. Since a digital image is composed of a fixed number of discrete, single-valued elements, a copy of these values can be made as precisely as the original. In fact, the 1000th generation of a digital image will have precisely the same image quality as the original. The difference between analog photographs and digital images has scientific and cultural consequences. Indeed, as digital imaging moved from being a laboratory curiosity into an applied technology, the uses of electronic images, their meanings, and their value as elements of factual discourse began to change.[1]

Early development of digital imagery coincided with the scientific aims of the space program. The public was in awe of images returned from the moon in 1964, images that were processed by NASA to remove imperfections. In 1968 digital enhancement was used to give dramatic clarity to the famous close-up of Surveyor 7's footpad resting in the moon dust. In the 1970s we began seeing ourselves on earth through the eyes of ERTS, Landsat, and Spot satellites. Later, the Voyager and Magellan missions returned spectacular images from much farther away in space.[1]

The raster-based cathode ray tube display was developed from the technology of the oscilloscope. The raster display scanned the cathode ray from side to side and top to bottom. For text processing these devices became the "ASCII terminal," now generally available for a modest cost. ASCII terminals use "character memory" to store the locations of dots representing the letters and numbers. As the cathode ray scans across the screen, these dot patterns are reproduced, forming the text being displayed. This method keeps the size of the terminal's memory relatively small, since only 256 patterns (the letters, numbers, and special characters) need to be reproduced on the screen.

As the cost of memory components fell and speeds were increased, displays were developed that allowed the programmer to access each dot on the screen individually. With these "bitmapped" displays, it became practical to display images. Early bitmapped displays were based on television technology and offered arrays of 525 by 480 black and white pixels. Current workstation displays typically offer arrays of 1280 by 1024 colored pixels, and more.

Meanwhile, the advancement of transistors and integrated circuits permitted the development of devices that could capture images to use in digital computers. Early devices that converted images into electronic signals were the television and the facsimile machines. These were analog, or continuously varying, signals. Later, methods were developed to digitize these analog signals, i.e., to convert the varying voltage into a sequence of digital values proportional to the voltage fluctuations. Today, electronic images are routinely captured and stored for a variety of purposes in business and industry. Insurance companies convert documents into electronic images for record-keeping. X-ray images are stored for medical and industrial uses. Television uses an array of digital image capture, generation, and manipulation techniques to keep our attention during and between the programs. Even the motion picture film industry relies on digital image generation, capture, and manipulation to make many movies more interesting.

3.4 Images vs. Graphics

Historically in computing, considerable work has been done on the generation of images from geometric descriptions. The computer-aided design (CAD) industry has evolved to a highly specialized skill, and utilizes scenes rendered from the geometric data necessary to build parts and molds to make products.[7]

The visible difference between a rendering of a visual scene or a real object generated by electronic imaging and one generated by computer graphics might be slight, but the methods used to build the analogies in the computer are significant. The choice of methods influences decisions on the architecture of the computer and on the programming methods used for display and analysis.[8]

A graphical representation of a scene is based on geometric objects and definitions, such as lines, spheres, and polygons. The surfaces of these objects are calculated, and the visual characteristics of these surfaces are provided, such as color, reflectance, transparency, etc. These geometric views are used in the design phases of architectural and manufacturing companies to inspect the appearance of the planned building or product. Since the geometric specification of the object can exist without the object, scenes can be created that have no actual counterpart in reality.[8]

By contrast, digital images are representations (or mappings) of real scenes and are generally formed as an array of picture elements (pixels) with attributes for each element, such as brightness or density.[9] For example, an image on a color television screen is formed by picture elements that have a red, a green, and a blue attribute. The ability of the eye and the brain to combine these picture elements into a scene allows one to "see" a mountain or a face when it appears.

The distinction between graphics and images is important to the selection of computers for imaging purposes.[10] Computer systems are evaluated and measured in a variety of ways, each designed to model some application of the system. Machines that perform graphics often specify their abilities in "vectors/second" or "filled triangles/second," whereas few standard measurements are presently available for measuring the performance of computers for image uses. Hardware accelerators for graphics may not improve image performance, and vice versa.[10]

3.5 The Workstation

By the mid-1980s, mainframe and minicomputer technology had matured, and personal computers were well established. Computer scientists realized that one large timesharing computer was not going to be the ultimate solution. The need for higher-performance systems attached to networks appeared in both the commercial and the university environments. Large collections of information were stored in central servers and they required faster computing speeds and higher graphical performance than personal computers could supply. University researchers were developing ways to combine microcomputer chips and high-resolution bitmapped video memory systems, since both of these technologies were falling dramatically in price. Several companies spun out of Stanford University, notably Sun Micro-Systems (SUN is an acronym for Stanford University Network), MIPS Technology, and Silicon Graphics Computers. Workstations from these companies, along with Apollo (later purchased by Hewlett Packard), IBM, and later, Digital Equipment Corporation, provide typical examples of interactive image processing and visualization imaging systems. Figure 3.2 is a photograph of the typical components included in a desktop workstation.

Workstations started with technology to accommodate 32 bits (a bit is a single digit of the binary numbers that computers use) in each word. Since these words were twice as large as the 16 bits used in personal computers, they were twice as fast for memory access (or four times as fast as early 8-bit PCs). Practical and affordable 32 bit systems became available as prices dropped on the chips, memories, and peripherals necessary to complete a workstation. Cumbersome memory management schemes needed to address larger volumes of data in personal computers were eliminated or replaced by hardware memory management schemes.

Another feature of workstations is that the memory, and often the disk drives, are "byte addressable." (A byte is 8 bits.) This simplified the programming task to manipulate images that were 8 bits deep, since the pixels could be addressed directly without any packing or unpacking schemes nec-

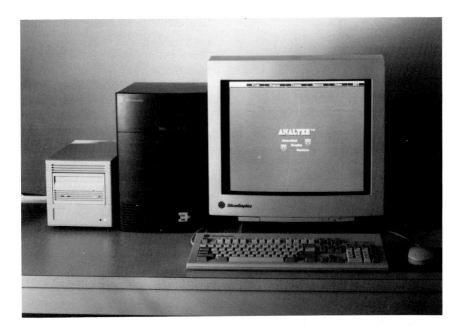

Figure 3.2. Typical modern workstation. This stand-alone system includes, from left to right, an external SCSI optical disk drive, the system chassis with CPU, memory, and disk, the graphics display monitor with keyboard below, and the mouse.

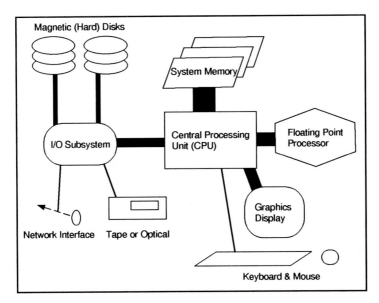

Figure 3.3. Main hardware components of a workstation. Line weights show relative speeds of interconnecting busses (thicker = faster).

essary to read and write the pixels in many mainframe computers. Figure 3.3 is a diagram of the main hardware components of a standard workstation computer.

3.6 Image Size

Since computers need to store, recall, and manipulate the picture elements of the images, the size of the image dictates the size of the computer needed to execute a particular operation in a given time. Kirsch's images of 176 by 176 pixels were relatively small by today's standards, but he is to be commended for managing 30,976 picture elements in a computer holding only 1500 words!

Digital images are at once both small and large. The size of each picture element is relatively small—8 to 12 bits for gray scale images, or 8 bits each for red, green, and blue for color images (24 bits). The number of picture elements can be quite large. For example, a CAT (computer-assisted tomography) image will normally be 512 by 512 picture elements, or 262,144 pixels, and these are often 12 bits per pixel. Typically, a CAT scanner will collect images at successive closely spaced locations yielding multiple CAT images or "slices." The total size of all of these images may then easily number in the tens of megabytes (1 megabyte = 1,000,000 bytes).

As the prices of computers have fallen, the sizes of computer memory and addressing capability have risen, allowing larger and larger images to be captured and manipulated by capture. In the medical imaging industry, image sizes and numbers have risen dramatically during the 1980s and 1990s. Figure 3.4 is a comparison of typical image sizes in both two and three dimensions.

3.7 Transferring Digital Images to the Computer

Whereas all digital medical image scanners incorporate computers as an essential element of their design, these computers only support image acquisition, reconstruction, and the limited viewing functions necessary to provide appropriate clinical evaluation. Advanced image visualization, manipulation and processing are often carried out on a separate workstation. This permits the computer designed for visualization and processing to incorporate additional features (such as large memory systems) that are not required in the scanner. Generally, image visualization and processing tasks demand more time and compute power than image capture and viewing. These tasks may need to happen simultaneously and independently, necessitating separate computers.

Other image acquisition systems, such as confocal and video based optical microscopes, often rely on relatively inexpensive personal computers to

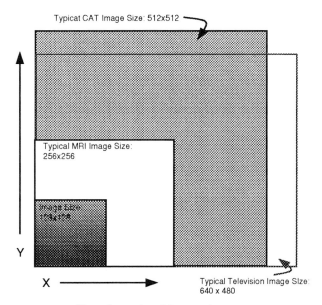

Typicat CAT Image Size: 512x512

Typical MRI Image Size:
256x256

Image Size
128x128

Y

X

Typical Television Image SIze:
640 x 480

Two dimensional Image sizes.

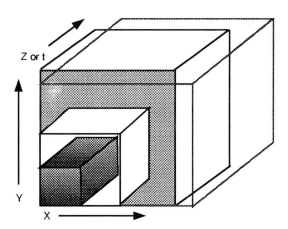

Z or t

Y

X

Three dimensional image sizes

Figure 3.4. Relative sizes of typical images. As the image size doubles in each dimension, total number of picture elements increases by 4 times in 2 dimensions (top), and 8 times in 3 dimensions (bottom).

capture and store digital image data. As with medical scanners, it is often desirable to be able to perform visualization and analysis functions simultaneously with image capture, so separate computer systems are required. Under such circumstances, the digital image data is transferred between computer systems which may have different architectures and operating standards. The problem is confounded by the variety of tape and disk media and networking protocols, many of which have no common data interchange capability.

The two basic methods of transfer are 1) compatible intermediate media, such as tape or removable disk, and 2) computer networks with compatible protocols. In either case, the image acquisition system and the visualization computer need to be configured with hardware and software that permits writing or reading images from the other system. This essential function should not be overlooked when selecting tape drives, optical disks, or networking systems to connect these computers.

Care must also be taken that all levels of the interoperating medium will communicate correctly and completely. For example, most systems will support Ethernet networks, but some may use TCP/IP protocols, while others use DECNET protocols. Similarly, rewritable optical disk subsystems use different file system structures for each system type.

3.8 Image Media

As the Jacquard loom used punched cards to store the weaving pattern, all computers employ a means to store data for later retrieval. All rely on some physical principle to record and retrieve series of digital bits by a reliable method. The earliest storage devices were quite similar to the loom, in fact. Punched cards and paper tape were common storage media in the 1960s and 1970s. Later, magnetic tape was developed in a variety of sizes and formats for computers. Currently, optical media are being developed for high-density storage of computer data. This medium is now available in read-only, write-once, and rewritable versions.

3.8.1 Magnetic Tape

For many years, the primary magnetic tape standard in electronic imaging was the 2400-foot reel of ½″ tape. Advances in technology increased the capacity of this medium from 800 bits per inch (about 10 megabytes on a reel) to 1600 bits per inch (20 megabytes) to 6250 bits per inch (over 100 megabytes). While this form of storage became ubiquitous in both data and image processing centers, the cost (approximately $25/reel in the mid-1980s), reliability (tapes are easily erased, and the tape drives are complex mechanical devices), and permanence (tapes needed rewriting every few years) made working with them relatively difficult as newer, more reliable media were developed. Reels of tape were also bulky. A year's worth of CAT scans from a busy radiology department (1 gigabyte per day, stored at a mean density of 25% of maximum capacity) required approximately 14,400 tapes, enough to fill a small warehouse. Nonetheless, in most medical imaging environments, the ½″ tape was the preferred medium to archive and transfer images to secondary image processing stations.

In the mid-1980s, magnetic tape cartridges were developed to store computer data (audio cassettes and cartridges were put to limited use for computer data, but were unreliable). This became the preferred method of off-line storage in workstations, as the manufacturers delivered the operating system software on cartridge tapes until about 1989. Early ¼″ tape standards offered a capacity of 40 or 60 megabytes per tape. The current standard tape cartridge holds 620 feet of ¼″ high-grade computer tape, and through a serpentine recording method, achieves 150 megabytes of storage on a single cartridge.

Later in the 1980s, the wide distribution and low cost of video tape media spawned a new set of standards for storing data. The ubiquitous VHS cartridge is still being developed as a data standard (under the name "Metrum"), with a single cartridge capacity of 18 gigabytes (1 gigabyte = 1000 megabytes). With this medium, a typical radiology department could store a year's worth of scans on 81 VHS tapes, small enough to fit on the shelf of a doctor's office. Since the hardware for VHS data technology is still relatively expensive, these devices are not likely to be attached directly to medical image scanners, but may find their way into large storage systems.

As standards emerged for the consumer camcorder market and the digital audiotape market, these technologies were adopted as the 8-mm and 4-mm (DAT) data standards, holding 5 and 1.2 gigabytes of data, respectively. These tapes are convenient for storing image data off-line, as they are quite small. Recording "standards" and schemes used by the various vendors may differ somewhat, however, frustrating achievement of the desirable goal of common exchangeable image data across many different computing platforms. Another tape format, called Digital Linear Tape (DLT), is an evolution of ¼″ cartridge tape developed as a proprietary format by Digital Equipment Corporation. This cassette, about 6 inches by 6 inches by 1 inch thick, stores 10 gigabytes on each cartridge, or 20 gigabytes if a drive equipped with data compression is used.

In spite of significant advances in tape technology, magnetic tape still degrades over time. Properly handled and stored tapes can retain their data for 5 to 7 years, but should be unwound and rewound periodically to help prevent "print through," an effect where the magnetic field of one layer of tape slightly magnetizes the next layer. If data are to be stored for longer periods, the tapes should be periodically rewritten to new media. Figure 3.5 is a photograph of various magnetic tape types and forms.

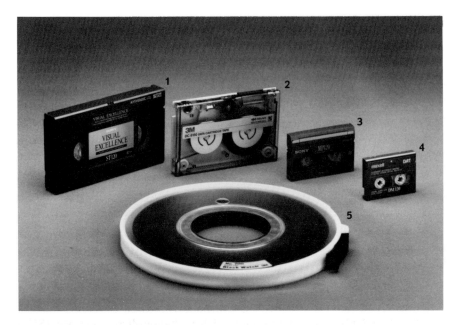

Figure 3.5. Magnetic storage media: 1) VHS ½″ tape cassette; 2) 150-megabyte ¼″ tape cartridge; 3) 5.0-gigabyte 8-mm tape; 4) 1.2-gigabyte 4-mm (DAT) tape; and 5) 120-megabyte ½″ 9-track reel.

3.8.2 Floppy Disks

For some imaging applications, the floppy disk may be suitable to transfer data between machines. The current standard size is 3½″ diskettes. Due to the variety of density standards and formatting standards, interoperability between different systems is difficult, but not impossible. Many workstation vendors now include diskette drives and multiformat reading programs with their systems.

3.8.3 CD-ROM

The audio compact disk, or CD, was the first mass digital medium. The abundance of hardware and the rapidly declining cost permitted the adoption of the CD in the computer marketplace. Like CDs for audio, most computer CDs are produced with the data already stored on the disk. These "read-only memory (ROM)" disks are becoming popular for reference materials and interactive computer games in the PC marketplace.

A simple CD-ROM holds about 600 megabytes of data and costs about $1 to produce in quantity. Because of this very low cost per byte for CDs, they have been adopted as a standard for the dissemination of system software in the workstation marketplace. As a result, nearly all workstation environments have one or more CD-ROM readers installed in their local area networks. The International Standards Organization (ISO) has provided the standard for data format on CDs since their inception, and interoperability is excellent. Since this medium has been designed for mass marketing, the equipment to produce CDs is quite expensive. Emerging technology is now making writable CD-ROMs affordable for computer data archiving. Subsystems which attach to workstations and PCs can write special CD-ROM disks which can be read in any CD-ROM drive. Care must be taken to ensure interoperability between systems due to a variety of substandards. Kodak's recent introduction of the "Photo CD" will likely help standardize the media and reduce costs.

3.8.4 WORM

A variety of vendors have developed other optical media for use in the computer marketplace. A write-once recordable media (WORM) drive was developed in both 12″ and 5½″ formats in the mid 1980s, and 12″ and 5½″ rewritable optical media later in the decade. This market suffered from poor standardization; optical disks from one vendor's rewritable media drive were usually unreadable in another vendor's drive. Standardization by the ISO in the early 1990s improved the situation somewhat, but did not eliminate the interoperability issue between computer vendors' file systems. Write-once media are valuable for long-term archival storage of data.

3.8.5 Rewritable Optical

Technological advances increased the standard capacity for rewritable optical disks to 1.2 gigabytes per 5½″ disk in 1993, at 600 megabytes per side. Assuming that interoperability issues will be overcome, optical media provide excellent intermediate storage media, as they can be rewritten if the data need not be stored, or written to WORM drives if they are to be archived. Rewritable optical media have been adopted as the preferred media for large mass storage devices, in "jukeboxes" holding over 100 disks.

Optical media are more permanent than magnetic media. Rewritable media are typically guaranteed to have a shelf life of over 10 years. The WORM disk, if stored properly, can remain viable for many decades. Figure 3.6 is a photograph of some optical media types.

3.9 Networks

Integrated networks of small but powerful computers have replaced central mainframe computer systems for many image processing tasks—even large ones.[11,12] In many ways, the network becomes the computer. Workstation computing systems can generally be configured into an integrated network

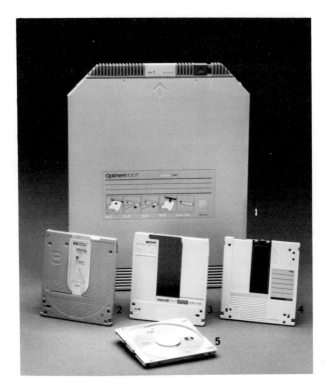

Figure 3.6.   Optical storage media: 1) 12″ 2-gigabyte disk; 2) 1.3-gigabyte rewritable disk; 3) 600-megabyte rewritable disk; 4) 900-megabyte write once (WORM) disk; 5) CD-ROM in data cassette for use with workstation.

in an intelligent way to meet both current and future needs of multidimensional biomedical image analyses.[12]

All components in a typical computer network run under a standard operating system (e.g., UNIX), are connected by standard cable (e.g., Ethernet), and have compatible network file communication protocols (e.g., TCP/IP). The overall system can readily grow or shrink simply by adding or deleting components to and from the network as appropriate. Workstations are configured to function independently of the network if desired, but can benefit from availability of other resources on the network if connected to it. The file servers can be readily expanded to support an increased number of applications, users, and programmers. The resources on the network, including all central processing units (CPUs), memory, disks, printers, etc., can be intelligently used to make any given computer seem bigger than it is.

The networking and distributed processing concepts provide several advantages over even large stand-alone systems:

1. Software development takes place in an optimized environment;
2. Dedicated image analysis computers provide high bandwidth between the

CPU and the display, a requirement for real-time image processing inter-
activity;

3. Compute-intensive tasks can be queued and batched on separate processors, avoiding interruption of interactive tasks;
4. Expensive hardware that has intermittent usage can be shared by all
   users (examples are printers and array processors);
5. Redundant software in the network is reduced by shared copies of operating systems and applications code;
6. System maintenance time is reduced;
7. All users of the network have "electronic" access to each other, allowing
   for sharing of data, programs, and even ideas (mail).

To provide optimal utilization and allocation of all the available compute
cycles, memory capacity, and disk space available, a network management
system (NMS) can be employed. The network may be viewed as a set of
common user interfaces connected to a large parallel processor architecture.
NMS enables each system in the network to share tasks with any other system in an efficient, transparent way. Such a scheme is depicted in Figure
3.7. Systems requiring service will broadcast requests, indicating the requirements of the service desired, such as memory allocation and CPU time.
Any other system in the network that has the required resources and/or services available may respond with a status packet. The calling system may
then assign the job to the system that best fulfills the requirements of the
job. Through careful software design, functions that require intense com-

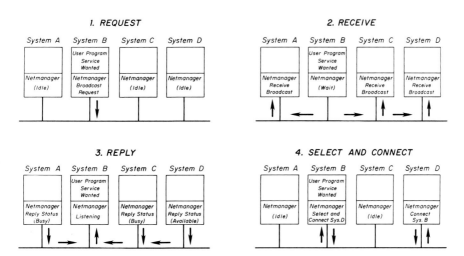

Figure 3.7. Diagram of typical operation cycle of network management software
system: 1) a nondirected request for service is made by one of the systems (system
B); 2) the request is received by all systems; 3) a status reply of availability is returned to the requesting system; 4) the system available (system D) is selected and
connected to provide the requested service.

putation can be distributed throughout the network, and the data can then be collected back into the calling system. Busy systems have the right to reject jobs, and load changes in any "usurped" system's status cause NMS to "dump" the job back onto the network for another system to handle. In the worst case, if no system resources are available to handle the request, the calling system would compute the task itself.

3.9.1 Ethernet and Token Ring

The "pure" definition of a workstation includes hardware for attachment to a network. The network provides intercomputer communication and multi-user access to "network-smart" devices, such as printers that contain computers. Networking is still early in its technological development life. Computers have needed to reach a relatively significant level of sophistication before they could stress today's higher-speed networks. With effective, careful connections of workstations, and intelligent devices and software, the network *becomes the computer.*

There are a variety of networking technologies and topologies in use today. As an image transfer medium, the important characteristic is the "bandwidth" of the network, or the rate at which bits of data can be pushed through the connecting wires (or fibers). The most common standard for networking in use today is Ethernet, which operates at a "base" band of 10 megabits per second. This networking technology provides relatively fast transfer rates (comparable with hard disk rates) on quiescent networks, but since it is a parallel technology (all systems talk to the same network at the same time) it can suffer from overload as the traffic increases. Busy Ethernet networks can sometimes be subdivided, or "subnetted," to localize traffic on separate segments of the Ethernet, but if the traffic pattern is random throughout the networked organizations, this will not help.

IBM developed a token-ring technology for networking, readily available in the mainframe environment. Although the slowest token ring rate offered was only 4 megabits per second, the forced sharing of the technology and lower network overhead permitted throughputs near that of Ethernet under some circumstances. However, token ring was not adopted as a standard in the workstation marketplace, and the cost of connection devices can make token ring more expensive to install than Ethernet. Newer token ring technology is now available that operates at 16 megabits per second.

Since the ability to carry a signal reliably over copper wires, used in both token ring and Ethernet, falls off as the frequency of the signal rises, faster networks were limited in their connection distances. The original Ethernet utilized a "thick" coaxial cable and would carry its signal for 1000 feet. Later, a "thin" Ethernet standard was developed (and readily adopted by the workstation community) which was considerably less expensive to install, but only had an effective distance of approximately 300 feet.

The parallel nature of Ethernet can cause many reliability problems. A break in the cable halts the network. The inexpensive nature of thinwire Ethernet, built out of wires and connectors like cable-TV, makes it prone to people tripping over exposed wires and "bringing down" (electronically) the entire room or building. This has been effectively solved by installing Ethernet "concentrators," which use "unshielded twisted pair" wire (UTP), and each workstation or computer is connected directly to the concentrator. Thus, a wire failure on one computer only affects that computer.

3.9.2 Ethernet Throughput for Images

Whereas the baseband speed of Ethernet is 10 megabits per second, the transfer of data through the network is partioned into packets of data. Each packet has an address, a description, and a checksum for the network. Since it is not practical to connect all computers on one Ethernet, another address is layered on top of the Ethernet address to permit Internetwork communication. This stacking of addresses is called the Network Protocol. The most common protocol in use for imaging workstations is TCP/IP. Although this protocol suffers from having been developed by network users in a rather haphazard fashion, it is in widespread use today, and nearly every computer manufacturer can provide an interface to TCP/IP.

Within the TCP/IP suite of standards, there are additional protocol layers that are added to the stack as each packet is built. Eventually, the data (such as an image) are added to the packet and the packet is placed on the network. The packet size in Ethernet is limited to 1500 bytes, though most packets are well under the maximum allowable size. The addresses, checksum, and other packet data, or "overhead," are about 64 bytes. Some high-reliability TCP/IP protocols also require that a reply packet be returned for every packet sent, and these acknowledgment packets are assembled and sent down the wire in some finite time. After this overhead is accumulated, the typical throughput on Ethernet ranges from 10 kilobytes per second (1 kilobyte = 1000 bytes) to 200 kilobytes per second, far short of the theoretical maximum of 10 megabits (or 1.250 megabytes per second). Some disk sharing protocols over Ethernet and TCP/IP (such as the Network Files System) can achieve rates of 400 kilobytes per second, adequate for some uses, but still too slow for transferring large quantities of image data.

3.9.3 Fiber Optic Networks

For transmission over long distances, glass fibers permit networks to be built throughout the United States at speeds approaching 1 gigabit per second. In many multibuilding campus facilities, fiber optic cables extend Ethernet between buildings. Until quite recently, the cost of fiber optic components made their use in small networks prohibitive. Several networking standards are appearing now that offer higher throughput at reasonable cost.

3.9.4 FDDI

Fiber distributed data interface, or FDDI,[13] currently uses an optical fiber to carry the data at a baseband rate of 100 megabytes per second. The "full" FDDI standard calls for a double counter-rotating fiber token ring system, which provides redundancy in case of failure (the cost of fiber cable itself is usually considerably less than the cost to install it). Switch-over devices detect the failure of one fiber and switch to the other automatically. Packet sizes in FDDI are also larger, up to about 4000 bytes, so the packet overhead is a smaller percentage of the total.

In workgroup installations, FDDI can be installed in a single ring, avoiding the duplicate fiber and the automatic switching. FDDI concentrators allow connection of multiple systems together on the same ring with improved reliability.

In some reports, data have been transferred over standard FDDI networks at speeds approaching 11 megabytes per second, and rates of 2 megabytes per second are easily achievable.[13] The ability to transfer data quickly seems to be more dependent on the workstation design, its operating system, and the FDDI interface card than on the network itself.

3.9.5 HIPPI and ATM

Even faster standards have been developed and are available for use in situations where the added cost can be justified. HIPPI (high-performance parallel interface) was developed as a protocol for transferring large amounts of data from supercomputers to analysis workstations or to image framebuffers. HIPPI is a limited use network, as the number of connections is relatively small. The maximum throughput is 1 gigabit per second, achieved through 4 parallel elements of 250 megabits each. HIPPI can easily achieve full motion video frame rates of TV-sized pictures.

ATM (asynchronous transfer mode) is a new technology, and components for it have only recently become available. ATM is designed to solve several problems in networking: 1) accommodate various speeds of long-distance networking segments, 2) synchronize multimedia signals in a network, and 3) attain higher speeds (the slowest ATM network is 640 megabits/sec).

Users who specify systems that rely on networks to transfer images between capture devices and workstations (or storage devices) need to be sure that the system will interoperate properly, that it will have adequate bandwidth to carry the needed data, and that is is designed to be as reliable as the budget will allow. Given the continual growth of image data volumes, it is prudent to install faster and/or redundant systems that can bear and share the future load.

3.10 Image Storage Systems

Once a means of transferring the captured data has been determined, the image data must be stored on the workstation or in a storage system readily accessible to the workstation (i.e., on its network). In some cases optical media can be used to store image data, although this will be too slow for many uses. The most common storage media will be magnetic disk or "hard" disk. In some cases, the data will only be stored in the memory of the computer, but this will generally be a short-term solution.

3.10.1 Magnetic Disk

The most common medium-term storage device is the magnetic hard disk. These disks have evolved from the 24-inch-diameter boxes used in the 1950s to the 3½"-diameter devices common in workstations of the 1990s and even to tiny 1½"-diameter drives in laptop computers. All modern disk drives use the "Winchester" technology of sealing the disk drive against contaminants. A lever arm containing several "heads," or magnetic sensors, rides on a very thin cushion of air over multiple disk surfaces spinning at 1800 rpm or faster. The disk surfaces are divided into tracks, and the tracks into sectors. A permanently recorded control track lets the electronics of the disk drive always know rotational position. A process called "formatting" labels all the tracks and sectors, substituting the addresses of good sectors for any that might be damaged. The read/write heads move in and out over the disks to access the recorded data.

Hard disk drives are generally fast, typically delivering 1 or 2 megabytes of data per second to a workstation's memory. Several standard hard disk interfaces have been developed, under the acronyms of SMD, EDSI, EISA, IPI, and SCSI. SCSI, for small computer system interface, is gaining favor most rapidly, and is available for computers of all sizes. The original SCSI interface was designed on an 8-bit transfer system, for a peak throughput of 5 megabytes per second, with up to seven drives per "port." SCSI-2 and SCSI-3 have appeared, offering "fast" (10 megabytes/sec) and "wide" (16-bit transfers) for peak performance of up to 20 megabytes per second. These devices can also be combined on multiple ports, or "striped," on some systems to further increase the peak throughput.

SCSI is available in "single-ended" and "differential" versions, referring to the topology of the data signal connections. Single-ended cables are limited to about 15 feet total, including the wires inside the boxes. Differential extends this to about 75 feet. Care must be taken when installing SCSI devices to be sure that the speed, width, and "endedness" are the same between the drives and the computer. Figure 3.8 is a photograph of various forms of SCSI magnetic disk drives.

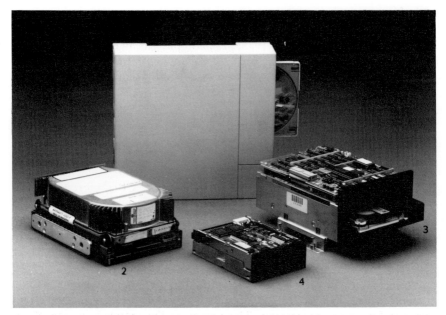

Figure 3.8. SCSI peripheral devices: 1) External CD-ROM disk drive, with CD-ROM in cassette partially inserted into slot; 2) internal 5 ¼″ "full height" disk drive; 3) internal ¼″ tape cartridge drive; 4) internal 3 ½″ "half height" disk drive.

3.10.2 File Systems

All computers organize data on disks in some hierarchy to make naming and retrieval fast and easy. This is referred to as the computer or disk "file system," since it places data in logical (not necessarily physically contiguous) "files." The hard disk is organized along the lines of the file system, although disk blocks may be assigned randomly to files as needed. After considerable use, disks are often "fragmented," that is, both free and used blocks are scattered throughout the disk. This reduces disk performance, since the heads have to travel farther to sequentially reach the blocks making up a single file. Workstations, combined with modern operating systems such as UNIX, reduce some of this overhead by: 1) reorganizing the data on the disk periodically (every night on some systems); 2) storing some of the often-used disk blocks in computer memory, called "caching"; 3) permitting the disk interface to write to the computer memory while the CPU does other things, called direct memory access, or DMA; and 4) permitting the CPU to attend to other jobs while waiting for disk transfers to be completed.

3.11 Memory Systems

Memory systems on modern workstation computers can be characterized in four domains: main system memory, cache memory, virtual memory, and shared memory. These domains each have specific functions and nuances that are important to understand for both the software developer and the application user.

3.11.1 Main Memory

The memory system of a workstation stores the operating system, the program(s) being executed, and the data being used. The CPU references memory constantly to load instructions to execute. Memory is read into and out of the CPU registers. Memory is also read and written by DMA capable peripheral devices, such as disk interfaces.

As the cost of memory has declined, the size of software systems to support the user environment on workstations has risen. In 1986, workstations were typically equipped with 4 megabytes of memory. In 1989, the amount was 8 megabytes. Today, 16 megabytes is the minimum for reasonable performance for image processing. The reason is the increase in size of the operating system and windowing systems that share memory with application programs.

Memory is generally modular in design. Single inline memory modules, or SIMMs, are the typical memory component in workstation equipment. SIMMs can range from as small as 256 kilobytes per module up to 32 megabytes per module. They are built from dynamic random access memory (DRAM) chips, and they can vary in speed as well as size. They are usually installed in banks of four SIMMs. Some systems permit the mixing of different-sized SIMMs in separate banks, some do not. Newer systems use memory interleaving schemes, in which different SIMMs can be addressed and data retrieved from them simultaneously to increase throughput. While memory can often be purchased from vendors other than the computer manufacturer, users should be wary of interoperability, timing, and warrantee issues, and should have the supplier guarantee that the memory will operate properly under all normal circumstances. Figure 3.9 shows different types of SIMM memory modules.

The memory bus consists of lines (or wires) for each bit of the data to be transferred, plus lines for each bit of the memory address. The number of lines (also called the width) for data transfers is usually the same as the number of bits in the CPU (32 bits on most machines, 64 bits on newer machines), although on machines with large cache and interleaved memory, more bits may be returned to "cache in" a single request. The width of the address lines determines the maximum amount of memory the CPU can address, although this computation is not straightforward, since memory may

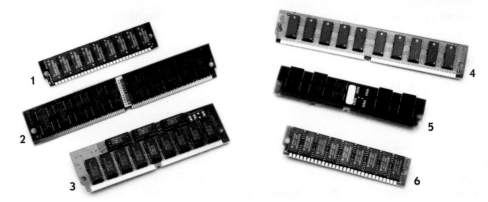

Figure 3.9. Single inline memory modules (SIMMs). Memory modules are generally not interchangeable between different brands of workstations. 1) 1-megabyte Sun; 2) 2-megabyte Digital; 3) 4-megabyte Silicon Graphics; 4) 4-megabyte Digital; 5) 4-megabyte Sun LX; 6) 4-megabyte Sun IPC.

be addressed in blocks or pages. For 32 memory address lines, the maximum memory address will be 2^{32} or 4 gigabytes. Although this seems like a large amount, some individual geographic images are that large, and newer systems can accommodate up to 16 gigabytes of main memory.

3.11.2 Cache Memory

Since the development of high-speed reduced instruction set computer (RISC) processors, memory speeds have been unable to keep pace with CPU speeds. To prevent this bottleneck against performance, most systems use one or more high-speed memory caches to store data and/or instructions from main memory. These cache systems are built close to the CPU physically, to keep the length of the signal leads short, and are built from static random access memory (SRAM), which is both faster and more expensive than DRAM. Information from memory is then loaded into the cache in "pages," a page being 512 to 8192 bytes in size. The effectiveness of this system is measured in the percentage of "cache hits," or references to data that already exist in the cache when running a program. Since the usage pattern of data in programs determines the cache hit percentage, the software can be designed to improve the number of cache hits. Good compiler design will include features that can optimize the use of cache.

Memory systems are accessed via a system communication channel called a "bus." In early workstations, the memory was accessed in the same bus as all of the rest of the system components. This sometimes caused the CPU to wait while the system bus was being used by peripherals to transfer data in or out of memory, to other peripherals, etc. Modern systems use a separate memory bus, which can run at a higher speed than the bus used by peripheral devices.

3.11.3 Virtual Memory

The cost ratio of main memory to disk memory has always been high. In 1994 this ratio is about 50 to 1, as main memory is about $50 per megabyte and disk memory is about $1 per megabyte. To extend the usable size of programs that would compile and run on computers with limited amounts of main memory, operating systems were developed with the concept of "virtual" memory. Under this scheme, a portion of the hard disk is reserved as "swap space," directly addressable by the operating system. As the amount of physical memory dwindles, programs that are loaded in main memory (but that are not currently scheduled to run) are "swapped out" to the reserved space on hard disk. The memory that was occupied is then freed up to be used by the programs that are running. This permits the system to run programs with data sets larger than main memory, making them "appear" as if they were entirely loaded in main memory. Since the transfer rates between disk and main memory are approximately 20 times slower than between main memory and the CPU, the trade-off is the time it takes to load back the data into main memory when it is required. When image data sets that are larger than available memory are being processed, the slowdown will be quite noticeable, particularly if the image processing algorithm is searching through the image data in a random way. This is referred to as "thrashing," since data blocks are often moved back and forth between memory and swap space on the disk. Ways to avoid this problem are to use smaller images, add more memory, and/or use efficient data accessing algorithms.

Varying "rules of thumb" are used to determine the appropriate amount of swap space for a particular computer. Some vendors recommend 2 times the amount of physical memory. Some have used a large fixed amount, regardless of the amount of physical memory. Trial and error is the best guide. Most recent versions of the UNIX operating system allow the system administrator to add to swap space by designating a file or disk partition to be added to the swap list. As a reasonable starting point, swap space should be at least as large as physical memory.

From the user's point of view, there is no distinction between real memory and virtual memory (aside from the speed trade-off mentioned above). As a result, the combination of real memory and virtual memory together is referred to as "system memory." This is the total amount of memory that can be allocated to the operating system plus all programs and data running on the system at any moment. Attempts to exceed this limit will result in failed programs, or in some cases, a system crash.

3.11.4 Shared Memory

Another important memory concept is shared memory. This is a portion of system memory that has been made accessible to more than one program at a time. It is often used to make specified amounts of data memory accessible so that programs can operate on the data without having to load and unload the data to disk, or to have duplicate copies of the same data in more than one place. The popular X window system uses shared memory (on newer systems) to share the visible part of a window between the X server (which represents the screen in software) and the X client program (which places images or objects inside the window). When both of these programs are running on the same computer, using shared memory significantly increases the performance of the windowing system.

Shared memory may also be used by imaging applications programs. In such cases, the image data are loaded into a shared memory segment, and various programs can then access and/or modify the data. Some versions of UNIX may require modifications of the operating system kernel parameters to permit shared memory segments to be large enough for those applications. Figure 3.10 illustrates the relationship between multiple CPUs sharing the same segment of memory while also utilizing separate private segments.

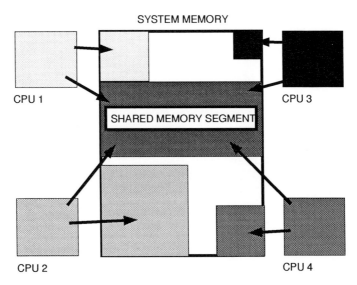

Figure 3.10. Four central processors utilizing a shared memory segment. Each processor also has a private segment of memory.

3.12 Central Processing Units

The Jacquard loom had no CPU. The stored data on punched cards were transferred directly to the output device, the loom. Conversely, Babbage's calculating engine had no storage. The machine had to be adjusted for a certain type of calculation, then "cranked." Computers, by definition, have storage and processing units. The processor is the heart of the system. It interprets the instructions of the stored program and executes operations on the data in memory according to the instructions.

As computers developed, the list of instructions that the CPU could execute was expanded to reduce the burden on the programmer and to save memory space. The types of instructions to be executed initially were simple ones, such as ADD, STORE, and SHIFT. By appropriately combining even these simple steps, complex mathematical operations could be performed, such as MULTIPLY and DIVIDE. Since these were fairly common operations, CPU designers subsequently added these commands to the hardware of the CPU itself. Larger instruction sets required larger numbers of bits in the instruction itself, and took longer for the CPU to determine the instruction and adjust the internal logic to execute the instruction. These instruction sets became so complex that systems designers were forced to put the instruction set of the CPU itself into a separate memory, referred to as microcode. Good microcode design was the key to faster and faster processors.

As single-chip microcomputers were developed in the late 1970s and early 1980s, the microcode became part of the integrated circuit. Although the chips were shrinking in size, the instruction sets were still getting larger. Examples of this kind of design are the Motorola 68000 series and the Intel 80x86 chips. While these chips were getting faster, their complexity required longer design times for new chips.

An IBM research project in the 1960s had put forth the idea that faster computers could be developed with a small set of instructions, since 90% of the operations that most CPUs performed were simple and well-defined. This reduced instruction set computer or RISC concept did not pay off in the 1960s, as it required faster memory, disk, integrated circuits, and compilers to achieve the desired performance gains. In the 1980s, however, RISC became technically and commercially viable. Microcomputer chip design and manufacturing techniques led to doubling the speed of components every 18 months. The RISC design was resurrected, placed in silicon, and became the heart of the IBM RT (RISC Technology) system. Sun Microsystems shifted away from Motorola 680×0 chips to its own SPARC (Scalable Processor ARChitecture) chip. MIPS, Incorporated won over Silicon Graphics and DEC with the R2000 chip design. Motorola announced the 88000 chip, adopted by Data General in their Aviion workstations, and Apollo showed a workstation built on their PA-RISC design. Later in the 1980s and early 1990s, Hewlett Packard acquired Apollo and their RISC technology,

DEC introduced their own RISC chip, the ALPHA, and Silicon Graphics both designed their own RISC chip and acquired MIPS. IBM introduced the POWER series chipset. Speeds increased from 12 to 25 to 200 MHz. Performance increased by 2 orders of magnitude. The promise of RISC architecture for quantum leaps in CPU performance has been realized!

Along with this shift to RISC, software compilers had to get smarter, too. It was not sufficient that the chips would run faster. The reduced instruction set philosophy required that the compilers be able to reorganize the instructions of the program (without altering the intent of the programmer) to execute in a more efficient manner. Otherwise, 50% of the power of small, fast chips would be wasted. Most workstation vendors have now achieved this by either developing or buying better compiler technologies.

The trend in the 1990s is once again to slowly add a few instructions to the chip as designs are produced. For example, Silicon Graphics has used the MIPS chipset starting with the R2000 chips in 1987. As newer versions of the chip have arrived, they have maintained forward compatibility (i.e., programs compiled on the R2000 chipset will still run today), but in order to take full advantage of the latest chips, the programs must be recompiled on the newer chips, and having been compiled, they may no longer run on the old machines. This is due in part to the migration from 32-bit CPUs to 64-bit CPUs, not only to the addition of new CPU instructions.

Along with the shift to RISC, UNIX emerged as the most prominent (fastest growing) operating system in the 1990s. UNIX had an advantage in that it was promoted by AT&T, a company whose business was not computers. Since UNIX was not proprietary to a computer maker, companies who had expertise in chip technology and graphics systems could adopt it and leverage their own expertise.

3.12.1 Supercomputers

In the 1970s, Cray Research developed the Cray 1 computer, the first successful "supercomputer." These machines were designed to operate efficiently on vectors, sequences of numbers that required similar operations. By using custom compilers and building a "pipeline" of multiple CPUs, the results of one operation could be handed directly to the input of the next processor, down the line, so that the mathematical operations were taking place in parallel as long as there were data to feed the input. The pipelines were built to perform floating point calculations (both large and small fractional numbers) and through the vector design achieved remarkable results. But the machines were expensive to build and maintain, they required special compilers, and often users had to design their programs to be "vectorized." Nonpipelined performance of these machines was no better than that of workstations, and they tended to be used by people with large, complex problems that required many iterative steps to converge to an answer (like weather forecasting). While the vector architecture was ideal for many image processing operations (an image is a vector of numbers), access to the machines was slow and expensive, and many image processing algorithms are not readily translated to vector form.

3.12.2 Mainframes

Mainframe computers are best characterized by their ability to respond well to large numbers of users and to maintain reasonable response times. These computers are built to have large and wide input/output channels, and although they can support large memory sizes and fast computation, their cost usually prohibits their use for routine image processing, especially in light of the favorable cost–performance ratio of workstations.

3.12.3 Special Purpose Processors

Numerous special purpose processing systems have been developed to solve a variety of image and computational problems.[14,15] They are best applied in an environment where a specific problem is to be solved repeatedly, such as a specific imaging task, or a computation performed routinely, such as CT image reconstruction from a scanning device. Special processors for these applications can be justified, along with the custom programming necessary.

Examples of special-purpose processors are graphics accelerators, vector accelerators, high-speed frame buffers, video adapters, array processors, and floating point accelerators. When these devices require custom programming, use of special program libraries, or custom hardware connections to achieve their performance gain, they will have limited lifetime in general purpose applications. In many cases, a later upgrade to a faster CPU in a general purpose workstation may provide the same performance, without special programming, and will have the possible added benefits of other programs that can be used on the workstation.

3.12.4 Workstations

Graphical workstations suitable for image processing are all running on RISC-based CPUs today.[12] Any inherent differences betwen RISC and CISC CPUs is hidden from the user by the operating system and the application programs. Thus, users can go straight to the applications level when selecting among workstation systems.

3.13 Graphics Displays

In order to view images, a graphics display device is needed on the computer system.[16] Although most workstation systems can be purchased without a graphics display for use as a file server, most vendors offer a selection of sizes and resolutions for their displays.

3.13.1 Color Displays

Color is now an accepted standard, and all vendors supply color displays for their systems. Monochrome (1 bit) and grayscale displays are available, but their use is now limited to specific applications. When used properly, color can add significant enhancements to the effective display of image data. Most imaging applications and windowing systems themselves now make generous use of color.

The least expensive color displays on workstations are 8-bit, or "color lookup table" displays. These systems use a single 8-bit value to specify each pixel, and through a list of color values, convert the 8-bit value into a 24-bit color (8 bits each of red, green, and blue). Since the table has one entry for each of the possible 8 bit values, the total number of colors that can be shown on the screen at one time is 256. This provides adequate "pseudo" color display for many applications. The hardware to hold the table and perform the conversion is far less expensive than the additional memory required to hold the full 24 bits required for "true" color display, and this accounts for the lower cost.

Twenty-four-bit displays include hardware to store 8 bits each for red, blue, and green for each pixel on the screen, allowing a full range of 16,777,216 separate colors to be displayed for each pixel on the screen, so-called true color display. Their cost is approximately 3 times that of 8-bit displays, and images displayed in 24 bits will require 3 times the memory to store and transmit the full data set. Users should note that while a full range of colors can be displayed on a 24-bit system, the number of grayscales provided is the same as for an 8-bit or grayscale system, 256 colors. This is due to the fact that the grays are generated only when the red, green, and blue values are equal ([1, 1, 1][2, 2, 2] etc.).

3.13.2 Display Size

The second characteristic that can be specified is the display size. The most common sizes are 16-inch (measured diagonally) and 19-inch displays. Most vendors offer the same resolution in both sizes. As a general rule, 19-inch displays are preferred if the location for the system has adequate space to hold the larger, deeper tube.

3.13.3 Display Resolution

The ability to display full images correctly depends on the number of pixels available in the display. Workstation systems most often offer a display resolution of approximately 1000 × 1000 pixels, with several variations according to vendor. Some vendors offer both higher- and lower-resolution displays, with the lower resolutions available in smaller screen sizes.

3.14 Operating Systems

An operating system is the principal software associated with modern computer systems. The operating system provides standardized interfaces to all of the computer's attached peripheral devices, and methods for starting and stopping application programs. Operating systems first appeared in the late 1950s and have since become a mature technology. Most operating systems in use today were developed in the 1960s.[5]

Early operating systems were proprietary and designed specifically for a single vendor's hardware. While this permitted the vendor to tailor the features of the operating system to the features of the computer, transferring application software to a new system, called "porting," required conversion of all of the system-related references in the application. Porting was an expensive task, so there was considerable pressure to adopt standard interfaces for operating systems.

3.14.1 UNIX

Nearly all modern workstations are supplied with UNIX as the standard operating system.[17] In addition, IBM PCs, Apple Macintoshes, Supercomputers, and Mainframes all have versions of UNIX available. UNIX is readily available, is becoming standardized, and offers many useful features to an industry which is rapidly evolving.

UNIX offers the following standard features:

1. Multiuser, multitasking functionality;
2. Standard X windowing system (see next section);
3. Standard networking capabilities;
4. Modular design;
5. Supports large memory and peripherals;
6. Shared memory, signals, interprocess communications

Because UNIX supports many users and tasks, it is a relatively complex operating system to set up and manage. Workstation vendors have made efforts to provide user-friendly tools to simplify the system administration tasks, but there is a limit to how much can be eliminated without reducing some desired functionality. In situations where a system is to be installed without networking, for a single user, the minimum tasks necessary are quite easy and inexperienced users need not be intimidated. In complex networked environments, experienced UNIX system administrators may be needed to complete and maintain the installation.

3.14.2 Window Systems

In the process of designing a new paradigm to speed the tasks of people who used computers for their daily work, developers at the Xerox Palo Alto Research Center (also known as PARC) built a graphical display based on an 808×608 point TV screen, featuring overlying rectangles that could hold text editors, system command shells, or other tools.[16] This PARC model was adopted by many companies, most successfully by Apple as the Macintosh interface. In the workstation market, all of the vendors developed a user "desktop" based on the Xerox PARC model as well.

Early window systems were designed around the graphics hardware and software delivered as part of the workstation, and were consequently proprietary in nature. A collaboration of vendors, including DEC, IBM, HPD, and others, along with MIT, developed a new system released to the public in 1986, called "X, A Windowing System." A key feature of this system was its ability to work over networks. A program called the "X Server" runs continuously on the workstation and provides a form of "canvas" upon which to draw. The server "listens" constantly for events on the network interfaces of the workstation. Other programs, which may run on the same workstation as the server or on another workstation on the network, are called "clients." These client programs generate and send X events to the server, which interprets them and displays the functions requested by the events. While this imposes another layer of software abstraction between the application program (an X client) and the screen (now represented by the X server), and consequently impairs performance to some degree, the benefits gained by interacting through a standard programming interface allow much faster porting of programs between various vendors' workstations. In addition, it is possible to achieve standardized functionality for programs in such an environment, often referred to as "look and feel." This is characterized by the way various features in the windowing system behave, such as menus, buttons, scroll-bars, etc. No single standard has yet appeared for an X Windows "look and feel," but the user community is applying enough influence on vendors to force them to adopt and follow common practices.

The X Window system includes a special client program called the "window manager." The purpose of this program is to control in an organized manner the various "resources" available from the server, such as color values, space on the screen, and whether a window appears "on top" or "on the bottom." Window managers also control the ability of windows to be "closed" or transformed into a small "icon." These icons permit many programs to be accessible at once on the entire screen or "desktop." The programs represented by icons are usually idle, awaiting a command from the user to be "opened" and operational again. Figure 3.11 is a photograph of a workstation monitor on which is displayed a multiple windows session using X Windows.

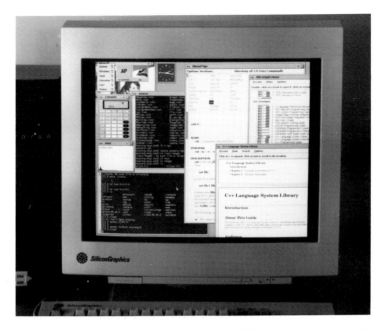

Figure 3.11.   Graphics display showing X windows. Various windows running a variety of programs can overlap each other on a single workstation screen.

The X Windows system has now been included as part of the UNIX operating system[17] and is available on all workstations. Many vendors provide X client tools to assist the user in his daily work, such as text editors, electronic mail interfaces, calculators, shell windows, file managers, print managers, etc. These value-added tools can greatly increase the efficiency of programmers and analysts using the workstation, because they can be collected into a "Desktop" or layout for the tools. Users can also benefit from having several windows open and active simultaneously; this is useful when several activities are occurring at once, such as the compile, edit, and debug procedures commonly used in developing programs.

The use of windows in image processing can similarly improve the efficiency of a working environment. For example, the parameters for an image processing function can be set and monitored in one window, the input data can be viewed in another, and the output data displayed in a third. Side-by-side comparisons can be generated and the windows opened and closed as needed to achieve the process required. Users may soon discover that this capability needs to be tempered with some restraint, however, as it is easy to lose track of the contents of a collection of 5 or 6 windows that otherwise appear the same.

Users who need to write programs to be used in an X Window display must be careful about the complexity of details involved in a windowing system. Although windows appear to be simple on the screen, the minute details "underneath," like the size of borders, color of menu backgrounds, shape of cursors, etc., all need to be specified for each program that interacts with the server. Many of these details can be specified by using X "toolkits" to write programs. "X Builder" programs are available that allow a programmer to interactively specify the size and location of various window elements, called "widgets," on the screen, and these builder programs then will generate C or C++ program fragments. The programmer can add additional functions to the fragments to complete the program.

3.14.3 X Windows Resources

Most X client programs permit the specification of a list of parameters that describe some of the details of the program as it appears on the screen. Users can place values for these parameters in an ".Xresources" file, in a standard location (usually /usr/lib/X11/app-defaults), or can allow the program to select its own defaults for its own appearance. These parameters control the placement of the window on the screen, colors of borders, etc.

Start-up files for X Windows, often named ".xinitrc" or ".xsession" in the user's home directory, control initialization and default characteristics for Windows systems. This file can be created or changed to modify the number, placement, size, and icon state of the windows when the user first starts up X. These start-up files may be superceded by newer window managers that remember the state and placement of windows on the screen when a user exits the system, and returns to the previous state upon reentry to the program.

3.15 Distributed and Parallel Processing

High-performance computing is accomplished essentially in three different ways: 1) high clock speeds on the CPU, 2) distributed load sharing, and 3) multiple CPUs computing simultaneously on parallel tasks. Higher clock speeds can also be used to improve both distributed and parallel computing; therefore this method is intrinsic to all methods and needs no separate explanation.

3.15.1 Distributed Computing

Many image processors have considered it attractive to utilize the apparent power of a collection of workstations connected by a network into a more powerful "metacomputer," whose combined computation ability would achieve a significant percentage of that for the total number of computers so connected. In practice, however, a completely successful scheme for such a distributed system has yet to appear.[18] The main problems with implementing such a scheme are the need to custom program the software to utilize the distributed power, and the reliance on networks and the availability of the collected workstations. Given the number of variables in any one installation, it would be difficult to offer such software commercially and to maintain it in the face of changing operating system versions.

There is still a place in the workstation environment for limited distributed processing, however. It is most common, and readily used, in the management of the network itself. Since networking requires a scheme of co-operating processes, control of the details of the network cooperation is generally distributed throughout the network through a distributed database. Most prevalent of these is the Network Information System (NIS) developed and licensed by Sun Microsystems. Through NIS each workstation can receive information about other workstations and users and other basic information and incorporate this information into its own administration.

Another widely available function is remote procedure calls, or RPCs. NIS functions are built on top of RPCs when performing transfer of data through the network. Some image programs may include the ability to perform RPCs to connect to other systems on the network for specific processing functions. The ability to provide efficient processing remotely is limited by the bandwidth of the connecting network. In most cases, network delays have outweighed the speed of remote processing.

A number of advances in computer science may provide more gains to future image processing by remote systems. These include faster networks, high-performance parallel computers, and the standardization and enhancement of RPC methods through the Open Software Foundation's Distributed Computing Environment (DCE) and other similar standards.

3.15.2 Parallel Computing

The concept of a parallel computer is similar to that of a distributed system without the network bottleneck. Many variations on parallel systems have been developed, including several specifically designed for image processing systems. These systems can provide significant performance improvements, but most require custom programming to achieve high levels of performance.

Most interesting are general purpose, shared memory, symmetric multi-processing systems, which contain two or more CPUs. As the name implies, the CPUs share a large memory area. Under UNIX, each processor acts independently, but under control of a single job queue. As each process on this type of system becomes ready to run on a CPU, each CPU is assigned to a process on an "as available" basis. Since the memory space is the same for all CPUs, no transfer of program or data need be made to begin execution on any processor.

While these systems are particularly effective for multiple users on a single system, or multiple separate jobs, some also offer parallel compilers, which attempt to effectively partition programs among the processors available. This has varying degrees of success, usually depending on the nature of the program, but can be very effective in some cases, and requires little additional effort on the part of the programmer.

In no case is the performance benefit gained by running a single program under parallel or distributed processing equal to the aggregate performance of a number of separate processors (i.e., a program that runs in 10 sec on one processor will not run in 1 sec on 10 processors). This occurs because the processors still need to communicate and synchronize their operations to complete the processing in the program. As a result, the efficiency gained by adding processors declines to about 80% in systems with eight processors. Advances in parallelizing compilers and symmetric multiprocessing operating systems, along with faster hardware, will likely increase this ratio in the future.

3.16 Shared File Systems

As the number of computers on a network increases, it becomes desirable to share data among the systems. The simplest abstraction for this is to extend the file system of the operating system to include the files of another computer. For example, in the PC DOS operating system, the disk drives are identified by letters, A, B, C, etc. A network sharable file system for DOS occupies an additional letter, such as E.

In the UNIX environment, the file system is organized as a hierarchical tree structure of directories and files, with the root (called simply "/") at the top. As additional disks are added to a system, they are "mounted" on directories that existed in the tree. For example, nearly all UNIX computers have a disk partition assigned to the "/usr" directory. This disk holds most of the UNIX operating system (the rest, stored in the "/" partition, usually holds only sufficient instructions to get the system up and running). Once the operating system is running and all the disks are "mounted," a user cannot distinguish between the disk partitions except in certain rare cases (such as limits to renaming a file to be in another disk partition with the UNIX "mv" command).

This distributed file capability has been implemented through a number of protocols. Most popular and widely available is the Network File System, or NFS, that was developed by Sun Microsystems in the mid 1980s. NFS is now available for all workstations, and although it is a somewhat dated protocol, has worked well in most environments. NFS places a program into the core of the operating system. As NFS mounted disks are accessed, this program may request data from alternate computers through remote procedure calls. As it turns out, NFS is a relatively efficient network protocol for Ethernet networks, since it uses an "unreliable" but fast portion of the TCP/IP protocol and large packet sizes. No data are lost, because NFS handles reliability after all the packets have been received. Since most Ethernet networks are inherently quite reliable, this scheme works well in most installations.

One recent addition to NFS is the "automounter," now available with most versions of NFS. This program uses a table of disks to be mounted by NFS, and the table can be distributed by NIS. In this case, when a new NFS partition is accessed and it is not mounted, the automount program will mount it. After an idle period (usually 5 or 10 min) the disk is unmounted. This helps reduce system and network overhead.[19]

Other file-sharing protocols include the Remote File System (RFS) developed by AT&T and the Andrew File System (AFS). AFS has better features for long-distance networking, such as file caching on the remote system.

3.17 Image Data Management

A single computer user may collect dozens or hundreds of image data files. Usually a scheme can be constructed to organize this number of images using a hierarchical directory structure as is provided with UNIX or DOS operating systems. The introduction of additional users or the increase of images to thousands requires more sophisticated schemes for the organization and management of the image data. This includes means of indexing and annotating image entries to reveal referential detail without actually loading each image.

No standards exist for such a catalogue at this time, though several commercial products exist to provide a picture archiving and communications system, or PACS.[20–25] Such systems have been developed to address the needs of medical image storage and retrieval, and are often based on relational database models with the patient being the primary reference. Considerable effort has been expended to design solutions to the problem of pseudorandom image selection in a busy radiology department, with emphasis on rapid transmission of electronic images, coupling of table-based data to image data, and appropriate security measures. Efforts are being made to integrate all types of imaging systems into a variety of transmission media to support general practitioners in their offices,[26] small clinics,[27] and large hospitals,[28] along with a variety of efforts in teleradiology and telemedicine,[29–31] which are designed to provide long-distance transmission of images and other medical data.

Several of the PACS designs attempt to integrate imaging workstations into the overall design of the PACS system. Such designs make reasonable trade-offs between system performance, standards, and cost in an attempt to arrive at practical solutions. For example, radiological image display on a workstation may suffer some loss in detail over the original film of the image, but radiologists trained in the physics of the display system may be able to compensate by using processing techniques or display adjustments or by referring to a film image when necessary to complete the analysis of the image.

Important advances have been made on PACS, on relational databases for radiology information systems (RIS), and on radiology display stations.[25,26] Standards have been developed to permit open interfaces between systems, which have included object-oriented analysis to develop information models. This permits identification, classification, and abstraction of relationships among images.[31] However, despite the variety of tools and standards available to users of medical images, no complete infrastructure is available to provide effective and efficient organization of these tools. The users of medical images require a diverse set of methodologies, languages, and semantics to effectively communicate with the imaging technologies they use. Medical specialties often have unique, well-developed notations and references that are required to support their needs.

It is envisioned that systems will be developed offering image database techniques that can provide some of the same benefits for image data that have accrued to numerical and textual data in the relational database arena. Such techniques will permit content-based searches to be made on image data, much as structured query languages (SQL) now offers the opportunity of content-based searches on lists of names. Some work has been accomplished in this area,[32] but the development of trustworthy image processing algorithms that can provide unassisted methods for segmentation, classification, and measurement, combined with tools to select and retrieve collections of images and apply these algorithms to them, will provide a new paradigm for image databases.

Such projects will combine the worthwhile database elements of PACS with the power of image processing and analysis tools. Current standards, commercially available products, and a flexible user interface will be incorporated into medical object-oriented databases. With such a database, one can extend to images the same characteristics that have been used in alphanumeric database management systems, that is, the ability to perform queries on images based on their content and context. This will be accomplished by applying image analysis software to the images in the system as part of the response to content/context-sensitive queries made by a user.

In the future, such a system will permit users to select images based on features and attributes such as anatomic name, pattern similarities, shape, color, dimensions, etc. Users will be able to ask questions of the system that include original images, processed images, stacked images, or even "sketches" that they provide with new user interfaces developed to support such queries. Images can be registered (translated and scaled to match another frame of reference) to common standards and comparisons made to reference images or templates.

The implied power of such a system will require the users to be able to store and recall the steps and methods used on the system itself. Therefore, the system will also incorporate the ability to store and retrieve sequences of image access and processing steps, that is, maintain an audit trail of all procedures performed in response to a query. This will facilitate the development of higher-level abstractions and query designs to address specific image database needs.

3.18 Some Image Processing Programs

Software for the display and analysis of biomedical imagery has evolved from single programs for specific tasks to comprehensive, integrated software systems which make available large sets of tools and algorithms. These integrated software systems take several forms, including image processing toolkits, interactive display and analysis programs with menu-driven user interfaces, and the more recently developed visual programming environments. The software systems available have a variety of functions, both application independent and specific to given applications, with varying degrees of flexibility, extensibility, and ease of use. Most software systems are available on multivendor platforms, with mixed degrees of performance based on platform capabilities and the efficiency of the code.

3.18.1 Image Processing Toolkits

Most toolkits for imaging are organized as sets of libraries containing high-level language (i.e., C, C++),[33] callable functions with a specific applications programmer interface (API) to define the data structures, and calling conventions used to access the functions in the toolkit. These toolkits are primarily used by software developers who integrate various functions from the toolkits with other software specific to the given application. These are then supplied with a user interface, either proprietary or standardized (e.g., Motif). Several levels of functionality may exist in the toolkits, from low-level functions that perform single, succinct tasks, to groups of functions that provide a higher-level procedure or multiple tasks. The granularity of the functions implemented in a software toolkit directly contributes to the extensibility of the toolkit and to the usefulness for higher-level application integration. The functions are completely interface independent, allowing implementation in any desired user interface. Such software toolkits include the AVW (A Visualization Workshop) software system from the Mayo Foundation (Rochester, MN) and the Imaging Applications Platform (IAP) from ISG Technologies Inc. (Toronto, Canada). The IAP software system developed by ISG is implemented as a set of servers, including a processing server that performs the image processing functions. This paradigm allows network access to one or multiple servers on machines with higher compute power than local workstations.

3.18.2 Interactive Display and Analysis Programs

Display and analysis functions accessible through an interactive user interface characterize the most common software systems available for biomedical imaging. These software systems may or may not be built from a common toolkit of functions, and generally restrict operations to a specific set of functions implemented in the system. Most are implemented using a single user interface paradigm, such as menu-driven systems. The restricted set of functions implemented in a specific user interface limits the flexibility and extensibility of these systems, and often these programs are written to be application specific. Yet, these software systems offer easy access to the underlying functionalty, allowing ready exploration given image data sets and rapid prototyping of potential solutions for given turnkey problems. Many have adopted standardized interface mechanisms and have been ported to many different vendors' systems. Software systems in this group have been under development for several years and have reached a high level of maturity, with widespread distribution and usage. Such software systems include ANALYZE™ from the Mayo Foundation (Rochester, MN), VoxelView from Vital Images (Fairfield, IA), PV-Wave from Precision Visuals (Boulder, CO), and IDL from Research Systems (Boulder, CO).

An example of a complete image display and analysis software package is ANALYZE™, a unique and powerful software package developed by the authors in the Biomedical Imaging Resource at the Mayo Clinic. This software can be used with many 3-D imaging modalities, such as X-ray CT, radionuclide emission tomography, ultrasound tomography, MRI, and light, electron, and confocal microscopy. The package is very comprehensive in its synergistic integration of fully interactive modules for direct display, manipulation, and measurement of multidimensional, multimodal image data. Several original algorithms for multiplanar reformatting, oblique and curved sectioning, multipanel cine loops, shaded surface rendering, and 3-D volume rendering provide interactive displays of high-quality images. The volume-rendering algorithms are optimized to be fast and flexible, without compromising image quality, permitting interactive definition, manipulation, and measurement of individual or multiple rendered objects. The inclusion of a variety of interactive editing and quantitative mensuration tools significantly extends the usefulness of the software. Advanced algorithms are included for automated 3-D segmentation, 3-D image registration and fusion, and 3-D feature classification. Arbitrary regions and/or volumes-of-interest can be manually specified and/or automatically defined for numerical determination and statistical analyses of distances, areas, volumes, densities, textures, and shapes. The system provides a powerful macro capability for generating highly tailored sequences of operations and routines for prototyping custom extensions and applications, as illustrated in Figures 3.12 and 3.13 (see color figures 2 and 3). Capabilities for interactive surgery simulation and radiotherapy planning are examples of such extensions and applications.

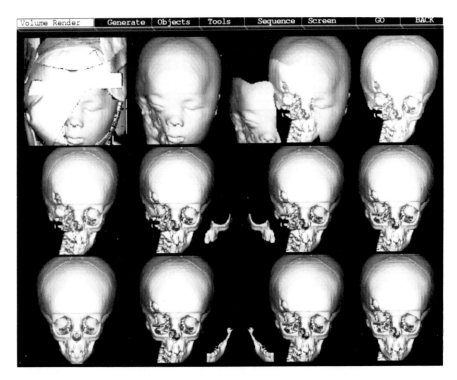

Figure 3.12. Illustration of capabilities of image computers and software packages for realistic 3-D simulation of surgical procedures (using ANALYZE™). Top row shows 3-D renderings of full head CT scan of patient with facial wound. Top left image is original data with bandage over wound. Middle row shows creation and placement of new cheekbone into damaged skull. Bottom row shows creation and placement of new jawbone into damaged skull. Bottom right image is completed simulation of surgical repair. See color figure 2.

ANALYZE™ runs on standard UNIX computers without special-purpose hardware. ANALYZE™ is being used on hundreds of imaging computers in a wide variety of biological investigations and medical applications in many institutions around the world.

3.18.3 Visual Programming Environments

In recent years, a new paradigm for accessing biomedical imaging functionality and developing programs to address specific applications has emerged. This paradigm is based on a graphical user interface presentation of the basic functions contained in the aforementioned toolkits, allowing the components of the toolkits to be connected and integrated graphically without the need to do programming in a standard programming language. Users of visual

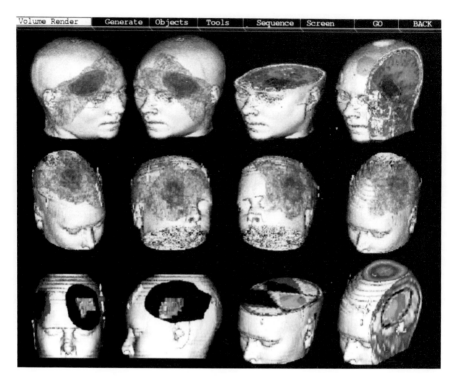

Figure 3.13. Illustration of use of display and analysis program (ANALYZE™) for 3-D radiation treatment planning. Top row shows simulated treatment beams through full head rendering and in cutaway views. Color is used to represent dose distribution to and around tumor. Middle row shows dose distribution from several beams from different angles of view. Bottom row shows simulated openings and cutaways to examine dose distribution in regional detail. Such 3-D planning facilitates optimal delivery of dose to tumor. See color figure 3.

programming environments build procedures from collections of functions using graphical representations of these functions and interconnecting them in a network-like architecture (this process is sometimes referred to as the "tinker-toy model"). The functions are available via a menu of modules which can be selected and placed in the current network. The interconnects between the modules define the data flow for the procedure, with each module having a set of potential input and output items to which the interconnects attach. A data model is specified to which the given image data must conform. Once constructed, these collections of modules that describe a procedure can be assigned data and executed, resulting in output that reflects the nature of the processing steps along the network path.

Systems of this type have sophisticated and interactive graphical interfaces that allow easy construction of the networks and allow for network editing and encapsulation. Even though such systems provide access to the entire collection of implemented functionality, permitting investigation and prototyping of solutions for applications without the need to write programs, most do not provide the ability to generate a turnkey operation independent of the network. This makes specific application development and distribution difficult. Examples of software systems of this type include AVS from AVS Inc. (Waltham, MA), Data Explorer from IBM (Hawthorne, NY), IRIS Explorer from Silicon Graphics Inc. (Mountain View, CA), and Khoros from the University of New Mexico (Albuquerque, NM).

3.19 References

1. Mitchell, W. J. *The Reconfigured Eye*. MIT Press, Cambridge, MA, 1992.

2. Kidder, T. *Soul of a New Machine*. Little, Brown and Company, Boston, 1981.

3. Aspray, W. (Ed.) *Computing Before Computers*. Iowa State University Press, Ames, IA, 1990.

4. Bashe, C. J., Johnson, L. R., Palmer, J. H., Pugh, E. W. *IBM's Early Computers*. MIT Press, Cambridge, MA, 1986.

5. Peterson, J. L., Silberschatz, A. *Operating System Concepts*. 2nd Ed. Addison-Wesley Publishing Company, Reading, MA, 1985.

6. Kernighan, B. W., Ritchie, D. M. *The C Programming Language*. Prentice-Hall, Englewood Cliffs, NJ, 1978.

7. Freeman, H. (Ed.) *Tutorial and Selected Readings in Interactive Computer Grpahics*. IEEE Computer Society, New York, 1980.

8. Ballard, D. H., Brown, C. M. *Computer Vision*. Prentice-Hall, Englewood Cliffs, NJ, 1982.

9. Castleman, K. R. *Digital Image Processing*. Prentice-Hall, Englewood Cliffs, NJ, 1979.

10. Ledeen, K. S. "Equipment for image processing—an overview." *Seminar Proceedings Computer Handling of Graphical Information*, Society of Photographic Scientists and Engineers, Washington, DC, 1970.

11. Robb, R. A., Stacy, M. C., McEwan, C. N. "A networked workstation approach to multidimensional biomedical image analysis." In: de Graaf, C. N., Viergever, M. A. (Eds.) *Information Processing in Medical Imaging*. Plenum Press, New York and London, 1988, pp. 349–374.

12. Robb, R. A. "Multidimensional biomedical image display and analysis in the Biotechnology Computer Resource Center at the Mayo Clinic." *Machine Vision and Applications*, 1, 75–96, 1988.

13. Stacy, M. "Report on FDDI for networking image servers to workstations." Mayo Foundation Internal Publication, June 1993.

14. Gilbert, B. K. "New computer technologies and their potential for expanded vistas in biomedicine." The 26th Annual Bowditch Lecture. *Physiologist*, 25, 2–18, 1982.

15. Gilbert, B. K., Harris, L. D. "Advances in processor architecture, display, and device technology for biomedical image processing." *IEEE Trans. Nucl. Sci.*, Vol NS-27, No. 3, June 1980.

16. Foley, J. D., Van Dam, A., Feiner, S., Hughs, J. *Computer Graphics: Principles and Practice.* 2nd Ed. Addison-Wesley Publishing Company, Reading, MA, 1990.

17. Sobell, M. *A Practical Guide to UNIX System V.* 2nd Ed. Benjamin/Cummings Publishing Co., Redwood City, CA, 1991.

18. Yemini, Y. (Ed.) *Current Advances in Distributed Computing and Communications.* Computer Science Press, Rockville, MD, 1987.

19. Sun Microsystems, Inc. "SunOS 5.1 administering NFS and RFS." Sun Microsystems, Mountain View, CA, 1992.

20. Huang, H. K., Mankovich, N. J., Taira, R., Cho, P., Stewart, B., Ho, B. K., Kangarloo, H., Boechat, M. I., Dietrich, R. B. "Picture archiving and communication systems for radiology." In: Lemke, H. U., Rhodes, M. L., Jaffee, C. C., Felix, R. (Eds.) *Proceedings of CAR '87.* Springer-Verlag, Berlin, 1987, pp. 487–497.

21. Jacobs, E., Lagerlund, A., Collura, T., Burgess, R. "A standard for the transfer of digital neurophysiological data." *Proceedings of the 14th International Conference of the IEEE Engineering in Medicine and Biology Society,* 1992.

22. Gray, M. J., Rutherford, H. "Functional specifications of a useful digital multi-modality image workstation." *Proceedings of the ISMII '84,* 8–12, 1984.

23. Birkner, D. A. "Design considerations for a user oriented PACS." *Proceedings of the ISMII '84,* 89–101, 1984.

24. Maguire, G. Q., Jr., Noz, M. E., Bakker, A., Bijl, K., Didden, H., de Valk, J. P. J. "Introduction to PACS for those interested in image processing." *Proceedings of the Xth IPMI International Conference,* Utretcht, The Netherlands, June 1987, pp. 403–412.

25. Huang, H. K., Taira, R. K. "Infrastructure design of a picture archiving and communication system." *Am. J. Radiol.,* 158, 743, 1992.

26. Múnoz, A., Dueñes, A., Gonzalez, M. A., Salvador, C. H. "General practitioner oriented workstation for a primary care communication system." *Proceedings of the 15th Annual International Conference of the IEEE Engineering in Medicine and Biology Society,* 1993.

27. Salazar, A., Forero, M., Goudin, S., Langevin, F., Fauchet, M. "A low cost image transfer system for small medical centers." *Proceedings of the 14th International Conference of the IEEE Engineering in Medicine and Biology Society,* 1992.

28. Ratib, O., Ligier, Y., Girard, C., Perrier, R., Logean, M., Vurlod, J. F. "A picture archiving and communications system based on an open and distributed architecture." *Proceedings of the 14th International Conference of the IEEE Engineering in Medicine and Biology Society,* 1992.

29. Bartsch, F., Gerweth, M., Schosser, R. "Remote expert consultation in radiology—the telemed project." *Proceedings of the 14th International Conference of the IEEE Engineering in Medicine and Biology Society,* 1992.

30. Gomez, E. J., del Pozo, F., Arredondo, M. T., Hernando, M. C., Sanz, M. "A telemedicine distributed decision-support system for diabetes management." *Proceedings of the 14th International Conference of the IEEE Engineering in Medicine and Biology Society,* 1992.

31. Bidgood, W. D., Horii, S. C. "PACS mini refresher course." *Radiographics,* March 1992, p. 345.

32. Arya, M., Cody, W., Faloutsos, C., Richardson, J., Toga, A. "QBISM: A Prototype 3-D Medical Image Database System." Bulletin on Data Engineering, Special Issue on Scientific Database, IEEE, March 1993.

33. Stoustrup, B. *The C++ Programming Language*. Addison-Wesley Publishing Company, Reading, MA, 1986.

4

Image Processing
and Visualization

The most beautiful thing we can experience is the mysterious. It is the source of all art and science.

Albert Einstein, *Letters*

4.1 Introduction

Locked within 3-D biomedical images is significant information about the objects and their properties from which the images are derived. Efforts to unlock this information to reveal answers to the mysteries of form and function are couched in the domain of image processing and visualization. A variety of both standard and sophisticated methods have been developed to process (modify) images to selectively enhance the visibility and measurability of desired object features and properties. Both realism-preserving and perception-modulating approaches to image display have significantly advanced the practical usefulness of 3-D biomedical imaging.

4.2 Image Processing

Numerous methods and approaches have been developed over the years to enhance or extract information from digital images. Many references are available[1-7] that describe these techniques, their advantages, and their limitations. Three general areas of image processing are briefly discussed here, namely algebraic, histogram, and filtering operations. These are only representative of the plethora of standard image processing methods used in biomedical imaging; but they demonstrate readily useful and practical extensions to 3-D biomedical imaging in particular.

4.2.1 Algebraic Operations

The algebraic combination of images (voxel by voxel) can be used directly for several simple but important image enhancement, display, and analysis tasks. Additionally, image algebra is the basis for more sophisticated image processing techniques. A comprehensive image algebra module is available in ANALYZE™ and was used to illustrate the following examples of algebraic operations on images.[8]

The most common use of image addition is to reduce random sensor noise in time sequence images of static or periodic phenomena. In Figure 4.1, seven gated MR images of the heart recorded at the same point in successive heartbeats have been summed to minimize the reconstruction artifacts in each original image. Image subtraction is an obvious first-order analysis of the difference between images. Subtraction of one time point of an image sequence from another reveals what has changed during the interval. Digital subtraction angiography is widely used to study arterial structures without interference from overlying or underlying structures. In Figure 4.2, identical versions of an original image are shifted one pixel in each of four directions and subtracted from the originals. The resulting images reveal edges (partial difference) in the four directions. Their sum is a rough approximation of an edge-strength image.

Image division is most often used to combine complementary image modalities. In Figure 4.3, the combination of T1-weighted and T2-weighted images better discriminates between tissue types than an image from either MRI sequence alone. In this case, the different tissue types that cluster in

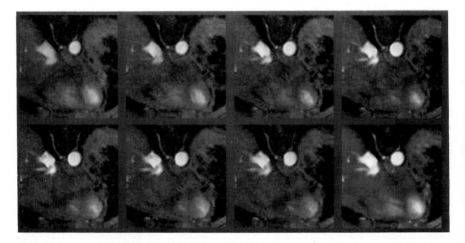

Figure 4.1.   MR images of the heart taken at the same time point in seven successive heartbeats (first seven images). The bottom right image is the sum of the other seven computed using image algebra in ANALYZE™. Note the clarity of structures and reduction of noise in the summed image.

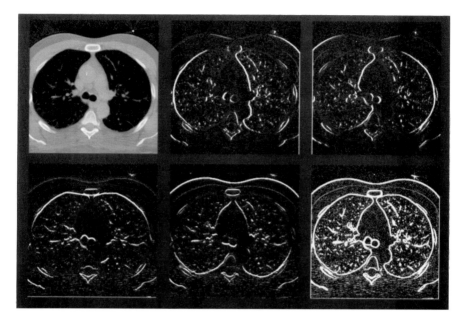

Figure 4.2. Four versions of the top left image shifted one pixel up, down, left, and right, respectively, were subtracted from the original to create the next four images. The sum of the four shifted images is an estimate of grayscale gradient magnitude, shown in the bottom right image.

the T1, T2 histogram space are spread along lines of differing slope, so the ratio image also shows a clear tissue type discrimination. Multiplicative image combining is primarily used to mask a grayscale image with a binary region. This can be used to composite useful images by combining modalities piecewise in 3-D space. In Figure 4.4, a set of adjacent X-ray CT sections

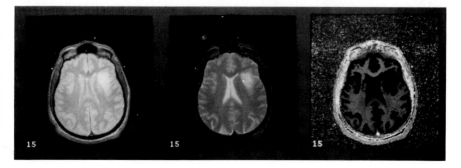

Figure 4.3. The T1 image (left) and T2 image (center) of the brain show white and gray matter in different ways, but the T1/T2 ratio image (right) shows this difference more dramatically.

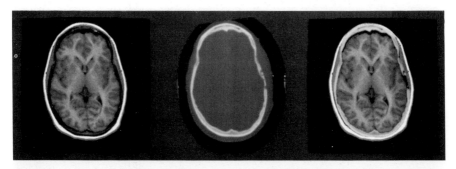

Figure 4.4. The MR image (left) has been combined with the bone field of the co-registered CT image (center) to produce the composite at right. The bone image was extracted as a binary image by threshoding and was multiplied by the grayscale image. The inverse of the binary bone image was multiplied by the MR image and the two segmented grayscale images combined additively.

and a volumetric MRI scan of the head have been coregistered. The skull has been segmented by thresholding the CT image and creating a binary mask of the skull alone. The brain has been segmented from the MR image using mathematical morphology, and a binary mask of the brain has been created from that image. The equation below describes the combination of grayscale information from both modalities to create the final image:

$$\text{output} = \text{MRI} * \text{MRI\_brainmask}$$
$$+ (\text{CT} * \text{CT\_skullmask}) * 250/2000 \tag{4.1}$$

The scaling constant (250/2000) is used to rescale the 16-bit CT image into the 8-bit range of the MRI.

4.2.2 Histogram Operations

The global statistical manipulation of grayscale values is based on histogram matching.[1,2] Figure 4.5 illustrates two images and their histograms produced in ANALYZE™. The left-hand image can be transformed to have a histogram similar to the right-hand image by creating a grayscale mapping function that consists of the forward application of the left-hand cumulative histogram function followed by the inverse application of the right-hand cumulative function as shown in Figure 4.6. Since the cumulative function of any histogram is a monotonic function, an inverse function exists and is monotonic.

If some ideal "flat" histogram shape is used for histogram matching, as in Figure 4.7, the process is called histogram "flattening" or "equalization," and the typical result is to maximize contrast in the single modality image.[1] Note that in both histogram matching and equalization, large areas of the grayscale range may be unused in the final image. This is required to achieve

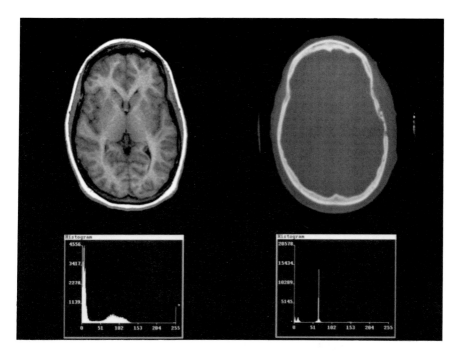

Figure 4.5. The MR image on the left has a multimodal histogram which indicates the multiple tissue types differentiated by MRI. The CT image on the right has a less complex histogram, indicating primarily the CT ranges of hard and soft tissues.

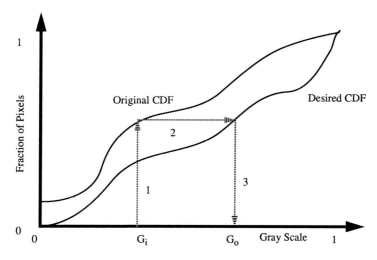

Figure 4.6. The cumulative density function (CDF) is the integral of the histogram normalized to the total number of voxels in the image. Cumulative histogram functions are always monotonic, and therefore are known to have an inverse. By mapping an original grayscale value against the original cumulative function, then against the inverse of the desired cumulative function, the original histogram can be made to resemble the desired histogram.

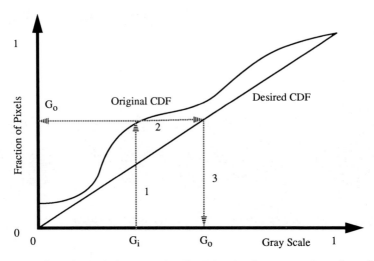

Figure 4.7. If the desired histogram is "flat," i.e. having an equal number of voxels at each gray level, the cumulative function is a simple diagonal line.

the contrast stretching which is usually desired. If the flattening step is being used to preserve contrast while moving from a high-resolution grayscale to a lower-resolution grayscale (as in scaling 16-bit data for display on 8-bit frame buffers) this "wasted grayscale" will tend to cause loss of detail. A slight modification of histogram flattening which effectively limits the maximum slope of the two cumulative functions can be used in this case to transmit maximum information content in the low-resolution image. Figure 4.8 illustrates the linear mapping between the minimum and maximum volumes of an X-ray CT image of the head and the 8-bit range of a display device (left), compared to an information preserving mapping (right).

Histogram matching provides a fixed global mapping that can be inverted to determine the rough value of an input voxel. The mapping is montonic, so that direction of voxel magnitude is preserved in the mapped image relative to the original image. This is generally a required characteristic if the images are to be objectively (i.e., numerically) analyzed after transformation. But if the purpose of the mapping is purely for visual enhancement, the local adaptive use of histogram flattening may bring out detail that was simply invisible in the original. The goal of adaptive histogram equalization[9,10] is to optimize the display of contrast gradients everywhere in the image, calibrated to the dynamic range of the display device. At the limit, adaptive histogram equalization constructs a region about each pixel and uses the local region histogram to remap the grayscale of only one pixel. The size of the region controls the amount of enhancement, with larger regions more nearly resembling the original. In practice, this algorithm is compute intensive, and a number of approximations are used.[10] Figure 4.9 is the same

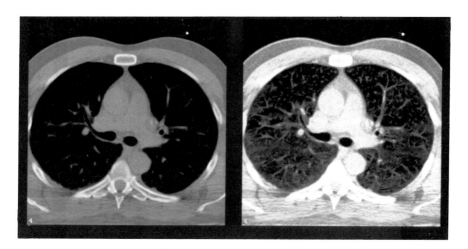

Figure 4.8. The image on the left is a conventional linear mapping from the original 16-bit range to an 8-bit range of a CT image of the chest. The right-hand image is the result of a slope-limited histogram-flattening process, again mapping to an 8-bit range using ANALYZE™. The relationship between the two images is nonlinear but monotonic, so that the direction of grayscale variation is preserved.

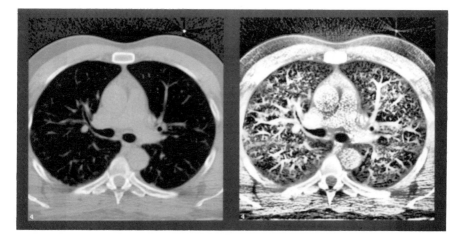

Figure 4.9. The image on the left is a linear mapping of the original 16-bit CT image to an 8-bit image. The right-hand image is the result of an adaptive histogram equalization process in ANALYZE™, again mapping to an 8-bit range. The process does not produce a global map of gray values, and may map identically valued original pixels to very different output values. The effect is to enhance contrast everywhere in the image with optimal mapping to the display range. The resultant is nonlinear and nonreversible relative to the original image.

image as in Figure 4.8 after adaptive histogram equalization in ANALYZE™. Note preservation of detail in both the lung and bone fields. Note also that large uniform regions tend toward a mid-level gray, and that there is no longer any global mapping function that allows recovery of the original grayscale value from the result. Adaptive histogram equalization is nonlinear and nonreversible. One must therefore be careful in making quantitative measurements from such images.

4.2.3 Filter Operations

Linear systems theory provides a wealth of image analysis and enhancement techniques.[1-3] Linear systems theory is based upon the supposition of linear relationships among all components of an image-forming system, which is often a reasonable assumption over the normal operating range of modern medical imaging systems.

Linear systems can be completely characterized by their response to impulse functions.[3] For an electrical system, an impulse is a finite amount of electrical energy that occurs over zero time. For an optical system, the impulse is a point source of finite luminosity in the object plane of the lens. For an X-ray imaging system, the impulse is a finite point source of radiopacity. In practice, these functions can be approximated by very short pulses and very small fluorescent or metal beads.

The impulse response (or point spread function, psf, for spatial systems) can be used to predict the output of the system to any arbitrary input by the process of convolution, essentially replacing each of the points in an image with its appropriately scaled psf. In the absence of noise, the psf can be used to correct for distortions produced by the system. In Figure 4.10, an original image is severely degraded through a noiseless system that fragments the image into several superimposed copies. Knowledge of the system's psf allows us to deconvolve the captured image and recover the original. The presence of noise in practical systems limits the extent to which the degraded image can be recovered, but there remains significant potential for image enhancement.

Most advanced image enhancement techniques are developed in the Fourier domain. Fourier's theorem states that any waveform (including the 2-D and 3-D spatial waveforms which are images) can be expressed as the sum of sinusoidal basis functions at varying frequencies, amplitudes, and relative phases.[11] It is fairly straightforward to understand that a musical instrument's unique timbre is composed of the unique combination of higher harmonics produced when a fundamental tone is played, but it is often difficult to visualize spatial frequencies. Figure 4.11 illustrates the 3rd, 5th, and 7th harmonic spatial frequencies present in an image. The slight irregularities in the patterns reflect the phase differences unique to this image which cause those harmonics to add and interfere with other components so as to put objects and edges at particular points in the image. Higher spatial frequen-

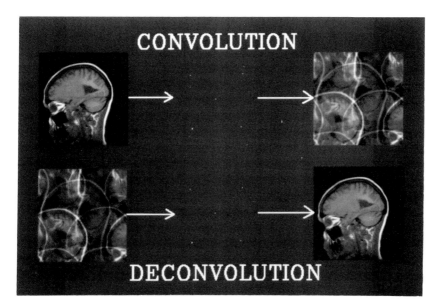

Figure 4.10. The original image at top left was degraded by convolution into the "multiple exposure" image at top right. Because the linear system is known exactly (no noise), the degraded multiple image can be perfectly restored to the original image using deconvolution.

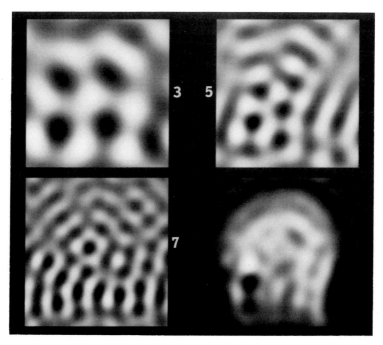

Figure 4.11. The 3rd, 5th, and 7th harmonic components of a sagittal MR section of the head. The irregularities in the sinusoidal patterns illustrate the phase information which puts features at particular places in the images. The lower right image is the sum of only the first 7 harmonic components, yet still begins to reveal the outline shape of the head (the original image had 128 harmonic components).

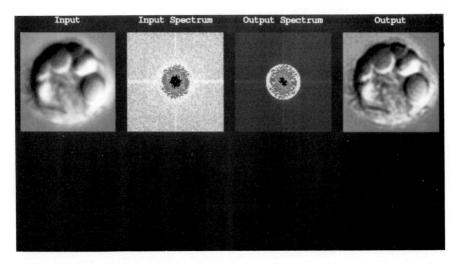

Figure 4.12. The original microscope image of an egg cell (left) is bandpass filtered to remove high-frequency noise and boost midrange frequency content. This will enhance features in the image (right) which are small, but larger than spot noise. See color figure 4.

cies relate to small features at sharp edges, and lower frequencies relate to absolute grayscale values and larger shapes in the image.

In the frequency domain, it is often possible to separate noise from signal.[2] In Figure 4.12 (see color figure 4), an image is first filtered (low-pass) to remove high-frequency noise, and then filtered (high-pass) to enhance

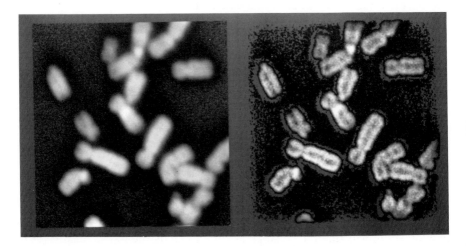

Figure 4.13. A photomicrograph of chromosomes is enhanced by a constrained iterative filtering technique in ANALYZE™. A guess at the enhanced image is iteratively modified until it matches the original image after being degraded by the theoretical impulse response of the confocal microscope.

features that are larger than noise events. (This sequence of visualizations is very helpful in designing effective bandpass filters for images, and is included in the Filter Design module of ANALYZE™.) More sophisticated approaches, such as Wiener filtering,[2,3] minimize the error between the Fourier-domain spectra of the original and recovered image. Figure 4.13 illustrates the use of a modified constrained iterative technique[12,13] applied to a 3-D confocal image of a metaphase spread of chromosomes. This technology, included in the 3-D FFT module of ANALYZE™, refines the theoretical psf of the imaging system and eliminates noise, enhancing the ultrastructure in the chromosomes.

4.3 2-D Image Generation and Display

There are many situations in 3-D biomedical imaging in which identification, generation, and display of the optimal image plane is critical, as the utility of 2-D images often depends on the physical orientation of the image plane with respect to the structure of interest. Most biomedical imaging systems have limited capability to create this optimal 2-D image directly, as structure positioning and scanner orientation are generally restricted. Therefore, techniques to generate and display these optimal 2-D images from 3-D volume images are particularly important, allowing the orientation of the 2-D image plane to ultimately result in a clear, unrestricted view of important features in the 2-D image. For example, the measurement of the cross-sectional shape of the left ventricular chamber of the heart may be necessary for proper functional assessment of cardiac ability.

4.3.1 Multiplanar Reformatting

The 3-D nature of volume images, when isotropic, allows for simple and efficient computation of images that lie along the nonacquired orthogonal orientations of the volume. This is accomplished by readdressing the order of voxels in the volume image, which can be done interactively when the volume image is entirely stored in the memory of an imaging computer. When the structure imaged has an anatomic reference, the orthogonal planes can be referenced by the anatomic terms for orthogonal orientation: transaxial, coronal, and sagittal. This is demonstrated in Figure 4.14 for a 3-D volume image of the head from a 3-D acquired MRI scan. The original plane of acquisition was the transaxial plane, as shown by the transaxial images in the top row. The orthogonally reformatted coronal sections from the back of the head towards the front are shown in the middle row, with sagittal sections from the right toward the left side of the head shown in the bottom row. Implementations of multiplanar reformatting techniques[8,14] on current

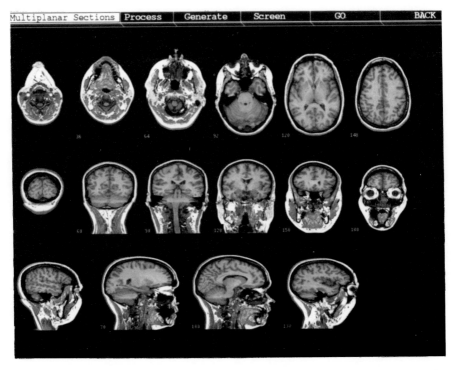

Figure 4.14. Multiplanar reformatting of a 3-D MRI volume image of the head with ANALYZE™. Multiple images in the original transaxial plane of acquisition (top row) and the orthogonally reformatted coronal plane (middle row) and sagittal plane (bottom row) can be interactively computed and displayed.

computer technology allow the interactive generation and display of these images, as in ANALYZE™. Display of multiplanar images usually consists of multipanel display of these images, as demonstrated in Figure 4.14. Display of a sequence of adjacent multiplanar images without position change on the screen provides an effective mechanism for visualization of section-to-section change in structures, often augmenting the visual synthesis of the 3-D structures. Another effective display technique for orthogonal sections of a volume image in ANALYZE™ is depicted in Figure 4.15. The volume image is displayed using a 3-D to 2-D transform, providing display of the orthogonal image data as if visualizing the actual cube of data at a particular orientation. A maximum of three of the six total orthogonal images in the volume image may be visualized at a time. With current computer technology, this volume image can be manipulated interactively to control orientation (middle sliders), while also specifying which orthogonal image along each orthogonal direction is displayed (lower sliders).

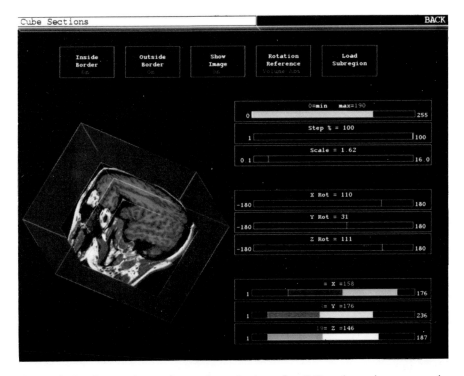

Figure 4.15. Interactive orthogonal sectioning of a 3-D volume image may be achieved using cubic volume display. Color coding along the outside edges of the volume (left) corresponds to sliders used to control interactive orthogonal sectioning (lower right), with angle selection sliders controlling the rotation of the cube (middle right).

4.3.2 Oblique Sectioning

The desired 2-D image may not lie along the orthogonal aspect of the 3-D volume image, but is more likely to lie along an arbitrarily oriented plane at some oblique angle to the orthogonal axes of the volume image. Oblique images are less intuitive and much harder to compute, as simple readdressing of the voxels in a given order will not determine or generate the proper oblique image. These two problems, specification of the orientation and efficient generation of the oblique image, require additional visualization and computation techniques.[14]

Specification and identification of the oblique image are often done using structural landmarks in the orthogonal image data. To accomplish this, several images need to be presented to allow unambiguous selection of these landmarks, usually through multiplanar orthogonal images, as shown in Fig-

ure 4.16. Two methods can be used for definition of the oblique plane orientation. Selection of three points on landmarks will uniquely define the
orientation of the plane, which may need to be rotated within the plane for
proper display orientation. Two selected points define an axis along which
oblique planes perpendicular to the axis can be generated. This does not
uniquely define a single plane, as the oblique image may be generated anywhere along the axis, but this method is often used when a stack of oblique
images needs to be generated through a structure, as with the left ventricular
sectioning problem. Interactive manipulation of the oblique plane orientation can be achieved if controls for angular rotation maneuvers are provided.
This is accomplished in ANALYZE™ using aeronautical maneuver terms
(i.e., pitch, roll, yaw) with angle increment specification and control buttons
for each maneuver, as shown in Figure 4.16.

Oblique sectioning, particularly when interactive, requires some method
of visualization for plane placement and orientation verification. One
method uses selected orthogonal images with a line indicating the intersec-

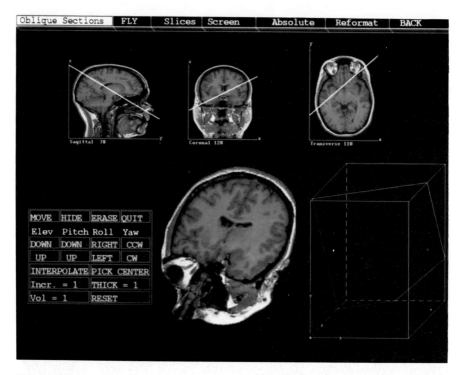

Figure 4.16. Arbitrarily oriented sections (bottom middle) cut obliquely through the
3-D volume image can be interactively selected and computed in ANALYZE™. Interactive orientation is controlled by aeronautical maneuvers (pitch, roll, yaw, ele-
vate) (lower right), with a graphical indication of the intersection of the oblique plane
on orthogonal images (top row) used as orientation reference.

tion of the oblique image with the orthogonal images, as shown in Figure 4.16. Another method depicts the intersection of the oblique plane with a rendered surface image, providing direct 3-D visual feedback with familiar structural features.

4.3.3 Curved Sectioning

Often structures of interest may have curvilinear morphology that multi-planar and oblique images cannot capture in a single 2-D image. This restriction of planar sections can be overcome using curvilinear sectioning techniques, as demonstrated in Figure 4.17 using ANALYZE™. A trace along an arbitrary path on any orthogonal image, as shown in the lower left, defines a set of pixels in the orthogonal image that have a corresponding row of voxels through the volume image. Each row of voxels for each pixel on the trace can be displayed as a line of a new image, as shown on the right, which corresponds to the curved planar structure lying along the trace. This technique is useful for curved structures that remain constant in shape

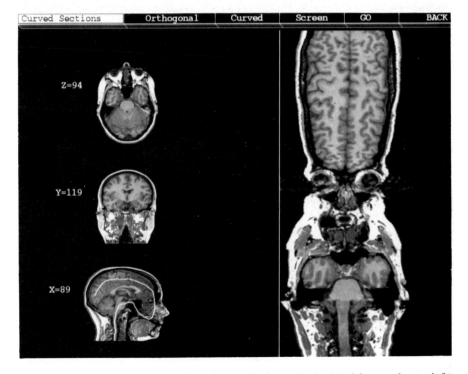

Figure 4.17. Tracing along an arbitrary path on an orthogonal image (lower left) interactively generates and displays a curved planar image sampled through the 3-D volume image along that trace (right).

through one orthogonal dimension (one degree of freedom), like the entire extent of the spine in sagittal CT images or curved structures in the orbit of the eye.

4.4 3-D Image Generation and Display

Visualization of 3-D biomedical volume images has characteristically been divided into two different techniques: surface rendering[15,16] and volume rendering.[17-20] Both techniques produce a visualization of selected structures in the 3-D volume image, but the methods involved in these techniques are quite different, and each has its advantages and disadvantages. Selection between these techniques is often predicated on the particular nature of the biomedical image data, the application to which the visualization is being applied, and the desired result of the visualization.

Surface rendering techniques characteristically require the extraction of contours that define the surface of the structure to be visualized.[16] An algorithm is then applied that places surface patches or tiles at each contour point, and with hidden surface removal and shading, the surface is rendered. The advantage of this technique lies in the small amount of contour data, resulting in fast rendering speeds. Also, standard computer graphics techniques can be applied, including standard shading models (Phong, Gouraud), and the technique can take advantage of particular graphics hardware to speed the geometric transformation and rendering processes. The contour-based surface descriptions can be transformed into analytical descriptions, which permits use with other geometric visualization packages (i.e., CAD/CAM software), and the contours can be used to drive machinery to create models of the structure.[21] Other analytically defined structures can be easily superposed with the surface rendered structures. The disadvantages of this technique are largely based on the need to discretely extract the contours defining the structure to be visualized. All other volume image information is lost in this transformation, breaking the connection back to the original volume information, which may be important for slice generation or value measurement. This also prohibits any interactive, dynamic determination of the surface to be rendered, as the decision has been made during contour extraction specifically which surface will be visualized. Finally, due to the discrete nature of the surface patch placement, this technique is prone to sampling and aliasing artifacts on the rendered surface.

Volume rendering techniques based on ray-casting algorithms have become the method of choice for the visualization of 3-D biomedical volume images.[14,22,23] These methods provide direct visualization of the volume images without the need for prior surface or object segmentation, preserving the values and context of the original image data. Volume rendering techniques allow for the application of various different rendering algorithms during the ray-casting process. No a priori surface extraction is necessary, as the entire volume image is rendered in this process, maintaining a relationship between the rendered image and the volume image data itself. This provides for the capability to section the rendered image and visualize the actual image data in the volume image, and to make voxel value-based measurements for the rendered image. The rendered surface can be dynamically determined by changing the ray-casting and surface recognition conditions during the rendering process. However, 3-D biomedical volume image data sets are characteristically large, taxing the computation abilities of volume-rendering techniques and the systems on which they are implemented. This is particularly true when the rendering process must preserve structure resolution with sufficient fidelity for appropriate visualization of the structures. Given the discrete voxel-based nature of the volume image, there is no direct connection to other geometric objects, which may be desired for interaction with the rendering or for output of the rendered structure to other devices.

4.4.1 Surface Rendering

Shaded surface displays are useful if there is a need or desire to visualize 3-D surfaces. This is the case in many situations of practical importance. Shaded surface displays have been successfully employed in craniofacial reconstructive surgery planning,[16,21] in studies of congenital and acquired cardiopulmonary disease,[24] and in analysis of pulmonary structure–function relationship.[25]

Shaded surface displays are a 2-D representation of a 3-D surface. The 3-D nature of the surface is conveyed with the aid of visual cues such as perspective, shading, texture, shadowing, and stereopsis. Generally, shaded surface displays are not well suited to "immediate" full visualization of the 3-D volume; that is, they require some preprocessing of the 3-D data to extract the desired surfaces. Shaded surface displays have proven popular in many applications, since, once the surfaces of interest have been determined, it is not difficult to quickly compute images for display. In most algorithms, the surfaces are described in terms of patches that join to form the complete surface.[26] Modern computational systems can process thousands of polygon patches per second. This speed permits satisfactory interactive capabilities in computer-aided design applications but does not satisfy the requirements of interactive display of biological/medical images. This is because a 3-D image of anatomic structures may contain up to 100,000 faces or more. Unless the number of faces can be greatly reduced, even state-of-the-art display packages do not really provide acceptable user interaction (response time needs to be of the order of seconds). Special-purpose hardware can achieve the necessary speed but increases the cost.

Several investigators have implemented methods for 3-D shaded surface displays of anatomic structures.[15,16,26,27] Some follow an approach similar to the techniques used in solid modeling. The main difficulty for display of biological structures is fitting tiles to a 3-D surface. This problem can be circumvented by defining the surface elements as the 3-D pixel (voxel) borders.[16] This makes the algorithm easy to apply to "real" data. However, the task of displaying a smooth surface from such elements is a problem. One approach is to employ a contextual shading scheme in which the shading of a displayed face depends on the orientation of its neighbors, its distance from the observer, and the incident angle of the light. Implementation of this type of algorithm has produced useful displays of 3-D images[26] but has also proven to be cumbersome, especially when the algorithm is used to detect and display soft tissues. The time required to segment the volume, isolate the desired surfaces (as is required by any 3-D surface display), and convert the faces to the program's internal description must be added to the display time. Even though these times are required only once for each volume, if several volumes are to be analyzed (as is almost always the case), they are too long for efficient analysis.

An improved approach[16] to 3-D shaded surface display has been implemented in ANALYZE™. Figure 4.18 illustrates the coordinate system used in the algorithm. The x, y, and l axes are fixed in object space. The object can be rotated in any direction relative to these axes prior to surface display. The output image is in the l, ξ plane, which is the display screen. For convenience of display, the algorithm places the l-axis on either of the vertical or horizontal axes of the display frame buffer. The z-axis is perpendicular to the l and ξ axes, i.e., it extends out of the display plane.

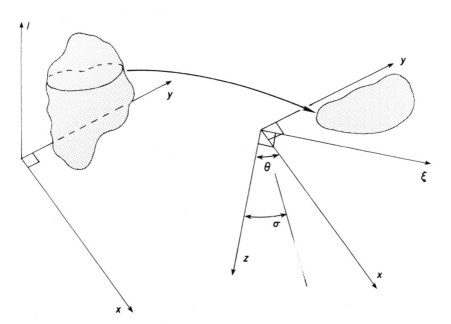

Figure 4.18. The coordinate system for 3-D surface display. The x, y, and ℓ axes are fixed relative to the object, whereas the ξ and z axes are fixed in display space.

To provide the optimal compromise between generality (flexibility) and efficiency (speed, accuracy, and "realism"), the following design constraints are specified for the improved shaded surface algorithm:

1. The object is illuminated by parallel light which is incident at an angle σ relative to the z=axis, where σ is referred to as the "highlight" angle. It is further stipulated that the view direction is always parallel to the z-axis. Thus, there is no perspective to be computed. As a consequence, the display generation task can be split into independent planes, each corresponding to one line of the output display.
2. Some smoothing of contours should be provided for aesthetic effect.
3. Depth cues, such as surface inclination and intensity diminution with distance, should be employed.
4. The algorithm should be fast and have modest memory requirements.

The sequential steps in the implemented algorithm are: 1) image segmentation, 2) contouring and smoothing, and 3) display generation. The input to the algorithm (i.e., the input to step 1) is a 3-D volume image. The segmentation step (1) produces a binary volume image in which all voxels are given a value of either 1 or 0. The nonzero voxels represent elements that are part of the structural shape (or shapes) to be displayed. Accurate segmentation of the 3-D volume is a nontrivial task. For example, it is usually possible to separate bone from soft tissue in a CT image by simple thresholding. However, it is much more difficult to separate one soft tissue from another (for example, brain tissue and the fluid-filled ventricles). The approach taken in the initial implemetation of the ANALYZE™ algorithm is to employ user-specified thresholds to separate the desired objects, followed by 3-D region-filling initiated from appropriate starting points selected by the user. Figure 4.19 illustrates thresholding multiple CT slices simultaneously through a volume image of the head to produce contours for rendering the surface of the skull and brain.

In the second step, each slice of the binary volume is transformed and stored in a contour format. The output of this stage is a list of points, equally spaced around each outward-facing contour of each slice, and each with an associated direction vector.

The third and final step is display generation. The user can specify the view angle, highlight angle, and several other parameters used to adjust the shading. Shading computation and hidden surface removal are performed in this step.

In a typical application of the algorithm, the user usually iterates on the last step until the desired object orientation and shading are obtained. The final object is generally a sequence of surface displays, such as a 360° rotation of the object in 2° or 3° increments. This rotation sequence is usually recorded as a "movie" on videodisk or video tape to enable playback off-line from the computer.

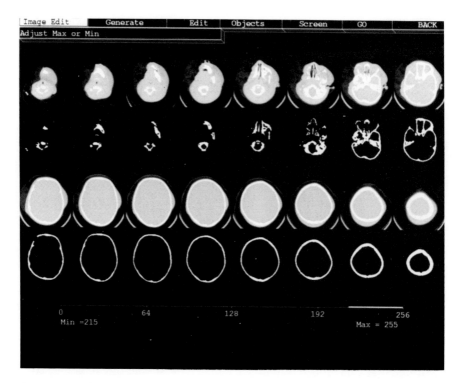

Figure 4.19. Simultaneous interactive thresholding of sequential CT slices through the head. A threshold (lower slider) is interactively applied to the CT sections (rows 1 and 3), creating binary images (rows 2 and 4) corresponding to each section which contain only bone. Using multiple sections through the volume provides a global view of the effect of the selected threshold over the entire volume image during the interactive process.

The structure of the algorithm allows incorporation of special display effects, such as dissection of the volume. This is implemented by inserting a preprocessing program to manipulate the binary volume prior to the contour extraction. For example, "volume dissection" is accomplished by producing new binary volumes such that the voxels in a region of interest are isolated and processed separately. The region of interest can be related to the entire volume at subsequent points in the analysis. Figure 4.20 illustrates surface rendering of the skull and brain from a thresholded CT scan of the head (as in Figure 4.19).

4.4.2 Volume Rendering

Most volume rendering techniques are based on ray-casting[28,29] through the volume image. Different algorithms[17-20] may be used during this ray-casting

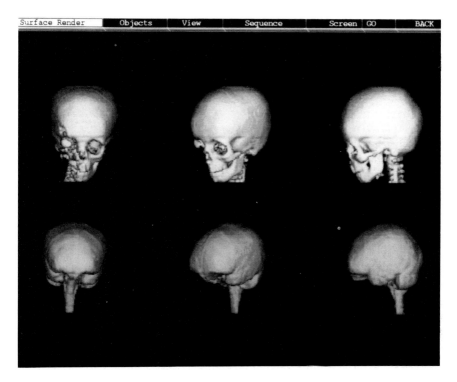

Figure 4.20. After contour extraction, shaded surface displays can be rendered for selected sets of contours using ANALYZE™. The shaded surface displays of the segmented skull (top row) are generated from exterior contours extracted from the thresholded images in Figure 4.19. The interior contours can be used to generate shaded surface displays of the brain (bottom row).

process. The algorithms may utilize different representations of the volume image space, usually through some decomposition step such as that in octree encoding.[30–32] The ray-casting technique provides the important advantage that the visualization is created directly from the volume image, with the selection of structures that will be rendered done during the ray casting process. A function of different attributes of the voxels in the volume image, such as density or gradient values (for surface segmentation) or spatial coordinates (for volume cutting), can be applied to control the rendering process and result in the desired output rendered image. The implementation[20] of volume rendering in ANALYZE™ has several features and advantages in comparison to conventional shaded surface display and other volume-rendering methods. It will be described in some detail.

Volume rendering display techniques have the characteristics of being able to display surfaces with shading *and* other parts of the volume simultaneously. An important advantage is to display data *directly* from the grayscale volume. The selection of the data that will appear on the screen is done during the projection of the voxels (also called ray casting). A function of different attributes of the voxels, such as their density or gradient values and/or spatial coordinates, can be invoked during the projection process to produce "on the fly" segmented surfaces, cutting planes anywhere in the volume, and/or selected degrees of transparency/opacity within the volume. Volume set operations (union, intersection, difference of volume) can also be invoked during the projection process.

The most common camera model consists of a source point (called *Eye*), a focus point (where the eye is looking), and a matrix of pixels (the *screen*)[28,29] The visible object to display (called *scene*) is in front of the camera within a truncated volume called the *viewing pyramid* (see Figure 4.21).

The purpose of a ray-tracing model is to define the geometry of the rays cast through the scene. To connect the source point to the scene, for each pixel of the screen a ray is defined as a straight line from the source point passing through the pixel. To generate the picture, the pixel values are assigned appropriate intensities "sampled" by the rays passing everywhere through the scene. For instance, for shaded surface display, the pixel values are computed according to light models (intensity and orientation of light source(s), reflections, textures, surface orientations, etc.) where the rays have intersected the scene.[33,34]

The goal of ray tracing in ANALYZE™ is to display a volume image interactively, without compromising image quality. In order to do this, careful and optimized coding of the algorithm was undertaken. Another advantage of the ANALYZE™ ray-tracing implementation is to interactively render an anatomic volume with different degrees of segmentation.

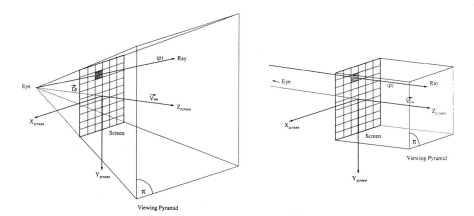

Figure 4.21. The camera models shown here depict the viewing pyramid for divergent rays (left) and parallel rays (right) used in volume rendering. The ANALYZE™ volume rendering program uses the parallel model as default, as it allows rapid ray casting through each pixel in the render screen using the same voxel increment for all rays.

Two classes of display have been implemented: transmission and reflection. An example of a transmission image is an X-ray radiograph; an example of a reflection image is a photograph. For the radiograph, the film is located behind the scene and only the rays transmitted through and filtered by the objects are recorded on the film. For the photograph, the film is located in front of the scene, so the film records the light reflected by the objects in the scene.

For most transmission-oriented displays, there is no surface identification involved. A ray passes through the volume and the pixel value is computed as an integrated function. Several different display models are in this family, including maximum intensity, voxel summation, and surface projection displays.

For all reflection display types, voxel density values are used to specify surfaces within the volume image. For example, if the value of a voxel intersected by a ray is between a specified maximum and minimum (a threshold), this voxel is defined as on the surface. Several types of functions can be specified to compute the shading, for example, depth shading, depth gradient shading, and voxel gradient shading.

In depth shading, the value of the display pixel is simply a function of depth, that is, the distance between the screen and the intersected voxel on the surface. In depth gradient shading, as shown in Figure 4.22, depth shading is used, but postprocessing is performed on the resulting image to enhance contrast. A sham normal function is computed for the current pixel depth and the neighboring pixel depths. Rather than computing a normal vector within the scene space, a sham vector is computed on the screen space where the z component of the normal is always equal to one.[33] In practice, the depth gradient model often produces artifacts due to discontinuities and noise of the gradient approximation. In order to reduce these artifacts, image smoothing is performed.

In voxel gradient shading, an improved computation of the normal vector associated with the voxel is used to implement the diffuse reflection lighting model without producing artifacts. A natural way to compute a normal vector at a point (voxel) is to compute the gradient associated with the point. In a 3-D volume image, this gradient can be computed using a 6, 18, or 26 neighborhood about the voxel,[19,34] as illustrated in Figure 4.23.

Another reflection-type display maps the grayscale threshold range to a continuum of opacity values between fully transparent and fully opaque and then composites a surface shading by accepting weighted contributions from all voxels having nonzero opacity. The main advantage of this display is improved rendering of features obscured by the partial volume effect, such as thin membranes, tiny cracks, and small surface features. This algorithm has two variants:

1. Fuzzy gradient shading back-to-front. The ray seeks a voxel of maximum opacity then returns toward the viewer adding a shading contribution for each voxel of nonzero opacity. The basic contribution of a voxel is its

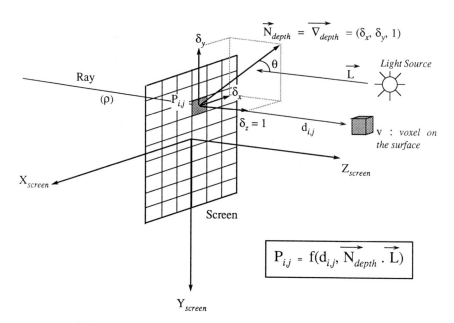

Figure 4.22.   Diagram of ray-tracing geometry for adding gradient shading to standard depth shading. The orientation of the normal vector N_{depth} is determined by the 2-D gradient in the computed depth image ∇_{depth}. The output pixel is then a function of the depth of the surface voxel, and the reflectance model for the normal vector $\tilde{N}_{depth}$ and light vector $\tilde{L}$.

voxel gradient shading. The contribution is then weighted by the voxel's opacity and the magnitude of the gradient vector at the voxel. The contribution is further weighted so that voxels nearer the viewer have a greater relative contribution than deeper voxels of identical opacity and gradient. This is the faster version of fuzzy gradient shading.

2. Fuzzy gradient shading front-to-back. The contributions of voxels of nonzero opacity are accumulated as the ray penetrates the volume. The ray only stops when it encounters a voxel of maximum opacity at a point of maximum gradient magnitude. The contributions of individual voxels are weighted similarly to those of the back-to-front algorithm. This version of fuzzy gradient shading usually produces superior renderings.

Several rendering algorithms have been implemented in ANALYZE™,[14,20] representing the two classes of reflection (surface) algorithms and transmission (projection) algorithms. The reflection algorithms model the image voxels as light reflectors and require the detection of surfaces within the volume. The basic reflection algorithms consider the first voxel along the ray path within the constraints of the rendering parameters (threshold, cutting depth, etc.) as the surface voxel to be rendered and differ in how the detected surface voxels are rendered into the output image. Advanced reflection al-

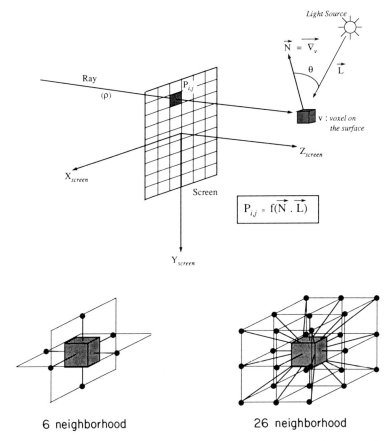

6 neighborhood   26 neighborhood

Figure 4.23. Diagram of full voxel gradient shading geometry using 6-voxel or 26-voxel neighborhoods. A computed gradient from the voxel values in the given neighborhood, ∇v is used to orient the normal $\vec{N}$. The output pixel is then only a function of the normal $\vec{N}$ and the light vector $\vec{L}$ in the reflectance model.

gorithms (e.g., fuzzy gradient) map the grayscale threshold range to a continuum of opacity values between fully transparent and fully opaque, compositing a surface shading value by accepting weighted contributions from all voxels having nonzero opacity. Transmission algorithms model the image voxels as light emitters and do not involve explicit surface detection. A rendered image pixel's value is computed as a function of the ray passing through a set of voxels. Each of these algorithms has an associated set of control parameters that alter the ray conditions and the rendered output pixel values. This provides a rich set of rendering functionality through which various structures from multiple modalities can be interactively visualized. Renderings produced by several of these algorithms are shown in Figure 4.24.

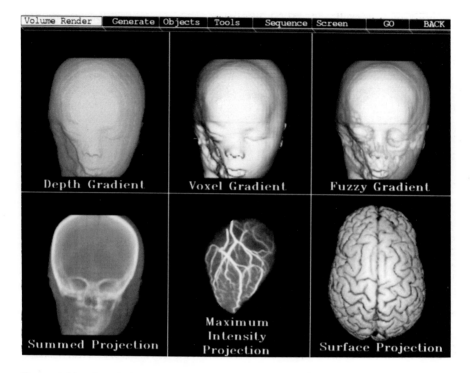

Figure 4.24. Rendering algorithms in the ANALYZE™ volume rendering program are divided into two classes: reflection (examples in top row) and transmission (examples in bottom row). The reflection algorithms render surfaces using several shading models, including depth gradient shading (top left), voxel gradient shading (top middle), and fuzzy gradient shading (top right). The transmission algorithms create projections, including summed voxel projection (bottom left), maximum intensity projection (bottom middle), and integrated surface projection (bottom right).

Figure 4.25 illustrates rendering of the brain from a full head MRI scan using a special "surface projection" algorithm. The MRI data are automatically segmented to remove the top of the head, and a projection rendering of just a few voxels capturing the surface of the brain parenchyma is performed. This provides a highly detailed and realistic rendering of the surfaces of the cerebral cortex. Figure 4.26 (see color figure 5) shows another voxel gradient rendering of a brain and major cerebral vessels, both segmented from a full head MRI scan. Figure 4.27 illustrates a particularly unique capability of ANALYZE™ volume rendering. A segmented brain is rendered as usual from MRI data (left) and compared with a special rendering type called radial cylindrical rendering (right), which has the effect of rolling out the entire 3-D brain surface flat, as in Mercator projections. This permits the entire surface around 360° to be visualized in a single display (like Mercator maps of the world).

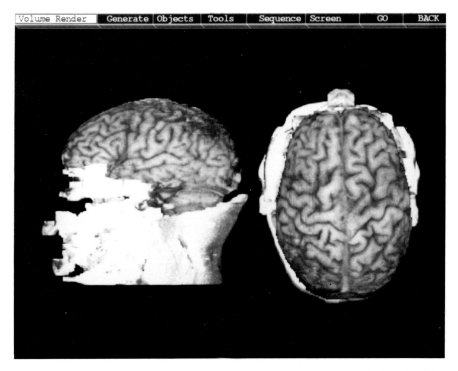

| Volume Render | Generate | Objects | Tools | Sequence | Screen | GO | BACK |

Figure 4.25. An example of the surface projection transmission rendering algorithm in ANALYZE™, demonstrating the capability for generating highly detailed and realistic rendering of the cortical surface of the brain. The brain was automatically segmented using 3-D morphological processing.

An option in the ANALYZE™ volume rendering module incorporates transparency in order to see two or more different structures in the display, each through the other. The basic principle is to define several structures with several segmentation functions, and assign transparency (or conversely, opacity) coefficients for each structure specified. The transparent effect for each pixel on the screen is computed according to a weighted function of the reflection due to the transparent structures, the light transmission through structures, and the reflection due to the opaque structures. The general model is illustrated in Figure 4.28. Figure 4.29 (see color figure 6) shows a transparent rendering in which the skin has been made translucent to reveal the brain underneath.

Figure 4.30 shows a volume-rendered display of the head (skin surfaces) from an X-ray CT scan of a trauma patient with facial wounds, showing cut planes along orthogonal views (top row), and a selective rendering mask within which skull rendering and X-ray-like projection renderings are inlaid (bottom row). Such visualizations provide the impetus for development of

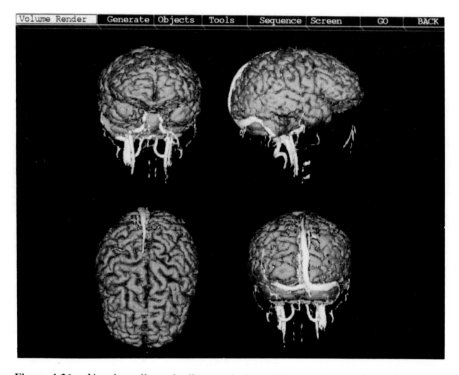

| Volume Render | Generate | Objects | Tools | Sequence | Screen | GO | BACK |

Figure 4.26. Voxel gradient shading rendering of the cortical surface of the brain and the major cerebral vessels. This rendering was created from two separate scans, one for the brain structure and the other to image the venous vasculature, which were then combined into this integrated rendering. See color figure 5.

simulated exploratory surgery and preoperative surgical planning, as will be illustrated in Chapter 7.

4.4.2.1 Rendering Multiple Structures

In visualization applications, it is desirable to visualize individual structures within the volume image and to discriminate specific structures. Using simple threshold discrimination along the ray path does not usually render sharp, unambiguous structures. An example is the cortical brain surface from an unsegmented MR volume image, as the soft tissue of the face falls in the same threshold range as the brain tissue. Prior segmentation of the brain would allow direct visualization of the cortical surface, but arbitrarily segmenting the data by removing everything outside of the brain forfeits the desirable effect of retaining correct anatomic relationships of the brain to other structures in the head. Therefore, other methods are used to partition the volume image into a set of structures without losing the structures within the actual volume image.[14,35]

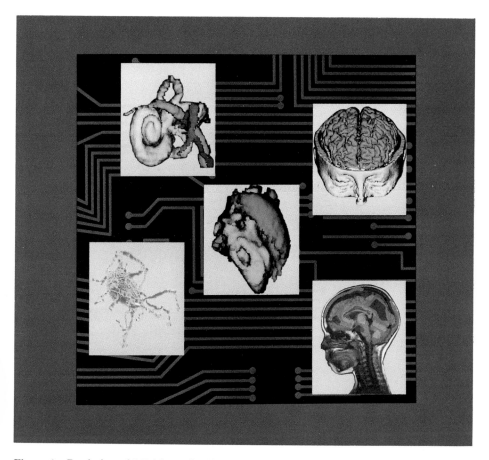

Figure 1 Depiction of 3-D biomedical images of structure and function of organs, tissues, and cells, made possible by modern electronic computing methods. See Figure 1.3.

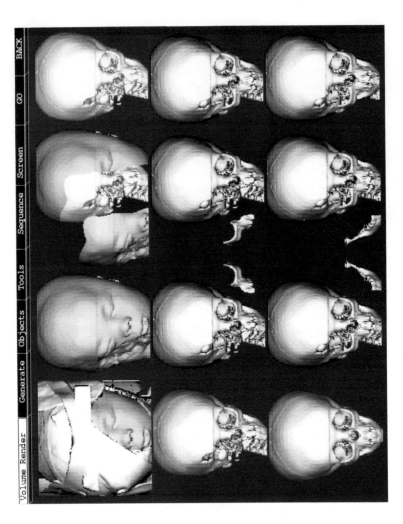

Figure 2 Illustration of capabilities of image computers and software packages for realistic 3-D simulation of surgical procedures (using ANALYZE™). Top row shows 3-D renderings of full head CT scan of patient with facial wound. Top left image is original data with bandage over wound. Middle row shows creation and placement of new cheekbone into damaged skull. Bottom row shows creation and placement of new jawbone into damaged skull. Bottom right image is completed simulation of surgical repair. See Figure 3.12.

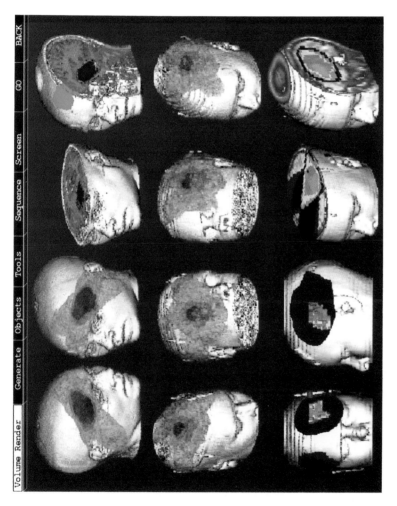

Figure 3 Illustration of use of display and analysis program (ANALYZE™) for 3-D radiation treatment planning. Top row shows simulated treatment beams through full head rendering and in cutaway views. Color is used to represent dose distribution to and around tumor. Middle row shows dose distribution from several beams from different angles of view. Bottom row shows simulated openings and cutaways to examine dose distribution in regional detail. Such 3-D planning facilitates optimal delivery of dose to tumor. See Figure 3.13.

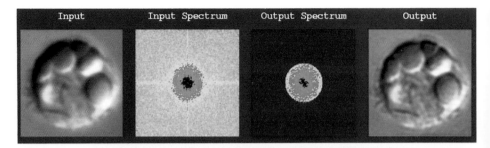

Figure 4 The original microscope image of an egg cell (left) is bandpass filtered to remove high-frequency noise and boost midrange frequency content. This will enhance features in the image (right) which are small, but larger than spot noise. See Figure 4.12.

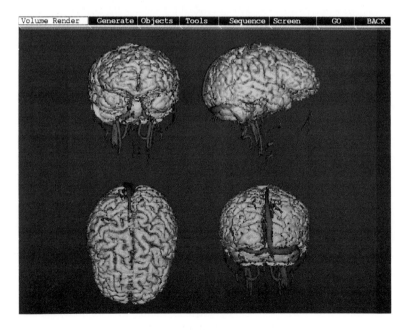

Figure 5 Voxel gradient shading rendering of the cortical surface of the brain and the major cerebral vessels. This rendering was created from two separate scans, one for the brain structure and the other to image the venous vasculature, which were then combined into this integrated rendering. See Figure 4.26.

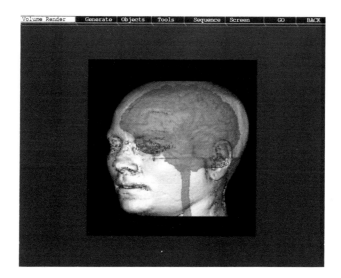

Figure 6 This ANALYZE™ rendered 3-D MRI volume image depicts an example of a transparency display for two surfaces. The transparent skin tissue allows the underlying brain structure to be seen, yet where there is no underlying brain, the skin surface is readily visible. See Figure 4.29.

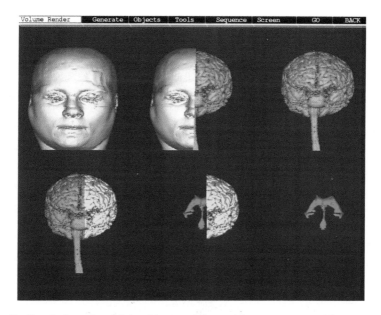

Figure 7 Rendering of multiple objects using an object map to partition the volume image in ANALYZE™ permits the assignment of independent object attributes, including visibility and color. As the visibility of selected objects is turned off, the voxels that constitute that object are removed from the rendering process, exposing the underlying structures. Each object has a separate color attribute, which can be interactively selected, as shown for the left brain hemisphere (pink/yellow). See Figure 4.31.

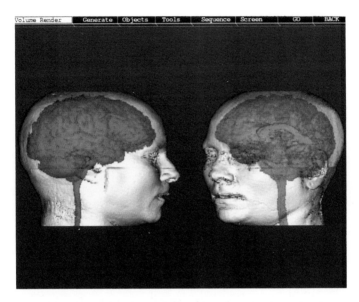

Figure 8 Multicolor transparent rendering integrates the voxels along a ray path weighted by a unique opacity coefficient for each object, as shown by the face-brain transparency on the left and the face-brain-ventricles transparency on the right. See Figure 4.32.

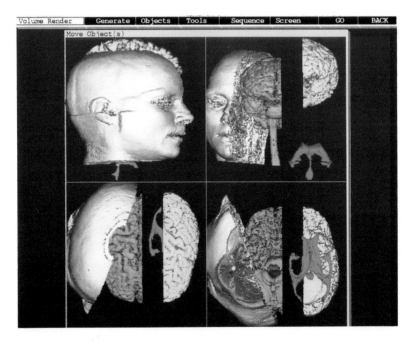

Figure 9 Each object maintains separate position and orientation attributes, allowing repositioning of the object within the full 3-D rendering space. These four panels show direct, interactive manipulation of each independent object using simple movements of the input device (mouse), important to surgical simulation and planning applications. See Figure 4.33.

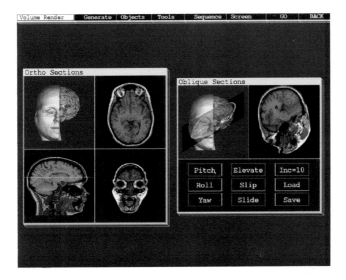

Figure 10 A 3-D rendered image provides a familiar visualization reference for investigation of the internal contents of the volume image. Orthogonal sections can be interactively selected and computed using a cursor placed anywhere on the familiar surface to define a point of intersection for the three orthogonal sections (left). Using such a familiar anatomic reference facilitates the positioning of an arbitrarily oriented oblique plane as it is interactively maneuvered in 3-space (right). See Figure 4.34.

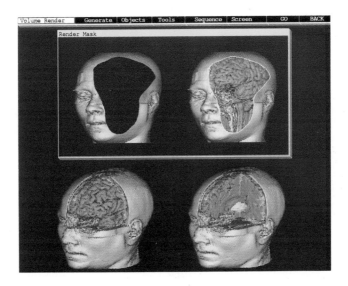

Figure 11 Various manipulation tools permit combined display of surfaces from multiple objects. Selection of a subset of rendering rays for separate rendering conditions may be accomplished by tracing on the rendered surface. The rendered display is updated by rendering only those structures selected within the region (top). Multimodal dissections can be imposed on the volume image, rendering interior structures in 3-D relationship to exterior structures (bottom). See Figure 4.35.

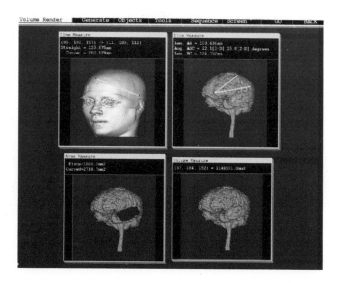

Figure 12 Measurement tools applied in the 3-D rendered space provide direct mensuration of important object parameters. Euclidean and curvilinear surface distance measurements are made by selection of any two points on the surface (upper left). Angle information can be computed from any three points (upper right). Surface area is measured using surface tracking to find and integrate over the exposed voxels in a user-defined region (lower left). Object volume is computed using region growing from a selected seed point on the surface and counting the connected voxels (lower right). See Figure 4.36.

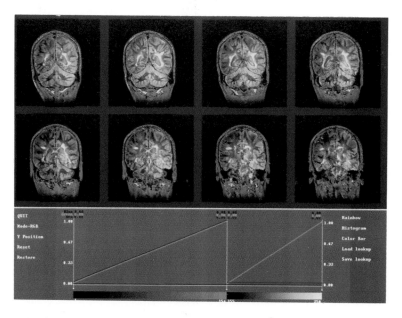

Figure 13 Grayscale thresholding is a straightforward way of segmenting structures that are readily differentiated by grayscale. This tool also provides remapping of grayscale values and may be used as an image enhancement function. See Figure 5.1.

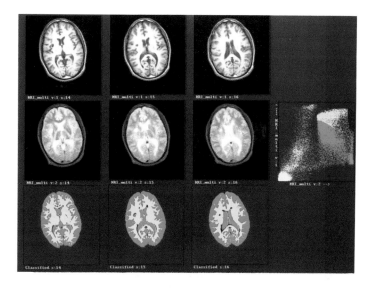

Figure 14 Manual classification of multiple tissue types from multispectral image data, in this case T1 (top) and T2 (center) MR images. The "clusters" of voxels (right) having unique T1 and T2 values allow simple definitions of regions in the T1/ T2 grayscale histogram to effectively segment spatially complex regions of the images (bottom). White matter (yellow), gray matter (blue), cerebrospiral fluid (green), and dense tissue (red). See Figure 5.8.

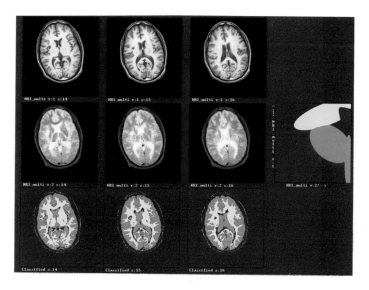

Figure 15 Automated classification of multiple tissue types (as in Figure 5.8) from multispectral image data using Gaussian maximum likelihood. The samples of different tissue types taken from regions of the image are analyzed and used to construct 2-D Gaussian distribution estimates (right) for each tissue type. The intersections of the Gaussians are the most likely boundaries for feature space clusters. See Figure 5.9.

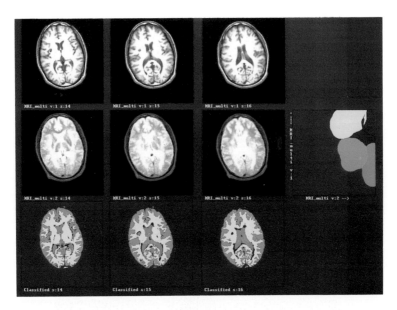

Figure 16 Automated classification of multiple tissue types (as in Figure 5.8) from multispectral image data using a nearest neighbor algorithm. The samples of different tissue types taken from regions of the image are compared to every voxel in the image. The voxel is classified to the type of its nearest neighbor voxel in feature space (right). See Figure 5.10.

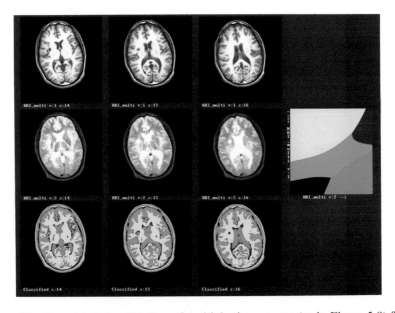

Figure 17 Automated classification of multiple tissue types (as in Figure 5.8) from multispectral image data using a neural network. The tissue type samples are used to train the network (by modifying the weight of the internode links) so that it correctly classifies the training sample. After training, the entire set of image voxels from new data sets can be classified by the network. See Figure 5.12.

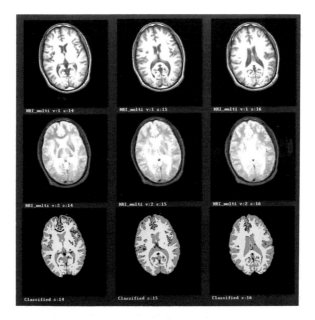

Figure 18   Automated classification of multiple tissue types (as in Figure 5.8) from multispectral image data using an unsupervised classifier. No samples of tissue types are taken. The algorithm simply looks for similarities and differences between groups of voxel vectors. See Figure 5.13.

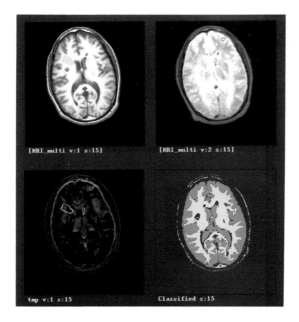

Figure 19   Images derived from the original by spectral analysis may be added recursively as additional spectral components. Here an edge strength image (lower left) has been added for classification. See Figure 5.14.

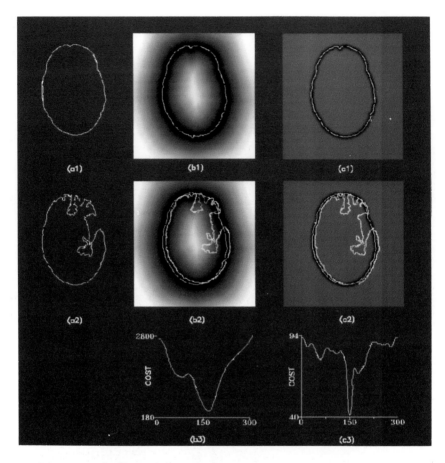

Figure 20 When matching difficult surfaces, greater robustness can be achieved by thresholding the Chamfer distance function. In this example a match contour (center row) with regions not present on the base contour (top row) is displaced by 150 pixels in x. Matching with an unthresholded Chamfer distance function locates an error minimum at approximately 160 pixels displacement (bottom row), because the high error associated with the nonmatching parts biases the low error of the matching region. By thresholding the Chamfer distance function (right column), the bias is removed, and the error minimum is found at the correct 150 pixels displacement. See Figure 5.30.

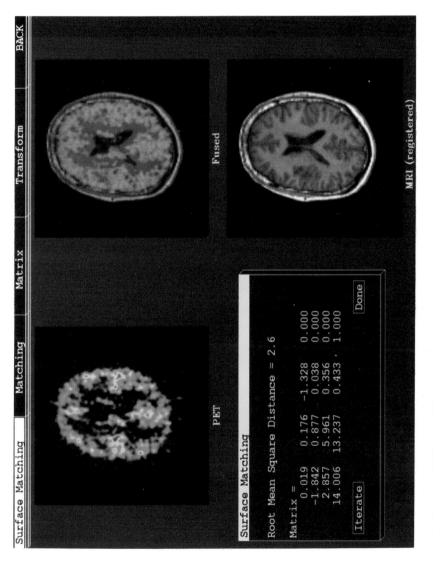

Figure 21 A selected slice from MRI and PET volume data demonstrating coregistration. Upper left is an original transverse PET slice from volume and lower right is a corresponding registered MRI slice, resectioned by computed transformation matrix shown at lower left. Fused images are shown at upper right. See Figure 5.33.

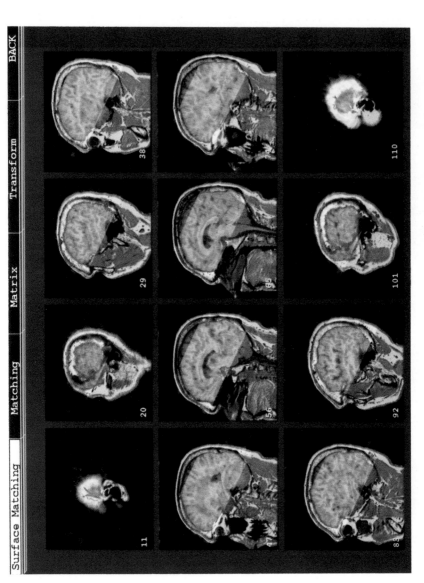

Figure 22 PET volume data transformed to match MRI volume data. Multiple slices from 3-D MRI and registered PET image are superimposed using color diffusion ("colorwash") technique to illustrate registration accuracy. See Figure 5.34. (From Jiang, H., Robb, R. A., and Holton, K. S., A new approach to 3-D registration of multimodality medical images by surface matching, *Proceedings of Visualization in Biomedical Computing 1992*, SPIE 1808, 210, 1992. With permission).

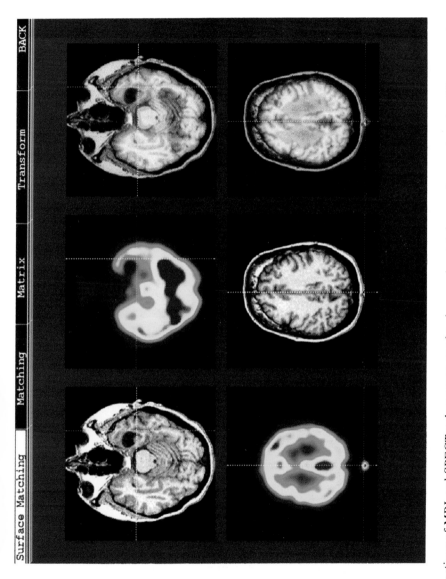

Figure 23 Sections of MRI and SPECT volume scan used as base and match images (top row); and a different section matching MRI to SPECT (bottom row). Registered, resectioned image is in center; fused images are at right. See Figure 5.35.

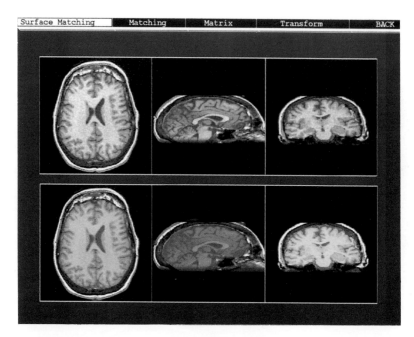

Figure 24 Three orthogonal section views of registered and fused MR and SPECT images. Segmented SPECT image with markers is superimposed on MRI. Markers are in good registration in all three orthogonal planes. See Figure 5.36.

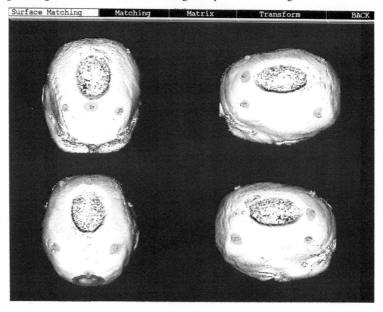

Figure 25 Four views of MRI head surface with superimposed overlapping markers from registered SPECT image. Registered MRI markers are visible beneath SPECT markers. Markers are in good registration on displayed surface. See Figure 5.37. (From Jiang, H., Robb, R. A., and Holton, K. S., A new approach to 3-D registration of multimodality medical images by surface matching, *Proceedings of Visualization in Biomedical Computing 1992*, SPIE 1808, 212, 1992. With permission).

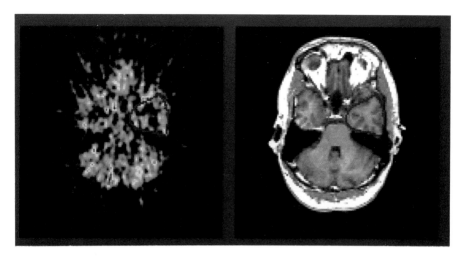

Figure 26 Defined regions of interest for measurement of coregistered data sets (MRI and PET). The desired anatomic region is specified in the high-resolution MRI, and the functional measurement made in the corresponding regions in the PET image. See Figure 6.7.

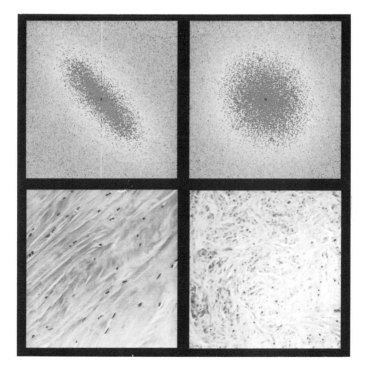

Figure 27 Fourier transform (color-scaled magnitude only) of anisotropic (left) and isotropic (right) photomicrographs of collagen show a clear Fourier feature related to the direction of anisotropy. See Figure 6.15.

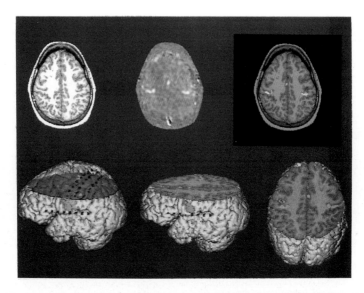

Figure 28 Functional images (upper row) integrated with ANALYZE™ depicting function in the motor cortex can be further visualized in full 3-D context (lower row), showing the location of the function (orange) in comparison to full 3-D brain anatomy (white) and tumor pathology (green). (Data courtesy of Dr. Clifford Jack, Mayo Foundation.) See Figure 7.2.

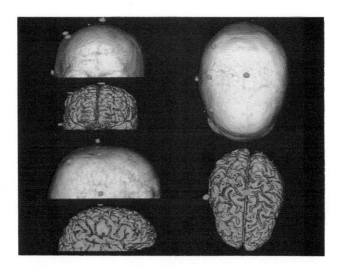

Figure 29 These volume renderings of 3-D acquired MRI data used for neurosurgical planning depict the soft tissue and brain structure of an epilepsy patient. The green structures visualized on the skin surface are capsules used as markers of EEG electrode positions indicating the electrical focus of the seizure activity (center marker). These can be projected from the skin surface to map the seizure focus to a specific gyrus in the brain parenchyma prior to surgery to aid the surgeon in optimally resecting the offending tissue. (Data courtesy of Drs. Frank Sharbrough and Clifford Jack, Mayo Foundation.) See Figure 7.3.

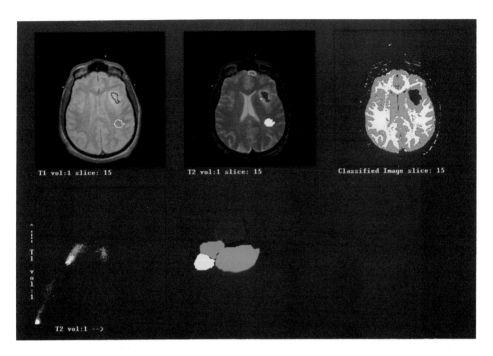

Figure 30 Manual classification of multiple tissue types from multispectral image data. The "clusters" of voxels having unique T1 and T2 values allow straightforward segmentation of the spatially complex regions of the images including white and gray matter (blue and yellow), cerebral spinal fluid (green), and tumor (red). The segmentation has identified all of the most likely tumor voxels as well as some obviously extraneous voxels with similar tissue characteristics. See Figure 7.6.

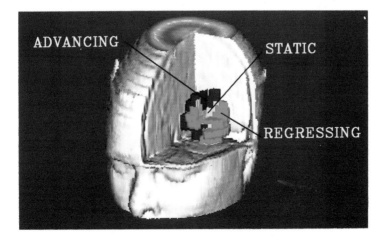

Figure 31 Since the tumor segments are in physical registration, determination can be made of which parts of the original tumor are regressing, which remain static, and whether or not new tumor regions are advancing (refer also to Figure 7.5). See Figure 7.8.

Ortho Sections

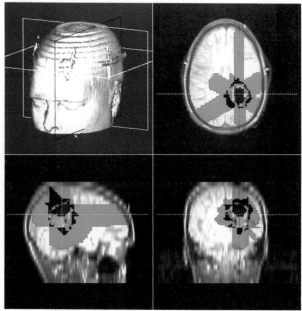

Figure 32 The dose distribution of a 7-beam non-coplanar radiation treatment therapy plan is shown as a color wash in the 3-D image volume rendered with ANALYZE™. Intersecting orthogonal planes may be displayed by picking a point of intersection on the skin surface or by pointing to the intersection point on any displayed section. See Figure 7.9.

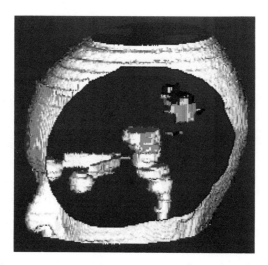

Figure 33 The same dose distribution of Figure 7.9 is shown on the surface of the tumor and on critical structures inside the head. Although most of the tumor volume is enclosed within the 90–100% prescribed dose region (orange), a small "tendril" of the tumor has escaped high dosage. One beam also brushes the brain stem, delivering only 30–50% prescribed dose (blue). See Figure 7.10.

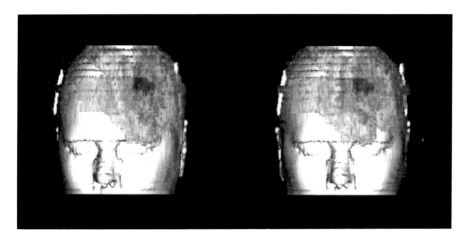

Figure 34 The same dose distribution of Figures 7.9 and 7.10 is shown as a stereo pair transparency. Rotational sequences of this type of rendering give a strong intuitive impression of the location and shape of the high-dose region, and thereby of the "goodness of fit" of the plan to simultaneous goals of tumor ablation and healthy tissue preservation. See Figure 7.11.

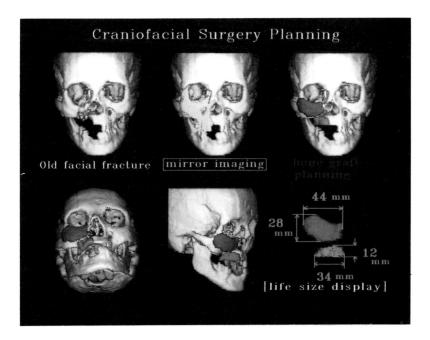

Figure 35 Presurgical bone graft planning with ANALYZE™ using mirror imaging (top row) and subsequent editing of the graft prostheses (top right, bottom left, and center), including accurate quantitative assessment of prosthesis size and shape (bottom right). See Figure 7.12.

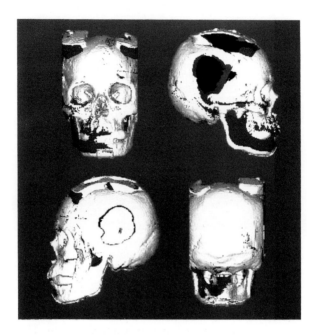

Figure 36 Two sets of 3-D CT scans of a dry skull were used to evaluate 3-D image effectiveness of analysis in orthognathic surgery. The first scan (red volume) was made with the mandible in its normal position. The second scan (white volume) had spacers placed between the temporal condyles and fossae. The right spacer was larger than the left, resulting in rotation and shifting of the mandible to the left. After coregistration, the two 3-D images are accurately fused into one skull, but the two jaws are in different positions, as expected. See Figure 7.14.

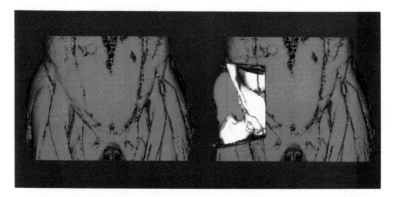

Figure 37 In orthopedic and biomechanical application, the muscles, tendons, and ligaments are often as important as the bone. From X-ray CT data, these soft tissue structures can be segmented with ANALYZE™ and rendered in their natural relationships to the bone (left). Sections of the overlapping musculature can be cut away to reveal the underlying hip bone, providing direct visualization of the relationship between these structures (right). (Data courtesy of Dr. David Lewallen, Mayo Foundation.) See Figure 7.16.

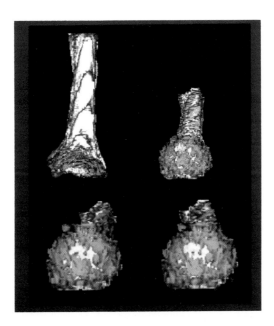

Figure 38 3-D rendering of the distal tibia of a physeal bar patient. Top row shows two views and shaft. Bottom row is stereo pair and shaft end. The bone is made transparent to expose the physeal plate (orange) and interior bar (white). These images are cross-fused (i.e., the left eye image is on the right and vice versa), so a 3-D image of the physis and bar can be seen by crossing the eyes. See Figure 7.17.

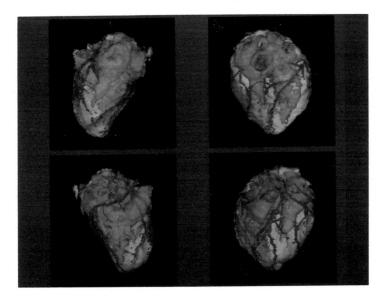

Figure 39 Transparent 3-D rendering of an intact heart scanned with the DSR showing the myocardium (pink), chambers (blue), and coronary arteries (red) from four different views. See Figure 7.18.

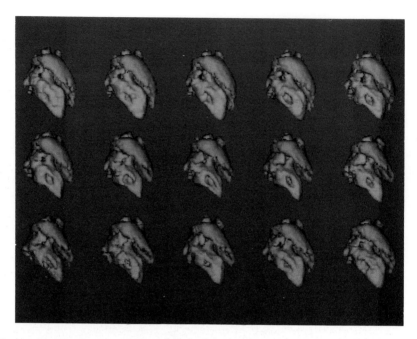

Figure 40 Multiple renderings throughout the cardiac cycle of an intact heart scanned by the DSR depicting the left ventricular chamber (red) and right ventricular chamber (blue) from end diastole (upper left) through systole (lower left) and back to diastole (lower right). See Figure 7.19.

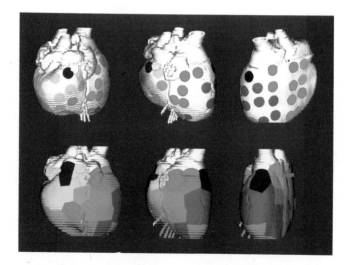

Figure 41 Heart surface colorized by evoked response activation delay. Each spot (top row) indicates the position of one of 54 electrodes on the surface of the heart. The color indicates the activation time at the electrode from early (red) to late (blue) in the heartbeat. The entire surface of the heart is colorized (bottom row) by interpolating an activation time for each point on the heart surface from the nearest two electrodes. See Figure 7.20.

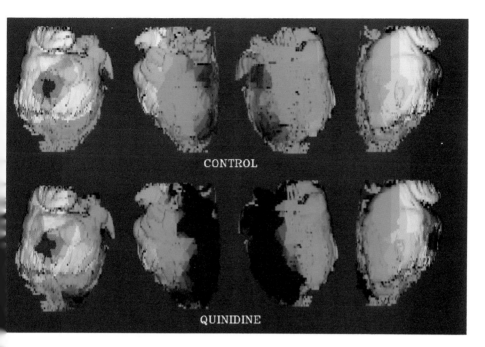

Figure 42 3-D volume renderings of fast CT scan of a heart colorized with activation time as recorded by 54 electrodes placed around the heart surface. The upper images represent a normal heartbeat, while the lower images represent a heartbeat after the administration of an anti-arrhythmic drug, which slows the heartbeat. See Figure 7.21.

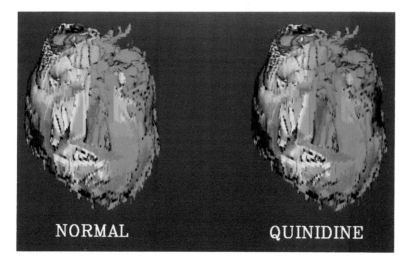

Figure 43 A cutaway view of the same data shown in Figure 7.21, showing the activation delay pattern on the interior surfaces on the heart. A "wedge" is placed in the center of the 3-D rendering to reveal the myocardial transmural activation patterns. See Figure 7.22.

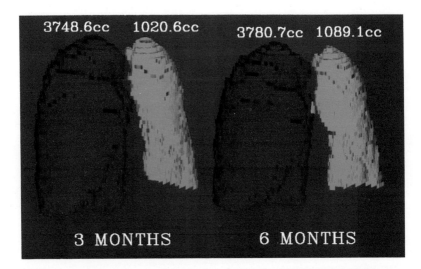

Figure 44 A volume rendering of the lung surfaces of a single-lung transplant patient 3 months (left) and 6 months (right) postsurgery. The transplanted left lung is noticeably smaller than the native right lung in both images, but volume measurement shows a 10% increase in transplant lung volume in 3 months, a favorable outcome. See Figure 7.23.

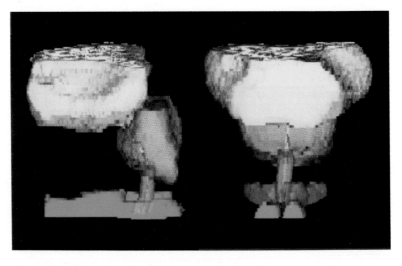

Figure 45 Transparent volume rendering of the urinary anatomy from 3-D MRI scan of pelvis. Segmented structures shown are bladder and urethra (yellow), prostate gland (green), external urinary sphincter (pink), and erectile support bodies (blue). Note that the external sphincter is fully visible through the transparent structures that would otherwise obscure it. See Figure 7.24.

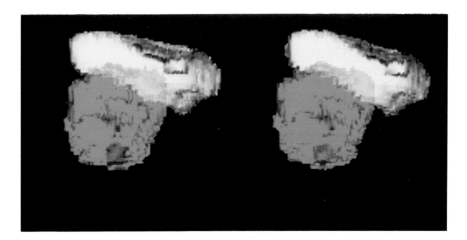

Figure 46 Stereo pair (cross-fusion) of transparent rendering of the bladder (yellow), prostate (green), and external urinary sphincter (red). Radical prostatectomy patients suffer temporary or permanent urinary incontinence due to damage to the external sphincter. This type of imagery may help surgeons visualize each patient's unique anatomic configuration and reduce such morbidity. See Figure 7.25.

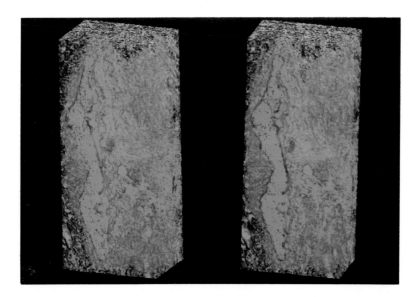

Figure 47 Stereo pair transparent rendering of a block of trabecular tissue reconstructed from microphotographs of 1-μm tissue sections. The green object is Schlemm's canal, a major drainage path for aqueous humor in the eye. The blue regions are aqueous humor in the spongy tissue coming from the anterior chamber of the eye. Pink material is solid tissue, either cytoplasm, cell nuclei, or collagen. See Figure 7.27.

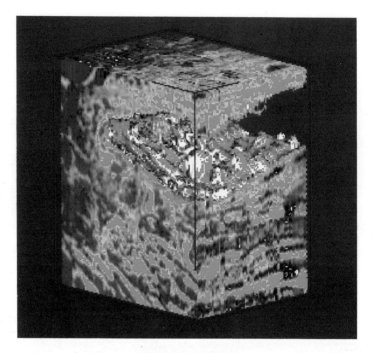

Figure 48 Opaque rendering of a block of trabecular tissue. Schlemm's canal is shown as a cavernous space. The "bumps" in the floor of the canal are cell nuclei. See Figure 7.28.

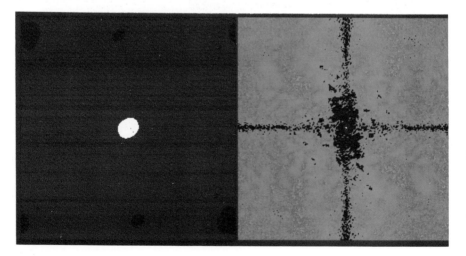

Figure 49 Color-coded Fourier transform of the psf of a normal cornea (left) and of an irregular cornea (right) of a patient after radical keratotomy. The violet color represents the first order of magnitude of attenuation in the modulation transfer function. Dark blue, light blue, and green represent the second, third, and fourth orders, respectively. See Figure 7.30.

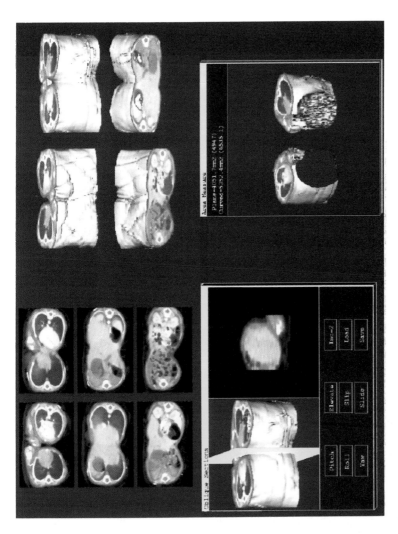

Figure 50 Full-body fast CT scans reveal several cross sections through connected body trunks of infant conjoined twins (top left). ANALYZE™ volume rendering of these CT scans can be rotated, tilted, etc. to visualize and study the connected bodies in 3-D (top right). Using a planar dissection tool (bottom left) the optimal approach to bisecting the bodies can be planned, directed at minimizing the surgical opening. The simulated bisection can then be used to accurately measure the area of the surgical openings (bottom right) to determine the amount of skin graft required to close the actual openings. (Data courtesy of Dr. Uldis Bite, Mayo Foundation.) See Figure 7.33.

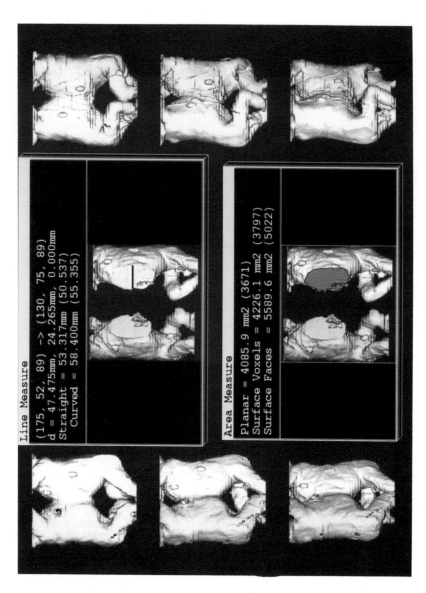

Figure 51 Another set of conjoined twins processed almost identically to those in Figure 7.33. Shown are simulated 3-D renderings of connected bodies, simulated bisection and segmentation, and measurement of area of surgical openings for calculation of skin graft. (Data courtesy of Dr. Uldis Bite, Mayo Foundation.) See Figure 7.34.

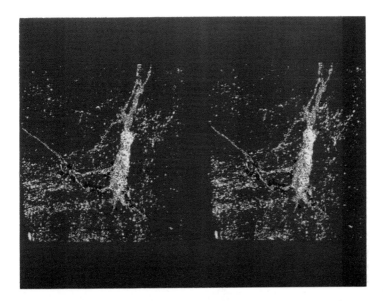

Figure 52 Multiple object stereo volume rendering from confocal microscopy of a neuron (yellow) from the inferior mesenteric ganglion bathed in a solution containing labeled VIP neurotransmitter (light blue), demonstrating receptor sites for VIP along the dendrites and somal body of the neuron (red). (Data courtesy of Dr. Joe Szurszewski, Mayo Foundation.) See Figure 7.35.

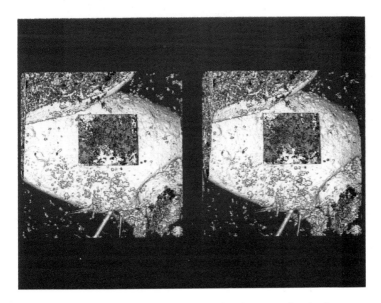

Figure 53 Multiple object stereo volume rendering from confocal microscopy of an amphipod appendage (white) infected with bacteria (red), with a cutaway view showing the relationship of the bacteria to the internal muscle (brown). (Data courtesy of Drs. Wilma L. Lingle and Dennis J. O'Kane, Mayo Foundation). See Figure 7.35.

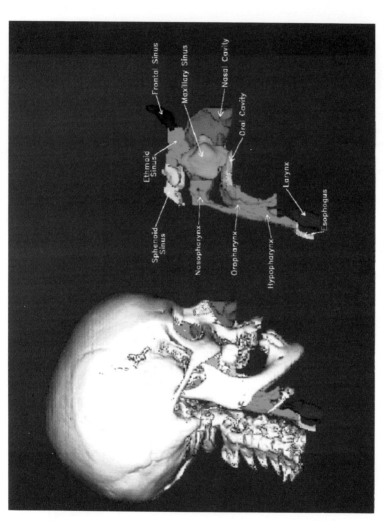

Figure 54 ANALYZE™ segmentation and volume rendering techniques can be used for the anatomic education of surgeons and physicians. For example, from cadaveric X-ray CT data of the head, the paranasal sinuses and other air spaces in the head can be segmented and rendered intact in the skull for localization to familiar anatomy (left), or without the skull to visualize internal spaces unobscured (right). Each sinus and air space can be assigned a different color and examined individually or in relation to the other spaces or structures, with labels identifying each component. (Data courtesy of Dr. Stephen Carmichael, Mayo Foundation.) See Figure 7.37.

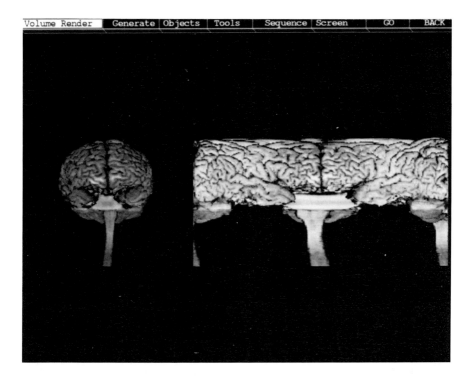

Figure 4.27. The rendered cortical surface of the brain (left) can be unrolled to obtain a full 360° view of the surface (right) using a radial cylindrical rendering technique in ANALYZE™. The central line of each rendering for 1° increments around 360° is displayed in the output image. This permits the entire 3-D surface of the brain to be visualized in a single display (like Mercator maps of the world).

A powerful concept for multiple object rendering and manipulation has been implemented in the ANALYZE™ software system. This method provides for interactive specification and manipulation of individual structures in the rendered volume image while preserving all data and relationships in the rendered display. The method provides functions that specifically classify voxels in the original volume image into user-defined objects, assigning names and attributes (e.g., color) to the objects and allowing for independent manipulation of each object in the rendered image. This is accomplished by using a complementary volume data set of the same size and dimension as the original volume image. This secondary volume data set is called an object map, as it partitions the original volume image into several selected objects. This object map only defines the partitioning of the volume image; rendering of any particular object is still accomplished using the voxel values contained within the original volume image. The partitions need not be spatially contiguous, i.e., the object map can be used to partition an image volume into localized function properties or physiological features as well as anatomic structures.

145

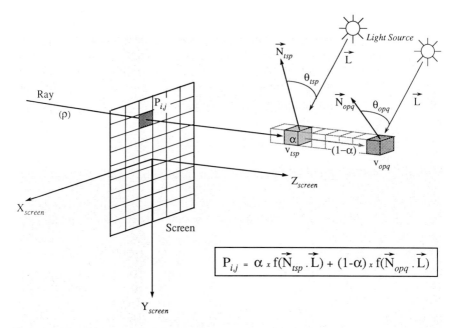

$$P_{i,j} = \alpha \times f(\vec{N}_{tsp} \cdot \vec{L}) + (1-\alpha) \times f(\vec{N}_{opq} \cdot \vec{L})$$

Figure 4.28. Diagram of the ray-tracing geometry used to render selected voxels transparent (or opaque). Two different surfaces are determined by separate prescribed ray conditions, with a transparent surface opacity coefficient α controlling the relative opacity of the exterior transparent surface versus the interior opaque surface.

An object map forms a one-to-one correspondence of the voxels in the original volume image to structures defined by the object map. In the ANALYZE™ implementation, the voxels in the object map are 8-bit values, with the specific values identifying a particular structure, of which there are a total of 256 possible objects. The set of voxels in the object map that have a specific value constitute the complex object without regard to the spatial connectivity of the voxels. Most volume images will be partitioned into anatomic structures, where the collection of voxels constituting a particular structure will often be spatially contiguous (e.g., brain, heart). Such objects are often segmented using region growing or morphological techniques that take advantage of spatial connectivity and bounding within a given threshold range, as the voxels constituting the structure of interest will most likely be of similar value and/or shape in the volume image.[36] Other objects may be a set of spatially disconnected voxels organized according to criteria other than anatomy or morphology. For example, a particular tissue may represent itself within a narrow threshold range in the volume but may be spatially disjoint throughout the entire extent of the volume image. It may be desirable to localize this tissue according to composition criteria rather than bounded regions. The partitioning of the volume image via the object map

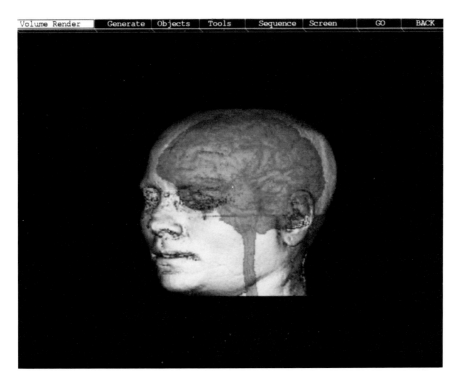

Figure 4.29. This ANALYZE™ rendered 3-D MRI volume image depicts an example of a transparency display for two surfaces. The transparent skin tissue allows the underlying brain structure to be seen, yet where there is no underlying brain, the skin surface is readily visible. See color figure 6.

provides for direct classification of sets of connected or disjoint voxels determined by any method that associates groups of voxels into particular sets. Currently, a single volume image voxel can only be associated with one object map voxel, classifying that voxel into a single object only. Future directions in this partitioning scheme will allow for hierarchical classification of voxels, permitting voxels to belong to more than a single object.

The construction of an object map can be accomplished by prerendering segmentation procedures or by interactive specification and editing directly on the rendered image. Prerendering segmentation of structures can be accomplished using many different segmentation techniques, including manual and semiautomated image editing, region growing, morphological processing, and multispectral feature space classification, all of which are described in Chapter 5. Each of these segmentation techniques partitions the volume image based on specific criteria, including spatial (e.g., region growing), intrinsic voxel value (e.g., thresholding), relative voxel value gradients (edge vectors), and association value of the voxels (e.g., multispectral classifica-

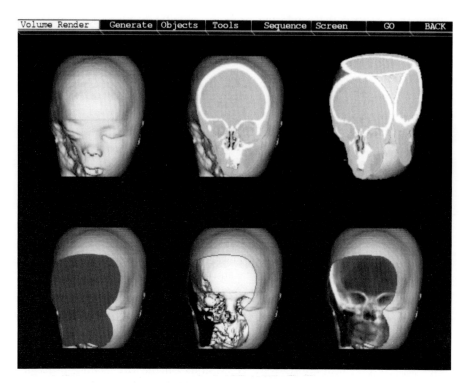

Figure 4.30.   Several interactive techniques in ANALYZE™ volume-rendering permit investigation of the internal contents of a volume image in conjunction with displayed 3-D surfaces. Clipping planes allow sectioning of the volume either along the viewing direction (top center) or along orthogonal aspects of the volume (top right). Regions drawn on the rendered image (bottom left) define a set of rays that can be rerendered with different parameters from the remainder of the surface. The ray conditions may prescribe a different surface inside the outer surface shell (bottom center), or a different algorithm may be used with the mask, permitting an integrated rendering from reflectance and transmission types of renderings (bottom right).

tion). Often these volume images are segmented into separate structures, which are then saved as multiple binary image files. These binary image files, representing binary masks for locations of voxels for the specific structures segmented from the original volume image, are used to generate the object map by assignment of all the voxels corresponding to nonzero values in the binary image file to a specific value in the object map. The multiple binary image files created from several different segmentations of the original volume image can be imported sequentially into the object map to build a partitioning of the entire volume image into multiple independent, yet congruent, structures.

Structures in the object map can also be defined directly from the rendered images. Given the wide variety of rendering parameters and algorithms that control the rendering process, specific combinations of these parameters and algorithms can often render a specific structure from the original volume without the necessity for a priori segmentation. For example, with X-ray CT data, the threshold criteria can be used to easily render bone directly, with voxels corresponding to other tissue types eliminated by using a sufficiently high threshold. Once rendered, the current candidate voxels in the volume image, which now constitute only the bone, can be used to create and save a specific structure in the object map. Note that this is no different than applying a threshold outside of the rendering program to segment the bone—only more convenient. However, other ray condition criteria can be used to further subdivide the rendering of the bone, such as clipping planes, permitting direct, interactive visualization and specification of specific bone structures and adding them to the object map during rendering. In this context, rendering is used as the segmentation tool, and once the structure is rendered independent of other structures, the voxels corresponding to the rendered structure can be assigned to an object in the object map. This technique is very powerful and dramatically facilitates the use of the object map concept in such applications as surgical simulation and treatment planning.

Objects can further be defined directly from the rendered image using manipulation tools to select regions of the rendered structures for assignment to a specific object. If a given object has been rendered separate from other structures using appropriate constraints on the ray-casting process, selection of a seed point on the rendered surface can be used to invoke a region-growing process that will find all connected voxels to that seed point in 3-D, conforming to the current rendering conditions, and assign those voxels to an object. This technique is frequently useful for eliminating disconnected structures not part of the structure of interest. Drawing and tracing operations on the surface can also be used to specify a set of voxels for segmentation. Definition of a region by tracing or drawing with a defined shape on the rendered surface selects a set of rays from the current viewing direction. Once these rays have been determined, voxels intersected by these rays can be assigned to an object. As the rays within the interactively defined region are interrogated for their intersections with voxels in the current rendering, the object map can be updated to include certain sets of voxels along these ray paths. It could include all voxels intersected along the paths (e.g., bore hole), only those voxels along the ray path from the first visible voxel to the next voxel that falls outside of the current ray conditions (e.g., a surface layer), or only the set of voxels that are the first ones encountered along the ray paths (e.g., a voxel layer), allowing the surface to be "shaved away" one voxel layer at a time. These voxel set specification techniques provide important interactive tools for the definition of multiple objects directly from the rendered image.

Often a specific anatomic structure may be subdivided further into selected components. For example, the brain may be further subdivided into its different lobes (e.g., frontal lobe, parietal lobe, temporal lobe), which may in turn be further subdivided into additional components (e.g., hippocampus, caudate nucleus). This hierarchical subdivision of a structure into its components may be accomplished in the object map model by building multiple object maps, each of which successively partitions the larger structure into its components. Several attributes (e.g., visibility, opacity, color) can be assigned to each structure, selected to either "hide" its independent relationship to other structures, to distinguish it, or to complement it.

Once structures have been defined in an object map, attributes can be assigned to each individual structure. Such attributes include visibility, color, spatial orientation, and opacity for transparent displays. The visibility attribute specifies the inclusion or exclusion of the voxels assigned to a specific object in the ray-casting process during rendering. This is the attribute that provides the important capability to render and visualize sets of voxels that would not otherwise be distinguishable using conventional rendering methods. When the visibility attribute for a particular object is turned off, the voxels corresponding to this object along any ray path are excluded from consideration in the rendering, regardless of the current ray conditions. That is, the ray tracing doesn't "see" them. If the visibility attribute is turned on, these voxels are included in the rendering process, and all current ray conditions apply to these voxels (e.g., threshold, clipping planes). For surface determination, the visibility attribute influences which surface is currently visible from the current point of view. In transmission rendering, the set of voxels projected can be restricted to only those objects which are currently visible, allowing selective projection of particular structures. Combinations of object visibility and ray conditions provide a powerful mechanism for visualizing independent structures in biomedical volume images. Figure 4.31 (see color figure 7) illustrates volume rendering using visibility attributes to control the display of multiple objects in the rendered volume.

The color attribute assigns a specific color to the object in the output rendering. Surface rendering depends significantly on the use of shading to depict 3-D depth effect along the surfaces. Therefore, the color assigned to a specific object is actually a set of colors that vary in intensity. This intensity variation is generated through an intensity ramp for a selected number of color cells in the lookup table, which maps the rendered image in the frame buffer to the color output on the screen. For 8-bit graphics displays, this lookup table function limits the selection to a total of 256 colors. Therefore the color ranges selected for each object should divide the 256 total available colors into an effective color partitioning to produce satisfactory rendering of each object. Generally, larger objects require more color intensity gradation along the edges of the surface in order to produce the desired 3-D effect, while smaller objects require less color gradations. On 24-bit systems this problem goes away, since the full color representation range of each of the red, green, and blue components of the color provides up to 16.7 million individual colors that may be displayed. This alleviates the problem

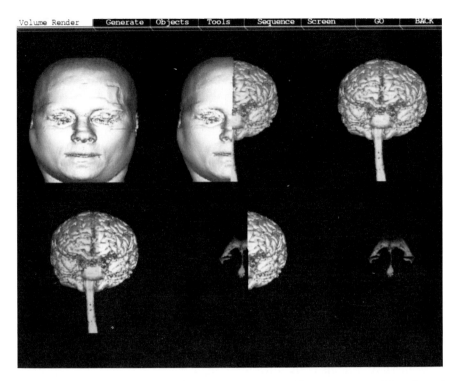

Figure 4.31. Rendering of multiple objects using an object map to partition the volume image in ANALYZE™ permits the assignment of independent object attributes, including visibility and color. As the visibility of selected objects is turned off, the voxels that constitute that object are removed from the rendering process, exposing the underlying structures. Each object has a separate color attribute, which can be interactively selected, shown for the left brain hemisphere (pink/yellow). See color figure 7.

of color partitioning for each independent object in the object map. Dithering algorithms exist for rendering a 24-bit RGB image to an 8-bit image with an associated color lookup table designed to effectively capture the color content of the rendering. Figure 4.31 illustrates the use of the color attribute in rendering multiple objects defined by an object map for the image volume.

The opacity attribute allows control of the weighted opacity applied to a particular object along the ray path when compositing the contributions of each object's voxel into a multicolored transparent rendering. Opacities are generally assigned in the range from 0.0 to 1.0, with 0.0 being completely transparent and 1.0 being totally opaque. Along the ray path, a voxel's contribution to the output pixel in the rendering screen is proportional to this opacity factor. This can be integrated into the output pixel using either the singular surface voxel for the object along the ray path, or every voxel along the path within the object can contribute a weighted opacity, thus integrating the opacity based on the thickness of the object. Figure 4.32 (see color figure 8) illustrates the use of the opacity attribute to produce a multicolor transparency in volume rendering.

For applications that require the movement of structures in the volume image, such as surgery simulation, spatial position attributes can be assigned to each independent object. Separate translation and rotation attributes for each object permit independent spatial manipulation of structures in the volume image. Translation provides for the positioning of an object at a specific 3-D location within the volume rendering space. The rotation attribute will allow the rotation of objects around a specified center of rotation. This rotation may be specified relative to the center of the specific object, rather than about the center of the volume, which is generally more useful. Sequences of images generated to show splitting and opening of selected structures often use independent object rotation where the center of rotation is defined at the back surface of each object from the current viewing direction. Increments for both the translation and rotation values allow for the

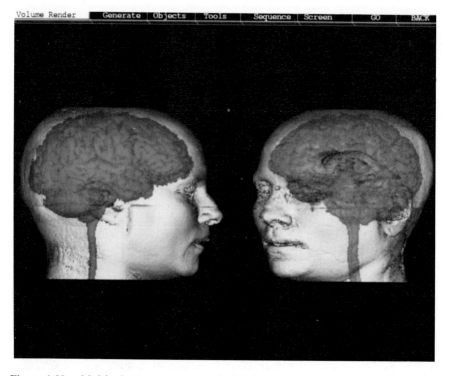

Figure 4.32. Multicolor transparent rendering integrates the voxels along a ray path weighted by a unique opacity coefficient for each object, as shown by the face-brain transparency on the left and the face-brain-ventricles transparency on the right. See color figure 8.

generation of sequences where different objects are moving and rotating to independent positions at various rates. Figure 4.33 (see color figure 9) illustrates independent spatial manipulation of separate objects during volume rendering.

For realistic simulation and planning functions, the ability to interactively spatially manipulate structures defined by the object map is an important capacity. As the position of an object is changed, the intersection of the object with the ray paths traversed from a specific viewpoint is determined. Only these intersecting rays are then recast, resulting in an "update" rendering of the object in its new position and a new rendering of the structures previously obscured by the object when in its old position. Since only the rays necessary to recompute the updated new rendering are cast, this operation is relatively fast, depending on the size of the object being moved, facilitating interactive, near real-time movement of the object. This operation requires an input device to control in 3-D the spatial position and rotation of a selected object on a 2-D screen. A technique that accomplishes this

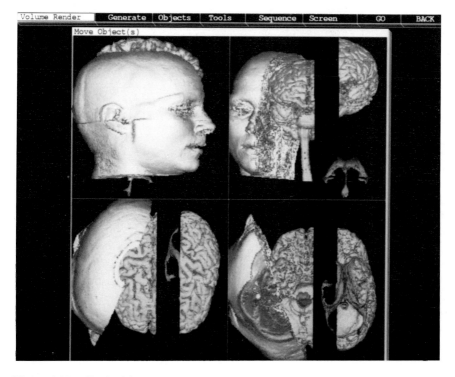

Figure 4.33. Each object maintains separate position and orientation attributes, allowing repositioning of the object within the full 3-D rendering space. These four panels show direct, interactive manipulation of each independent object using simple movements of the input device (mouse), important to surgical simulation and planning applications. See color figure 9.

by use of a standard workstation mouse is a multipanel, multiviewpoint display of the rendered structures. In any one viewpoint, the coordinate transformation from the *x-y* location of the mouse to the coordinates of the volume in the viewpoint is fixed (e.g., mouse *x-y* corresponds to volume image *y-z* when rendered from the sagittal viewpoint). Display of multiple viewpoints that present the updated rendered structures as directed by 2-D manipulations provides full and intuitive control of 3-D movement of the structures. Figure 4.33 illustrates interactive movement of objects during volume rendering. Specialized six-degree-of-freedom input devices may also be used to control structure movement, and direct 3-D displays (stereo, head mounted, etc.) may be used to visualize them, as in emerging virtual reality systems.

In certain simulation and planning applications, it is sometimes necessary to create a new object that is a copy of the original defined object, allowing the original object to remain in place while "practicing" with its copy. This is particularly useful in craniofacial surgery applications, where contralateral placement of mirrored objects is a good first estimate in designing a prosthesis or surgical implant. In such cases, a copy of the normal object on one side of the head is created as a completely new object and then mirrored across the desired orthogonal plane to place the object in approximately correct size, shape, and orientation on the abnormal (damaged, diseased, etc.) side of the head (see Figure 3.12 in Chapter 3).

4.4.2.2 Interactive Investigation of Rendered Space

Direct visualization of 3-D images using volume rendering provides significantly useful information in many biomedical imaging applications. However, the volume rendering process also provides an intuitive and accurate reference for further manipulation and analysis of the image data. The rendered image as placed on the graphics viewing screen contains a set of pixels each of which, for most rendering algorithms, corresponds to the rendered output value for a single voxel along the ray path (or a selected voxel within a set of voxels). The location of this voxel in the volume space is stored in an array, often referred to as the Z-buffer, associated with the current view of the rendered image. This defines a map between the original 3-D volume image and the pixels displayed in the output rendering. This map can be used for direct and interactive access to the volume image. Interactive investigation and analysis techniques operating directly in the rendered space have facilitated several advanced applications in 3-D biomedical imaging, including surgical simulation and treatment planning (see Chapter 7). These tools, which interact directly with rendered images, can be divided into three primary categories: display tools, manipulation tools, and measurement tools. All three categories are included in ANALYZE™.

Display tools use the rendered image as a visualization reference for directed display of the content of the volume image. Previously described 2-D section display techniques include multiplanar display, which allows multi-planar reformatting of the volume image and display of 2-D sections from either transaxial, coronal, or sagittal orientations, and oblique sectioning, which interactively computes and displays arbitrarily oriented 2-D sections through the volume image. Both of these techniques can be improved by using a 3-D rendered image for enhanced localization and interactive image generation. For multiplanar reformatting, a point selected on the rendered surface defines a 3-D location within the volume through which three orthogonal images can be extracted and displayed. On modern workstations, the point selection can be made interactively while all of the orthogonal sections are rapidly updated (without any apparent delay to the user). This provides an important investigative feature where the rendered surface can be used to direct the accurate localization and visualization of internal structures lying in orthogonal 2-D sections, much as seen at the diagnostic consoles of clinical imaging systems, but without the aid of the familiar 3-D reference image. The rendered image can similarly be used as a familiar reference for the spatial positioning of an arbitrarily oriented oblique plane sectioning through the volume image. In the description of oblique sectioning earlier in this chapter, 2-D orthogonal planes were used as an indicator of the intersection of the oblique plane, with anatomic features as a reference for the positions and orientation of the plane. This requires experience and education and some foreknowledge to be effective. But rendered surfaces provide natural and familiar 3-D anatomic landmarks for oblique plane positioning and orientation, and novices learn to use such displays quickly and effectively. Interactive manipulation of the oblique plane as the display of the plane updates its intersection with the rendered image provides powerful 3-D visual cues as to the true orientation of the plane in relation to the structures in the volume image. As the oblique plane is changing orientation in response to user manipulation with the input device (mouse), the oblique image along the plane from the volume image is rapidly computed and displayed. Special display techniques can be employed for enhanced visualization of the plane within the 3-D rendering, such as making the rendered surface transparent while superimposing the actual image data along the intersecting plane, allowing visualization of internal structures in arbitrary sections as they actually reside within the volume. Figure 4.34 (see color figure 10) illustrates examples of tools for orthogonal and oblique sectioning within a 3-D rendered surface.

Manipulation tools can be used to directly edit 3-D volume images. These techniques include removing selected voxels from rendering consideration, allowing multiple surfaces to be visualized within a single rendering, and integrating multiple rendering algorithms together into a single 3-D visualization. Defining subregions of the volume data for rendering can be accomplished either by specifying the region(s) through which the rays are cast or by specifying discrete regions of the volume image itself. Drawing and tracing on the rendered image can be used to directly define a region of the

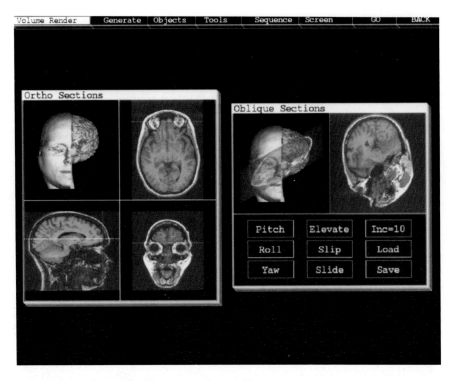

Figure 4.34. A 3-D rendered image provides a familiar visualization reference for investigation of the internal contents of the volume image. Orthogonal sections can be interactively selected and computed using a cursor placed anywhere on the familiar surface to define a point of intersection for the three orthogonal sections (left). Using such a familiar anatomic reference facilitates the positioning of an arbitrarily oriented oblique plane as it is interactively maneuvered in 3-space (right). See color figure 10.

render screen through which a unique set of rendering rays will pass. Once a set of rays has been so specified, subsequent renderings can be restricted to the region containing these rays. Changing rendering conditions allows multiple surfaces and/or different volume properties to be rendered and displayed together when they would not have otherwise coexisted in a single rendering. For example, changing the rendering algorithm to apply only within the bounds of selected regions permits multiple rendering algorithms to selectively apply in single volume renderings. This is important when, due to differential properties, separate structures require different rendering algorithms to achieve the desired composite visualization. Subregions of the full 3-D volume space can be used on an object-by-object basis to define sets of voxels that are not rendered into the output image. Establishing several sets of subregions, each of which is applied to a given set of objects, permits enhanced and penetrating visualization of the associative relationships among objects in the volume image. Figure 4.35 (see color figure 11) illustrates manipulation tools for defining selected masks for differential rendering and for multioriented dissection through multiple objects.

The connection between traditional surface rendering techniques and volume rendering can be made through extraction of contours from a volume rendered object. Often a contour-based data set representing the rendered surface is useful for purposes other than or in addition to direct visualization. For example, traditional CAD/CAM systems may be used with contour-based data to further model the surfaces and to interpose other geometric structures within the surfaces (e.g., beams of radiation in 3-D radiation treatment planning applications). Contour data sets can also be used in machines that can produce actual models or implants to be used in surgery, including numerically controlled milling machines and stereolithography devices.

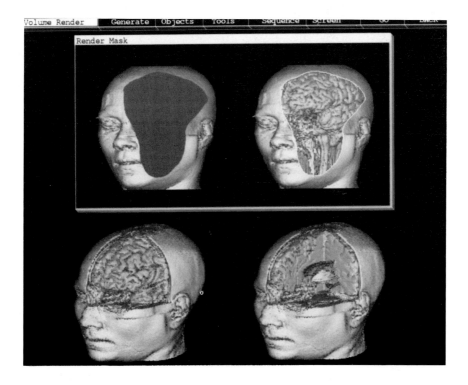

Figure 4.35. Various manipulation tools permit combined display of surfaces from multiple objects. Selection of a subset of rendering rays for separate rendering conditions may be accomplished by tracing on the rendered surface. The rendered display is updated by rerendering only those structures selected within the region (top). Multimodal dissections can be imposed on the volume image, rendering interior structures in 3-D relationship to exterior structures (bottom). See color figure 11.

Multidimensional measuring tools can be used on rendered structures for direct quantitative analysis of various properties of these structures. This is possible because of the aforementioned well-characterized associative mapping between rendered pixels on the rendering screen and a set of voxels in the volume image. As previously indicated, a single pixel in the rendered image corresponds in most cases to a single voxel in the volume image, and therefore points selected on the rendered surface as displayed on the screen can be used to sample the 3-D coordinates and associated voxel values from the volume image. Selection of two points anywhere on the displayed surface provides two 3-D coordinates that can be used to compute measures of distance. The simple Euclidean distance can be readily computed between these two 3-D points, but curvilinear distance along the surface is more difficult to determine. One method for surface distance determination uses all of the render screen points underlying the line between the two selected points as surface points, and sums all surface element distances between those points. Each of the points underneath the line has an associated 3-D coordinate, and the distance between successive points under the line can be estimated by simply computing the Euclidean distance between the 3-D coordinates that correspond to these points. This works well when the surface underneath the line is sampled in the Z-buffer at a high enough frequency, which will occur when the surface is not rapidly changing in depth. At the periphery of the object where the surface may change precipitously, the corresponding 3-D coordinates for each surface point change significantly in distance, and the accuracy of the integrated distance measure is affected.

Similar techniques can be used to measure surface area on the rendered image. Definition of a region via tracing or drawing on the displayed surface defines a set of pixels in the render screen, which again have corresponding 3-D coordinates. The planar surface area for the region as if it was cut through the surface is simply computed by counting the number of pixels in the region and multiplying by the pixel size. Computation of the actual curved area along the surface is more difficult and involves several estimation techniques. One method is analogous to the way in which linear distance measures are made on the surface. For each 3-D coordinate corresponding to the pixels in the rendering, the linear distance in the screen x and y directions can be computed. Integrating these distances in both directions and averaging provides an estimate of the area along the surface. However, this technique only uses those 3-D coordinates which have an associated visible rendered pixel, and does not account for infolding, invaginations, or tunneling of the surface. It also is too coarse for areas where the depth gradient of the surface is rapidly changing. To circumvent this problem, surface tracking algorithms need to be used to identify all candidate surface points within the defined region. The set of 3-D coordinates of voxels defined by the set of pixels in the region of the rendered image can serve as seed points for searching for other connected surface voxels. In this context, a surface voxel is defined as any voxel that has at least one of its six faces adjacent to a voxel that is outside of the current rendering conditions (i.e., an open face that would be rendered if the voxel was visible). The searching algorithm starts at the seed points on the visible surface and searches within the bounds of the defined region for such voxels, stopping at the boundary of the region and at voxels that have no surface face (this keeps the tracking algorithm on the surface and restricts it from going deep into the structure). Once all of the surface voxels have been identified, the total surface area can be estimated in different ways. One estimate is the count of the total number of surface voxels found in the search process. For objects that do not change shape significantly (i.e., smooth surfaces), this estimate is sufficiently accurate. However, for complex, sharply undulating surfaces, this method will consistently underestimate the surface area. A better estimate may be the total number of exposed surface faces for each voxel identified as a surface voxel. For each surface voxel, at least one and often several more orthogonal faces of the voxel will be a surface edge (i.e., the voxel next to it along that face is not a rendered voxel). For example, in a rectilinear solid, the voxels along the edges of the solid should contribute two faces to the total surface area, while the corner voxels contribute three faces. This method would accurately measure the surface area for this rectilinear solid, but most surfaces derived from biomedical images do not have these flat planar surfaces. This method of surface area estimation would generally overestimate the total surface area of biological structures. A more accurate estimation of surface area uses the surface gradient of surrounding voxels to determine the orientation of an oblique cutting plane subdividing every surface voxel, in order to compute the amount of surface area each voxel contributes to the entire surface area. One estimate of the orientation of this plane is the surface normal computed in the reflectance model used for the surface rendering. A planar facet positioned at the center of the voxel and oriented relative to this normal can be used to compute the amount of intersection between the planar facet and the voxel. Integrating over this localized voxel surface area for every voxel may give the best estimate of surface area for the entire surface. Selection of algorithms for surface area measurement, therefore, is quite dependent on the local shape properties of the surface region to be measured.

Volume measures for rendered structures are much easier than either linear distance measures or surface area measures. Volume can be computed by simple selection of a seed point and region growing to find all connected voxels within the current ray conditions (recall that ray conditions are multiple constraints placed upon the ray-tracing process during rendering, including algorithm type, clipping planes, thresholding, region masks, object visibility, opacity, etc.). The count of the total number of voxels found in the region-growing process multiplied by the known voxel volume provides the

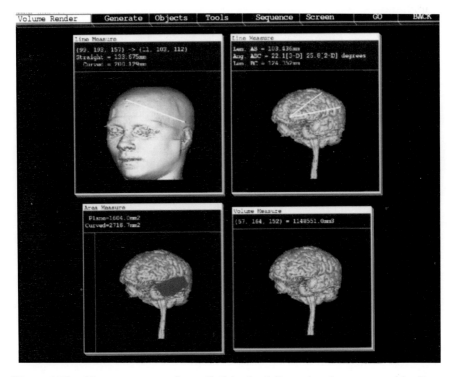

Figure 4.36. Measurement tools applied in the 3-D rendered space provide direct mensuration of important object parameters. Euclidean and curvilinear surface distance measurements are made by selection of any two points on the surface (upper left). Angle information can be computed from any three points (upper right). Surface area is measured using surface tracking to find and integrate over the exposed voxels in a user-defined region (lower left). Object volume is computed using region growing from a selected seed point on the surface and counting the connected voxels (lower right). See color figure 12.

estimate of volume for the rendered structure of interest. Figure 4.36 (see color figure 12) illustrates multidimensional measurements of distance, area, and volume in volume-rendered images.

4.4.2.3 Rendering Multiple Modalities

In many biomedical imaging applications, it is common to utilize multiple modalities or multiple scans from a single modality to get more complete information about the desired structures. With capabilities for effective co-registration of these multiple modality scans (if they are not registered when acquired), rendering techniques are challenged to present information from all modalities in a simple integrated display. The object map concept lends itself directly to this need, permitting objects in a common object map to be defined from multiple modalities in order to integrate the visualization of structures acquired from different modalities.

As an example, X-ray CT and MRI are often used in conjunction with one another to image the bone and soft tissues, respectively. The bone is best visualized in the CT, which provides high signal for bone vs. low signal for bone in the MRI. Conversely, soft tissue structures, like the brain, are best visualized by the MRI, as the dynamic range in the CT for these tissues precludes accurate segmentation. Once these structures have been segmented from their respective modalities, a common object map can be constructed that contains the objects from both modalities. Upon rendering, the voxel sets are rendered according to their assignment to an object from one of the modalities. An example of such an integration of MRI and CT data is presented in Chapter 7.

An example where the multiple data sets come from a single modality is dual fluorescent dye studies in confocal microscopy. Two different fluorescent dyes may be used to tag specific structures of interest in the tissue to be scanned. The images formed from these two different sets of confocal data are automatically in coregistration, and each is segmented separately (by color spectral analysis) for the unique structures tagged by the dye in the particular scan. In order to integrate these two scans for direct visualization, a common object map is formed with the two segmented structures imported into this map. An example of this technique is described in Chapter 7, Section 7.15.

Integrated function and structure may be accomplished using the object map to define the voxel sets that constitute both. Correlated 3-D MR and PET images may be used to visualize structural detail from the MRI through "anatomic" object maps for the brain, while establishing "functional" objects within the bounds of the anatomic objects corresponding to levels of radiopharmaceutical activity from the PET.[37] This allows direct visualization of the functional activity in accurate correspondence with the full 3-D anatomic detail of the brain. Another example of this using functional MRI is given in Chapter 7, Section 7.2.

Finally, the object map may also include objects that do not come from imaged structures at all. These objects may be defined by other means, such as by geometric modeling of analytical solids or of projection beam paths for radiation treatment planning (see Figure 3.13 in Chapter 3).

As visualization and rendering techniques for 3-D biomedical images continue to be refined, advanced data organizations and operations will continue to evolve from the powerful concept of object maps. Multiple object maps correlated to multiple modality scan data will emerge to allow complete visualization and investigation of the multimodal data from common rendering algorithms. Object maps established for each attribute or property of a structure will permit highly integrated renderings using multiple algorithms. Rendering of multimodal data can also be separated from the analysis task, so that structural modalities like MRI can be used directly as a visualization reference, while the analysis takes place in the correlated functional modalities.

4.5 References

1. Castleman, K. R. *Digital Image Processing.* (Ed.) A. Oppenheim, Prentice-Hall, Englewood Cliffs, NJ, 1979.

2. Jain, A. K. *Fundamentals of Digital Image Processing.* (Ed.) T. Kailath, Prentice-Hall, Englewood Cliffs, NJ, 1989.

3. Lim, J. S. *Two-Dimensional Signal and Image Processing.* (Ed.) A. Oppenheim, Prentice-Hall, Englewood Cliffs, NJ, 1990.

4. Katsaggelos, A. K. *Digital Image Restoration.* Springer-Verlag, Germany, 1991.

5. de Graaf, C. N., Viergever, M. A. *Information Processing in Medical Imaging.* Plenum Press, New York, 1988.

6. Colchester, A. C. F., Hawkes, D. J. *Information Processing in Medical Imaging. 12th International Conference, IPMI '91,* Wye, United Kingdom, Proceedings, No. 511, Springer-Verlag, July 1991.

7. Barrett, H. H., Gmitro, A. F. (Eds.) *Information Processing in Medical Imaging. 13th International Conference, IPMI '93,* Flagstaff, AZ, No. 687, Springer-Verlag, June 1993.

8. Robb, R. A., Hanson, D. P., Karwoski, R. A., Larson, A. G., Workman, E. L., Stacy, M. C. "ANALYZE™: A comprehensive, operator-interactive software package for multidimensional medical image display and analysis." *Comput. Med. Imag. Graph.,* 13, 433–454, 1989.

9. Pizer, S. M., Amburn, E. P., Austin, J. D., Cromartie, R., Geselowitz, A., Greer, T., Romeny, B., Zimmerman, J. B., Zuiderveld, K. "Adaptive histogram equalization and its variations." *Comput. Vision Image Proc.,* 39, 355–368, 1987.

10. Austin, J. D., Pizer, S. M. "A multiprocessor adaptive histogram equalization machine." In: de Graaf, C. N., Viergever, M. A. (Eds.) *Information Processing in Medical Imaging.* Plenum Press, New York, 1988.

11. Bracewell, R. N. *The Fourier Transform and Its Applications.* 2nd Ed. McGraw-Hill, New York, 1978.

12. Agard, D. A., Hiraoka, Y., Shaw, P., Sedat, J. W. "Fluorescence microscopy in three dimensions." In: Taylor, D. L., Wang, Y.-L. (Eds.) *Methods in Cell Biology. Vol. 30.* Academic Press, San Diego, 1989.

13. Kriete, A. *Visualization in Biomedical Microscopies.* VCH Publishers, Germany, 1992.

14. Robb, R. A., Hanson, D. P. "A software system for interactive and quantitative visualization of multidimensional biomedical images." *Australas. Phys. Eng. Sci. Med.,* 14, 9–30, 1991.

15. Herman, G. T., Udupa, J. K. "Display of three-dimensional discrete surfaces." SPIE, 283, 90–97, 1981.

16. Heffernan, P. B., Robb, R. A. "A new method for shaded surface display of biological and medical images." *IEEE Trans. Med. Imag.*, MI-4, 26–38, 1985.

17. Drebin, R., Carpenter, L., Harrahan, P. "Volume rendering." *SIGGRAPH '88*, pp. 65–74, 1988.

18. Levoy, M. "Display of surfaces from volume data." *Comput. Graph. Appl.*, 8(3), 29–37, 1988.

19. Höhne, K. H., Bernstein, R. "Shading 3-D images from CT using grey-level gradients." *IEEE Trans. Med. Imag.*, MI-15, 45–47, 1986.

20. Robb, R. A., Barillot, C. "Interactive display and analysis of 3-D medical images." *IEEE Trans. Med. Imag.*, MI-8, 217–226, 1989.

21. Vannier, M. W., Marsh, J. L., Warren, J. O. "Three-dimensional computer graphics for craniofacial surgical planning and evaluation." *Comput. Graphics*, 17, 263–273, 1983.

22. Höhne, K. H., Bomans, M., Pommert, A., Riemer, M., Tiede, U., Wiebecke, G. "Rendering tomographic volume data: adequacy of methods for different modalities and organs." In: Höhne, K. H., Fuchs, H., Pizer, S. M. (Eds.) *3D Imaging in Medicine.* Springer-Verlag, Berlin, 1990, p. 197.

23. Robb, R. A. (Ed.) *Proceedings of Visualization in Biomedical Computing 1992.* Vol. 1808. Chapel Hill, NC, October 13–16, 1992.

24. Sinak, L. J., Hoffman, E. A., Julsrud, P. R., Mair, D. D., Seward, J. B., Hagler, D. J., Harris, L. D., Robb, R. A., Ritman, E. L. "The dynamic spatial reconstructor: Investigating congenital heart disease in four dimensions." *Cardiovasc. Intervention Radiol.*, 7, 124–137, 1984.

25. Hoffman, E. A., Sinak, L. J., Robb, R. A., Ritman, E. L. "Non-invasive quantitative imaging of shape and volume of lungs." *J. Appl. Physiol.: Respir. Environ. Exer. Physiol.*, 54, 1414–1421, 1983.

26. Udupa, J. K. "Display of 3-D information in discrete 3-D scenes produced by computerized tomography." *Proc. IEEE*, 71, 420–431, 1983.

27. Cook, P. N., Batnitzky, S., Lee, K. R., Levine, E., Price, H. I., Preston, D. F., Cook, L. T., Fritz, S. L., Anderson, W., Dwyer, S. J., III. "Three dimensional reconstruction from serial sections for medical applications." *SPIE*, 283, 98–105, 1981.

28. Roth, S. D. "Ray casting for solid modeling." *Comput. Graph. Image Proc.*, 18, 109–144, 1982.

29. Kajiya, J. T. "Ray tracing—tutorial notes." *ACM SIGGRAPH '83*, 1983.

30. Gargantini, I. "Linear octrees for fast processing of three-dimensional objects." *Comput. Graph. Image Proc.*, 20, 356–374, 1982.

31. Meagher, D. "The manipulation analysis and display of 3D medical objects using octree encoding techniques." In: Scarabin, J. M., Coatrieux, J. L. (Eds.) Special Issue on Computer Graphics. *Innov. Technol. Biol. Med.*, 8, 23–36, 1987.

32. Sandor, J. "Octree data structures and perspective imagery." *Comput. Graph.*, 9, 393–405, 1985.

33. Gordon, D., Reynolds, R. A. "Image space shading of 3-dimensional objects." *Comput. Vision Graph. Image Proc.*, 29, 361–376, 1985.

34. Barillot, C., Gibaud, B., Luo, L. M., Scarabin, J. M. "3-D representation of anatomic structures from CT examinations." *Proc. SPIE*, 602, 307–314, 1985.

35. Höhne, K. H., Bomans, M., Tiede, U., Riemer, M. "Display of multiple 3D-objects using the generalized voxel model." *Med. Imag. II. Proc. SPIE*, 914, 850–854, 1988.

36. Höhne, K. H., Hanson, W. A. "Interactive 3D-segmentation of MRI and CT volumes using morphological operations." *J. Comput. Assist. Tomogr.*, 16, 285–294, 1992.

37. Valentino, D. J., Mazziotta, J. C., Huang, H. K. "Volume rendering of multimodal images: Application to MRI and PET imaging of the human brain." *IEEE Trans. Med. Imag.*, 10, 554–562, 1991.

CHAPTER
5

The Calculus of Imaging

What we have here is an insurmountable opportunity.

Yogi Berra

5.1 Introduction

Modern 3-D biomedical imaging presents a paradox—the potential and promise for major advances in both science and medicine increase significantly as higher-fidelity images are produced—but achieving this potential is dependent on two difficult and very important challenges in 3-D biomedical imaging: 1) automated and accurate segmentation of structures and features of interest and 2) automated and accurate registration and fusion of multimodality or multispectral information. These objectives may be referred to as the "calculus" of imaging science. To segment is to differentiate; to register and fuse is to integrate. And just like the differential and integral calculus, image segmentation and fusion are piecewise interdependent and inversely related; solutions for one lead to solutions for the other. For example, segmented image surfaces may provide the information required to fuse individual 3-D images into spatially registered multispectral sets of images, which in turn, offer richer possibilities for robust and automatic segmentation of more complex image structures by multispectral classification of the congruent image set.

High-level symbolic analysis of images requires the differentiation of voxel data into objects representing the spatial localization of some structure and/or features of interest. Just as the digital image is a mapping of some physical property in real space into voxel space, segmentation is a mapping of symbolic information from voxel space into object space. Ideally, the desired segmentation would be automatic, robust, and rapid. Much work has

165

been directed toward this goal, with encouraging results.[1-7] However, the objects of interest, whether structural or functional, are often only partially identifiable in any single image modality, and may have to be partially estimated by empirical models or by using the a priori knowledge of a human expert.

Registration and integration (fusion) of multiple images of the same object(s) recorded from different domains (modalities) offer significant possibilities for analysis and understanding of biological structures and living organisms. Multimodality images obtained from different medical imaging systems generally provide complementary characteristic and diagnostic information. Synthesis of these image data sets into a single composite image containing these complementary attributes in accurate registration and congruence would provide truly synergistic information about the object(s) under examination. Important work toward this goal has been achieved,[8-12] although the work is still incomplete.

5.2 Segmentation

Much of the recent research in 3-D medical image processing has focused on complete automation of image segmentation.[13-15] However, the degree of difficulty in automating a particular segmentation task is often directly proportional to the scientific or medical importance of the result! In practice, effective use of medical images still requires a certain amount of manual image editing, and it is important that such tools be as intuitive, responsive, and efficient as possible.

Grayscale thresholding is a common technique used for segmentation of medical images, even as part of more sophisticated segmentation techniques. In this approach, only image pixels within a defined grayscale range are considered as part of the desired object(s). Once an appropriate threshold is determined for a set of similar images, it can often be used for all images in the set with only minor adjustments. Experimental determination of standard or calibrated thresholds and the adjustments needed for nonstandard images requires a responsive interactive tool. Such a tool in ANALYZE™ is illustrated in Figure 5.1 (see color figure 13).

The wide variation of absolute grayscale across multimodal medical images, and the varying contrast differentials that characterize structures of interest in such images, require regional analysis for effective segmentation by thresholding methods. Region growing is one useful approach when structures of interest have relatively homogeneous interiors and reasonably well-demarcated boundaries.[16] Such images can be segmented by placing a "seed" point within the interior of the structure and "growing" out to the grayscale-bounded and connected border of the structure. Figure 5.2 illustrates the use of such a tool in ANALYZE™.

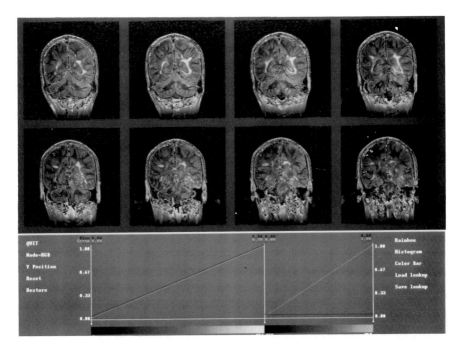

Figure 5.1. Grayscale thresholding is a straightforward way of segmenting structures that are readily differentiated by grayscale. This tool also provides remapping of grayscale values and may be used as an image enhancement function. See color figure 13.

Manual tracing is the last, and often the only, method of choice in image segmentation. "Last" because of the time and expertise needed for the task; "only" because no other method may work on difficult images. Intuitive image editing tools make the task easier in such cases. The ability to quickly correct a part of a trace as shown in Figure 5.3, or correct a region-grown trace, as shown in Figure 5.4, becomes an absolute necessity if much manual segmentation is required. Conversion of traces to spline curves[16] with control points that can be dragged around to correct traces (see Figure 5.5) is a useful enhancement to manual image editing.

The propagation of the results from manual and/or semiautomated segmentation techniques on one tomographic slice to adjacent slices in a 3-D volume image further reduces the time taken to edit a volume image manually. Bounded region growing may be used for several sections before requiring adjustment, or region growing directly in 3-D can be effective for segmenting relatively large, high-contrast (well-defined surfaces) objects in the volume image.

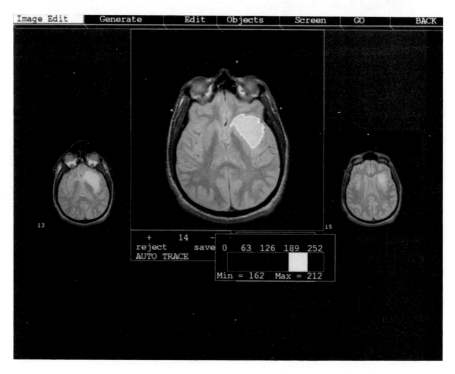

Figure 5.2.   Interactive seeded region growing controlled by grayscale threshold values. This tool works well for segmenting objects of fairly uniform grayscale.

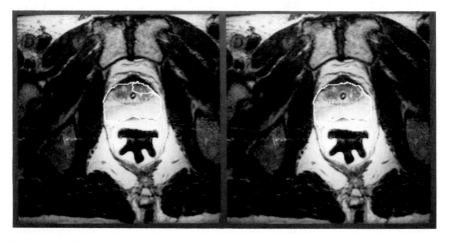

Figure 5.3.   Manual trace on image showing interactive correction by operator of part of trace.

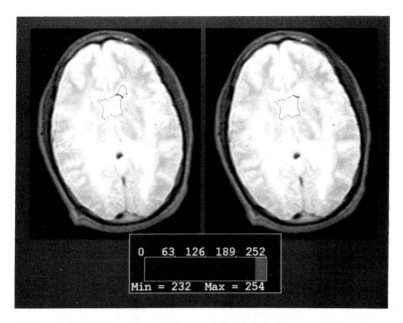

Figure 5.4. Artificial (hand-drawn) limits placed on region-growing tool extend its utility for complex image segmentation.

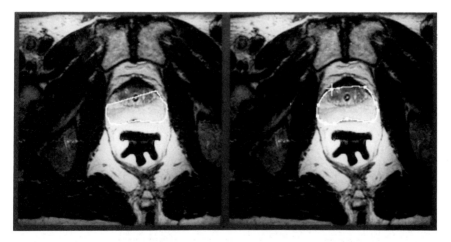

Figure 5.5. Converting hand-drawn traces to spline curves automatically smooths the curve. Interactive adjustment of the spline control points allows easy correction of a trace.

5.2.1 Multispectral Classification

Some semiautomated ways that images can be segmented include edge identification, shape matching, and texture analysis.[14] If different images of the
same object(s) are recorded containing different characteristic properties or
features of the object(s), then this spectrum of features can be used to segment the objects from the set of images. Such techniques fall into the domain
of multispectral classification methods,[5,17] and they are powerful, sophisticated approaches to robust image segmentation, particularly when multimodal images are available. To illustrate, if an image contains a solid field
of tissue type "A," the values in the image will have a statistical distribution
similar to that shown in Figure 5.6. Normalized, this image histogram is a
probability density function (pdf) for tissue type "A," i.e., the function gives
the probability that an image voxel will be a particular value given that it is
tissue type "A." We can similarly calculate the pdf for tissue type "B,"
tissue type "C," and so on.

 If we then scan an image field that consists of a region of type "A" tissue
consisting of ¼ the entire volume, surrounded by, say, tissue type "B," the
histogram should reflect the sum of the two originally determined pdfs
scaled by the proportional distribution of the tissue types. Such histograms
are often referred to as "feature space." These scaled functions are the a
posteriori pdfs, i.e., they are the probability of a pixel representing tissue
type "A" (or "B") given the grayscale value of the pixel. The point of intersection of these two pdfs (the minimum between the two modes of the histogram), as shown in Figure 5.7, is the threshold point at which each pixel
will be assigned to type "A" or type "B" by the criterion of maximum
likelihood.[18]

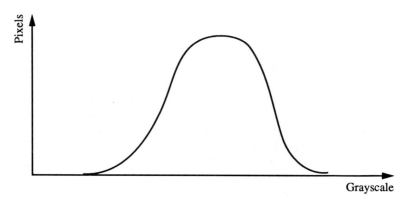

Figure 5.6.   The grayscale values in a visually uniform region often show a nearly
Gaussian distribution.

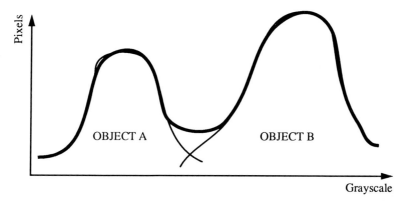

Figure 5.7. Bimodal histograms suggest two underlying distributions relating to two different tissue types. The point where the distributions cross is the most likely threshold for separation of tissue types.

If we sample a number of voxels known to be type "A" and a number known to be "B," and assume the distribution of each class to have some fundamental shape (e.g., Gaussian), the parameters of which are well represented by the training sample, we can calculate the threshold of greatest likelihood to use for all similar images. Such a system is known as a supervised parametric statistical classifier.

The significant value of this technique is that it has reduced a spatially complex segmentation into a simple threshold operation. Of course, the technique requires adequate discrimination of the tissue types of interest associated with the image modality used. The combination of modalities (e.g., any combination of MRI, CT, PET, SPECT, etc.) increases the potential differentiability of tissues by multispectral classification in proportion to the number of spectra used. As the number of feature dimensions increases, the simple grayscale thresholding operation generalizes into a multidimensional region definition. The advantage remains that the original spatially complex region having complex boundaries is represented in the feature domain as a compact cluster or shape with simple boundaries. With only two feature dimensions, it is often very effective to manually draw segmentation boundaries in feature space. In Figure 5.8 (see color figure 14), a manual segmentation of the 2-D histogram space (feature space) of T1- and T2-weighted MR images has resulted in a reasonable spatial segmentation of gray and white matter in the brain. This figure illustrates how a spatially complex region is transformed into a simple compact region in feature space. Manual segmentation becomes increasingly difficult to perform as the number of feature dimensions increases. However, manual segmentation can be effective for higher feature dimensionality by using multiple threshold ranges, derived perhaps by addressing only two dimensions at a time. But

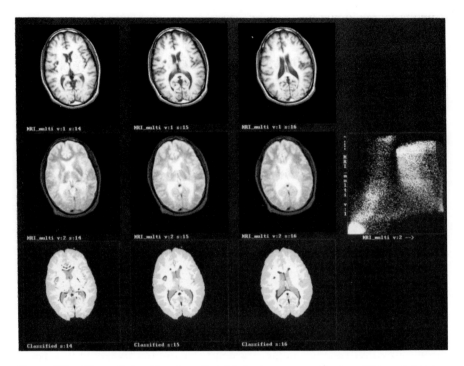

Figure 5.8. Manual classification of multiple tissue types from multispectral image data, in this case T1 (top) and T2 (center) MR images. The "clusters" of voxels (right) having unique T1 and T2 values allow simple definitions of regions in the T1/T2 grayscale histogram to effectively segment spatially complex regions of the images (bottom). White matter (yellow), gray matter (blue), cerebrospinal fluid (green), and dense tissue (red). See color figure 14.

such "tricks" will restrict feature space regions to rectilinear shapes, comprising potential achievable accuracy in the segmentation.

The 2-D spectra case can be used to illustrate other feature-space segmentation algorithms. Figure 5.9 (see color figure 15) illustrates the maximum-likelihood Gaussian classifier described above. In two dimensions, the Gaussian clusters constructed from the tissue type sample statistics can be visualized as elliptical spots with a Gaussian profile. The "valley" between two different spots is the boundary of classification. Gaussian classification can be undertaken in a measurement space of arbitrary dimension, with an associated computational burden.

Figure 5.10 (see color figure 16) illustrates a nearest-neighbor algorithm solution to the same two-spectra classification problem. Nearest-neighbor algorithms compute the Euclidean distance in measurement space from each pixel to all of the class samples. The class of the nearest neighbor is used as the classification result. Note that the boundaries between measurement

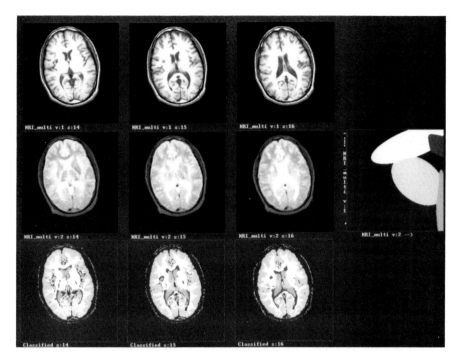

Figure 5.9. Automated classification of multiple tissue types (as in Figure 5.8) from multispectral image data using Gaussian maximum likelihood. The samples of different tissue types taken from regions of the image are analyzed and used to construct 2-D Gaussian distribution estimates (right) for each tissue type. The intersections of the Gaussians are the most likely boundaries for feature space clusters. See color figure 15.

space regions consist of circular arc segments. Neural networks can also be used to segment regions of a feature space.[19,20] Figure 5.11 illustrates the structure of a three-layer back-propagation network used as a classifier. Neural networks are "trained" by applying test vectors and comparing the classifier output to the known class of the vector. The weightings of internal interconnections are then modified based upon the error of the classifier. This process is repeated until the network converges to correct answers for the test set. The trained neural net may then be used to classify unknown vectors. Figure 5.12 (see color figure 17) illustrates the response of a trained neural network to the MRI T1/T2 images shown previously.

Finally, algorithms can be created that find "interesting" clusters and groupings in the measurement space without being "trained" on preclassified samples. The "chain data" method uses the Euclidean distance between the measurement-space position as its clustering criterion. As successive voxels are compared, those nearer than a threshold distance are grouped into

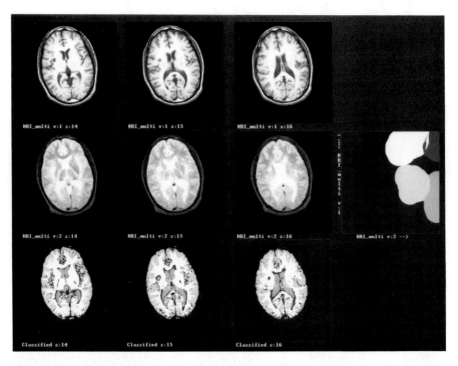

Figure 5.10. Automated classification of multiple tissue types (as in Figure 5.8) from multispectral image data using a nearest neighbor algorithm. The samples of different tissue types taken from regions of the image are compared to every voxel in the image. The voxel is classified to the type of its nearest neighbor voxel in feature space (right). See color figure 16.

classes. Class means are calculated and used for later classification decisions. Figure 5.13 (see color figure 18) illustrates the performance of such an algorithm on the test data used previously. Such an approach lends itself to modified recursion, since classified images derived from the original spectra of features may be used as additions to the spectra for further classification.

A simple example of this concept is the extraction of an edge image (as in Figure 5.14; see color figure 19) from the original data. Since this image primarily contains boundary information, it may be used to preferentially weight different statistical characteristics of border and central volume voxels in the image classification. Another example of this recursive concept is to use successively blurred versions of an image as multiple spectra. Since each blurred version of the image has information concerning only a restricted range of scale, this allows the scale of the object (or its persistence through blurring) to become a part of the classification process. Images defined by the operation of local operators (texture measurements, mean/median, deviation, etc.) also may be used as additional spectra. After an initial

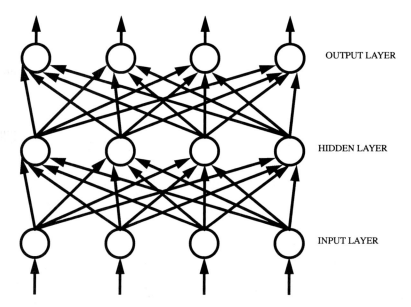

Figure 5.11. Three-layer Kolmogorov network. The hidden layer transforms the input domain to an output domain where output classes are simple connected regions.

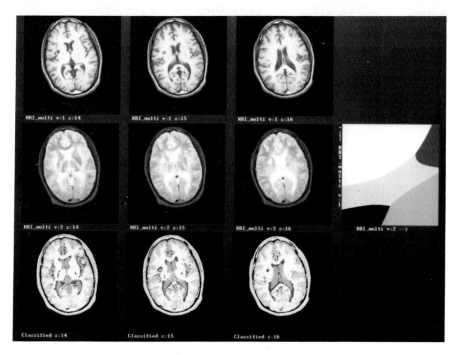

Figure 5.12. Automated classification of multiple tissue types (as in Figure 5.8) from multispectral image data using a neural network. The tissue type samples are used to train the network (by modifying the weight of the internode links) so that it correctly classifies the training sample. After training, the entire set of image voxels from new data sets can be classified by the network. See color figure 17.

175

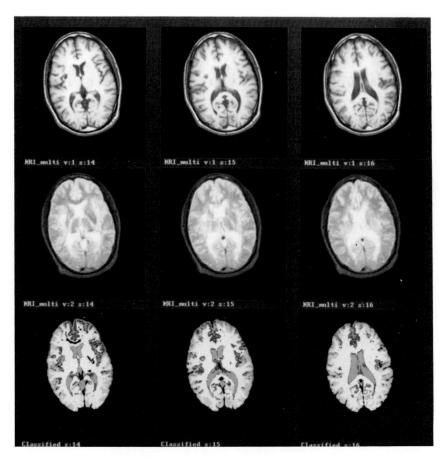

Figure 5.13. Automated classification of multiple tissue types (as in Figure 5.8) from multispectral image data using an unsupervised classifier. No samples of tissue types are taken. The algorithm simply looks for similarities and differences between groups of voxel vectors. See color figure 18.

segmentation has been performed in feature space, the spatial distribution of classes can be used to refine the segmentation.

One advantage of purely statistical classifiers is that they produce a numerical estimate of the likelihood of each classification. This may be used first to target low-confidence voxels for further processing, and then again to compare a given voxel's class confidence with those of its immediate neighbors. Simple rules could be used to switch the classification of a low-confidence voxel if it is completely surrounded by high-confidence voxels of a different class. More general rules might compare the confidence of a voxel's being in a given class with the average confidence value of neighboring nonclass voxels. This process can be iterated until no more reclassi-

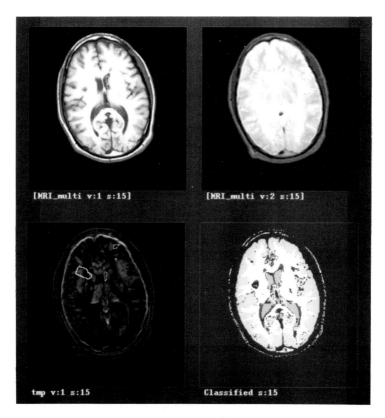

Figure 5.14. Images derived from the original by spectral analysis may be added recursively as additional spectral components. Here an edge strength image (lower left) has been added for classification. See color figure 19.

fication of voxels occurs, i.e., until the image is completely statistically segmented.

5.2.2 Mathematical Morphology

Although there may never be one all-purpose automatic segmentation tool which is successful on all types of objects for all modalities in biomedical imaging, there are some approaches that are promising in a wide variety of cases. As seen in the last section, techniques that do not rely *solely* on edge-strength analyses but rather can include other features show significant promise for automated segmentation. One such approach is multispectral analysis; another is the application of mathematical morphology.[21,22] Math morphology segmentation predominantly depends on shape features. It has been shown that use of morphological operators, when combined with edge-strength methods, such as thresholding and region-growing operations, can achieve excellent segmentation results quickly and without intensive user interaction.[6] Furthermore, once a sequence of steps has been devised to accomplish an accurate segmentation for a certain type of image data, the same set of steps will usually produce accurate segmentations for other data sets of the same type.

5.2.2.1 Basic Morphological Operations

There are two fundamental morphological operations, *erosion* and *dilation*.[21] Erosion is often thought of as a shrinking or reducing operation, while dilation is the complementary swelling or enlarging operation. This reducing or enlarging is achieved by peeling "layers" off an object and by adding layers back on an object. In binary morphology, a grayscale image is first reduced to a set of ones and zeros, typically by thresholding. Another smaller set of ones and zeros, called a structuring element, is then applied to the image by translating it across the image with its center on every point of the image. The structuring element has an analytically defined geometry (i.e., shape and size). Let I represent the image, $I(x)$ represent the value of the image at location x, $I'(x)$ represent the morphologically processed result, and $E(x)$ represent the structuring element centered on the image at location x. Erosion is defined by the following equation:

$$\{\forall x : \text{If } I \cap E(x) \neq E(x) \rightarrow I'(x) = 0$$
$$\text{else if } I \cap E(x) = E(x) \rightarrow I'(x) = 1\} \tag{5.1}$$

Figure 5.15 illustrates an erode operation, whereby small objects are removed, layers are peeled off of larger objects, and connections between thinly connected objects are broken. Holes in an object are also enlarged.

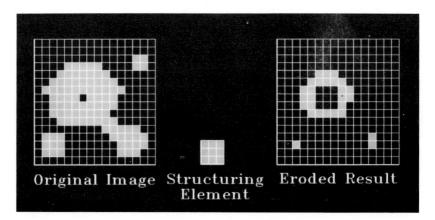

Original Image   Structuring   Eroded Result
Element

Figure 5.15. Example of binary erosion of an image with a 3×3 structuring element.

Dilation is defined as follows:

$$\{\forall x : \text{If } I \cap E(x) \neq \varnothing \rightarrow I'(x) = 1$$
$$\text{else if } I \cap E(x) = \varnothing \rightarrow I'(x) = 0\} \tag{5.2}$$

Figure 5.16 illustrates a dilate operation, whereby holes and cracks in an object are filled in, and layers are added to objects.

The erode and dilate operations when used in succession are very powerful. Two common morphological operations, called *open* and *close*, are simply combinations of the two operations.[22] A morphological open is defined as an erosion of an image followed by a dilation, with the same structuring element used in both operations. An open operation will delete small objects and break thin connections between objects without the loss of layers on other objects. The open function is illustrated in Figure 5.17. The result is the same as would be obtained by a dilation of the results shown in Figure 5.15, which was the output from an erosion. Similarly, a morphological close is defined as a dilation of an image followed by an erosion using the same structuring element. The close operation fills small holes in objects. Figure 5.18 shows the results of a close. These results are obtained by applying an erosion to the results in Figure 5.16. Note that when open or close operations are being done, the structuring element must have odd x and y dimensions to prevent mistranslation of objects.

5.2.2.2 Applications of Mathematical Morphology

There are many cases in medical imaging where an object is approximately definable by a certain threshold value or range, but other objects remain "connected" to the desired object due to lack of sufficient contrast differences between them. Typical segmentation approaches in such situations

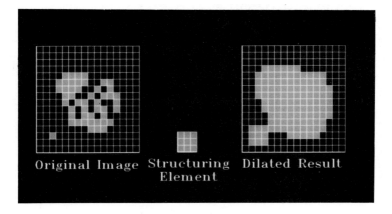

Figure 5.16. Example of binary dilation of an image with a 3 × 3 structuring element.

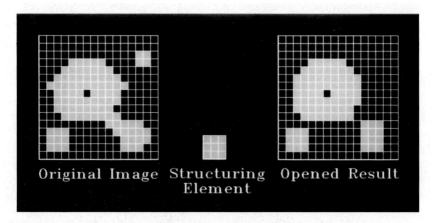

Figure 5.17.   Example of a binary open-erosion followed by dilation.

usually include manual or semimanual tracing techniques following thresholding and/or region growing. This process can be time consuming and requires an expert to interact with the data. Mathematical morphology can often be successfully applied to such cases, eliminating or significantly reducing the need for manual intervention.

As an example, data from a 3-D acquired MRI scan of the human head will be used to demonstrate segmentation of the brain from the rest of the data using mathematical morphology. As shown in Figure 5.19, trying various threshold ranges cannot completely isolate the brain from the soft tissues (e.g., skin). Therefore a semiautomated procedure will be described in detail.

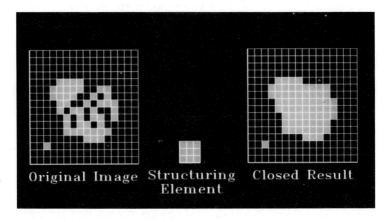

Figure 5.18.   Example of a binary close-dilation followed by erosion.

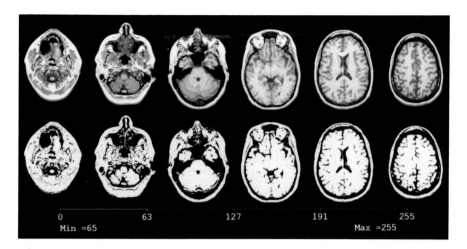

Figure 5.19. Display of a user-selected threshold range for the brain. The brain tissue is represented by the white pixels.

Erosion and dilation operators can be applied to this data set in an attempt to remove the skin and preserve the brain. First, after selecting the appropriate threshold range and reducing the data to binary representation (by setting the voxels within the threshold range to one and all other voxels to zero), erosion is applied to the data set. The grayscale results of the morphological operators can then be viewed by multiplying the original grayscale image by the morphological processed binary image. Figure 5.20 shows the application of various size structuring elements to one transverse slice of the MRI scan just above the eyes. Notice that a large enough structuring element can be chosen that will remove all of the skin from this slice. Also notice that a large portion of the brain has been removed in the process. Outside layers of the brain, as well as interior portions adjacent to voids in the original threshold data, have also been removed. Figure 5.21 illustrates applications of the dilate operator in an attempt to bring back these removed portions of the brain without adding the skin. Typically the structuring element for the dilation is the same size as the one used for erosion, which results in an opening of the data set. In this case the dilate cannot bring back all of the desired parts of the brain, because of the holes in the original threshold data. These holes caused the erosion to remove whole portions of the brain that the dilate operation could not recover (see Figure 5.21). This requires a retreat of a few steps to choose a more appropriate threshold for the data. The learning point here is, for preparing data for morphological processing, that the threshold range need not be the one that best represents the object in question, but rather should be defined so that a "break" between the desired object and undesired objects occurs without leaving unwanted voids (zeros) in the object to be segmented (see Figure 5.22). With

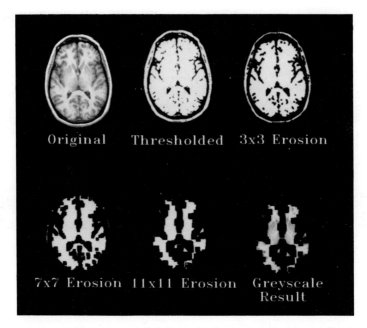

Figure 5.20. Erosions of increasing size can be applied to the original image until only brain tissue remains.

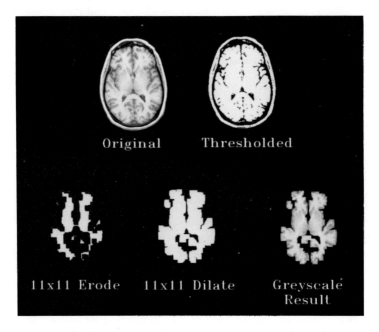

Figure 5.21. Attempted recovery of eroded brain tissue by dilation does not work if threshold is not selected correctly.

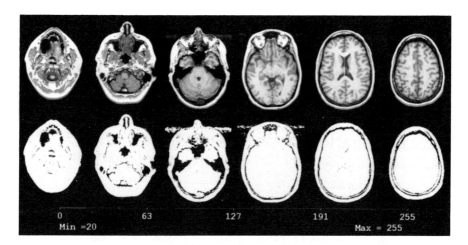

Figure 5.22. A proper threshold range for the brain, which barely separates it from the other tissue, will permit recovery by dilation of eroded brain tissue.

an appropriate threshold, a structuring element can be found so that the skin will be removed from the slices with an erosion, and a following dilate will bring back all of the brain, as shown in Figure 5.23. If this opening is applied to all of the slices of the scan above the eyes, and the resulting data are then rendered with a volume-rendering program, the segmentation can be viewed in three dimensions, as shown in Figure 5.24. This slice-by-slice iterative process on threshold selection and structuring element definition using morphologic opening operations can be successful in segmenting the brain over a wide range of MRI brain scans.

Although this approach has yielded good results on adjacent 2-D slices, the segmentation problem can be formulated so as to accomplish a direct, automated 3-D segmentation of the brain. First, an initial candidate threshold can be intelligently selected from the 3-D histogram of the volume image. Second, 3-D structuring elements, 3-D erodes, and 3-D dilates can be used to achieve the segmentation. This is accomplished by using spheres and cubes instead of circles and rectangles as structuring elements, and translating these through voxel space rather than pixel space. Third, the amount of erosion necessary to separate one object from another is greatly reduced by performing 3-D region growing in conjunction with each erosion. In this way, erosions can be repeated until the desired object is no longer connected to any other structure within the defined threshold range, and the unconnected voxels can be discarded. Once the connection is broken, further erosions are not required. Fourth and last, the selected threshold range that contains the desired object can be used to constrain the dilation process. In other words, the dilation operator is limited in adding back only voxels that were contained in the originally thresholded data. Since this formulation is a strong

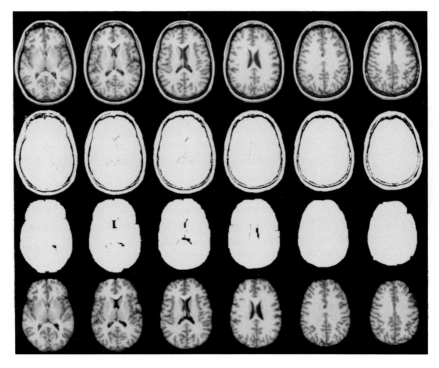

Figure 5.23. Original MRI transverse images (first row), thresholded images (second row), and results of a morphological erosion (third row) followed by dilation (fourth row). The brain is correctly segmented in all images.

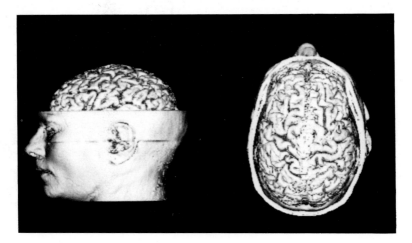

Figure 5.24. Volume rendering of the MRI scan after an open was performed on the top 80 slices.

potential candidate for fully automated segmentation of an important class of 3-D medical images (MRI brain scans), it will be described in some detail so that others may reproduce it.

The first step in this proposed 3-D segmentation approach is to threshold the data. In this process, the amount of erosion required is to be reduced by adding a 3-D region-growing step after each erosion, so a threshold range that includes the entire desired object, the brain, is used (the same as illustrated in Figure 5.19). Other structures are included as well at this first step. Threshold selection can be automated based on the image histogram (selecting a range based on peak mode and/or central tendency). After thresholding, a region-growing step is performed where voxels connected by 6-neighbors to a user-selected seed point on the brain are kept and all other voxels are discarded (set to zero). If this region-growing step does not separate the object from the other data in the threshold range, an erosion using a $3 \times 3 \times 3$ cube as a structuring element is performed. Note that the size of the structuring element can be increased if the user knows that the data will require a large amount of erosion to separate the desired object. After the erosion has been performed, the region-growing step is repeated to see if the connections between the brain and other tissue have been broken. The erosion and region-growing steps are repeated until this condition is met. Figure 5.25 shows the volume-rendered binary volume after the region-growing and erosion steps that result in the separation of the brain.

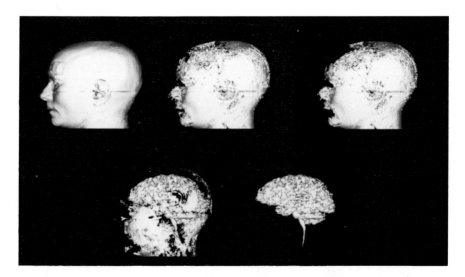

Figure 5.25.   Volume rendering of original data (top left) and binary rendering results after successive erosions (top center, right, and bottom) with a $3 \times 3 \times 3$ structuring element and region-growing operations.

Once the object has been successfully separated, a series of dilation steps is required to bring back the layers of the brain that were "peeled away" in the erosion process. In this dilation process, a modified dilation, called "conditional dilation," is used. In this process, each voxel to be added back to the volume through dilation must also meet the requirement of being contained in the originally thresholded data. This makes sense, because the threshold range originally selected was chosen to contain the grayscales of the object. This type of dilation proceeds slower than an unconditional dilate, because fewer voxels are added back to the volume each time a conditional dilation is performed. This means that more conditional dilates than erosions are required to correctly segment the data. The results of a series of conditional dilates are shown in Figure 5.26 by viewing the volume-rendered binary data. One can easily see the layers being added back to the brain in each step. The question arises when to stop the dilation process. One approach is to continue until the object "looks right," i.e., the process is interrupted when iterative display of the object being segmented has smooth edges and appears complete. The other approach, which is more objective, is to predefine a 2-D slice through the volume image in which the desired object is not connected to any other data. A count of the total pixels in the object on that slice before the iterative operation begins serves as the terminator criterion. The dilation process continues until "completeness" is achieved, defined as an arbitrarily close (e.g., within 2%) number of object points recovered on the segmented slice relative to the termination value.

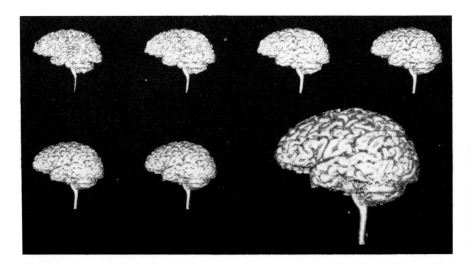

Figure 5.26. Application of conditional dilates to eroded object. The brain tissue is restored one level for each dilate. Bottom right image is rendered from grayscale data using final segmented binary volume (bottom center) as a rendering mask.

For robustness, several predetermined slices covering the object range could be used in checking for completeness during the dilate iterations.

There are other morphological techniques that may aid in the segmentation and visualization of medical images. The process of removing holes in an object is often very useful. The removal of holes can be used to fill in an object or to separate one object from another. For example, bone in MRI scans has an intensity range that overlaps the intensity range of air. Because the skull is a relatively thin structure compared to the brain, erosion or opening is not an available option for its segmentation. Instead, to separate bone from air, a threshold for the skin, which can be easily determined, can be defined. After thresholding, the holes (skull) on the slices of the volume can be filled by the following technique. First, the threshold image is complemented, or inverted (i.e., the ones of the threshold volume are changed to zeros, and vice versa). Next, through region growing techniques, all of the connected components and their sizes are calculated. Since the volume was inverted, the bone and air are now represented by ones in the volume (i.e., they are "positive" objects). At this point the background must be determined and removed. There are many case-specific ways for determining the background, one of which is to assume it is the largest connected component in the image (not always true, but a reasonable guess). After removal of the background "object," the remaining ones in the volume represent the holes, including the skull. This processed volume is added to the original threshold volume and then multiplied within the original grayscale volume to produce a bone-specific data set. Volume renderings of the bone and ventricles segmented from an MRI scan with this technique are shown in Figure 5.27.

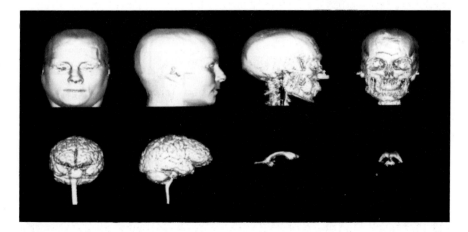

Figure 5.27.   Skin, bone, brain, and ventricles segmented from MRI scan using 3-D morphological operations. The brain was segmented using erosion, region-growing, and conditional dilate operations. The bone and ventricles were segmented by filling the holes within the skin.

In summary, careful use of the erode, dilate, conditional dilate, open, and close mathematical morphology operators can result in accurate and automatic segmentation of structures in 3-D medical images. The approach simply requires that the structure in question can be bounded by a specified threshold range, even if the desired structure is loosely connected to other structures in the volume within the specified threshold range.

5.3 Registration and Fusion

The full scientific, medical, and educational value of multidimensional, multimodality imaging remains largely unexplored, and has been impeded primarily by inadequate capabilities for accurate and reproducible registration and segmentation of multiple 2-D or 3-D images. With regard to registration, 2-D tomographic images taken at different times cannot be guaranteed to represent the same spatial section of the patient, and the 2-D images themselves do not contain the information required to either measure or correct the misregistration. The use of 3-D images makes full six-degrees-of-freedom registration possible not only for images taken at different times, but for images from different modalities.

A general approach to registration of multiple images has three steps: 1) defining corresponding features between the different image data sets, 2) finding the matching transformation, and 3) transforming one (or more) of the images to bring it (them) into spatial registration with another. External and internal anatomic landmarks have been used by several researchers as matching features within multimodal images.[11,12,23-25] Accurately locating these landmarks across modalities is an inherently manual process, presenting significant difficulty even to highly trained experts. Fiducial markers introduced at scanning time have been used for multimodal image registration with some success, but this technique requires the use of an immobilizing frame that is not removed between scans, and the technique is not applicable to serial studies. Complex moments calculated for each image data set[26,27] can be used as matching features, but exactly corresponding subvolumes must be defined. Matching of surfaces extracted from common objects[28,29] shows greater potential for automated registration of serial as well as multimodal images, but many proposed techniques can only accurately measure misregistration in a limited set of geometrically tractable anatomic situations. Most suffer the classical problems associated with a global minimum search and usually require manual intervention.

In searching for an image matching transformation, rigid body motion is often assumed in order to simplify the process. A rigid body is defined in classical mechanics[30] as "a system of mass points subject to the holonomic constraints that the distances between all pairs of points remain constant throughout the motion." It allows three translational and three rotational degrees of freedom, and knowing these parameters, any rigid body motion can be restored.

To illustrate this, if three rigidly connected points in 3-D space are rotated about a common origin, and the coordinates of each point are known both before and after the rotation, the three pairs of triplets resolve a rotational matrix that may be used to calculate the rotated coordinates of any other rigidly connected points, as shown in Figure 5.28. If a translational compo-

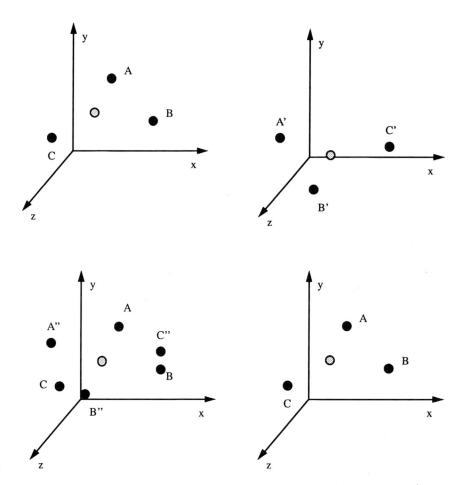

Figure 5.28. Three-point rigid-body solution. Upper left, original points and centroid. Upper right, rotated and translated points and centroid. Lower left, match centroids by translation. Lower right, solve rotational matrix:

$$\begin{bmatrix} x_A & y_A & z_A \\ x_B & y_B & z_B \\ x_C & y_C & z_C \end{bmatrix} \times \begin{bmatrix} & M & \end{bmatrix} = \begin{bmatrix} x_{A''} & y_{A''} & z_{A''} \\ x_{B''} & y_{B''} & z_{B''} \\ x_{C''} & y_{C''} & z_{C''} \end{bmatrix}$$

nent is also possible, a fourth point is needed to form the homogeneous coordinate matrix, as shown in Figure 5.29. The analytical solution depends upon the accuracy of point coordinate specification, rigid-body motion, and the knowledge of exact correspondence between coordinate pairs.

Both physical markers and anatomic landmarks may be used for attempted analytical registration. For greatest accuracy, physical markers should be attached to unchanging rigid structures such as bone. They should also be equally visible in all modalities to be used. Patient health and comfort, however, require the markers to be attached temporarily to the skin—often over small tattoo marks for long-term treatment, or over specific bony structure landmarks. Marker materials are generally incompatible between modalities, and so markers must be removed and reattached or slipped in and out of carriers.

All of these factors introduce so much real and apparent elastic motion between the points that an analytical solution is generally impossible. However, if the correspondence between points in two different modalities and/or two different points in time is known, a functional measure of registration error (such as the sum of Euclidean distances between corresponding pairs of points) can be searched for a global minimum, thus finding a compromise rigid-body rotation that minimizes the chosen measure of error.

Given the possible amount of random elastic motion each physical marker may take, it is not particularly likely that a best-fit solution of three points

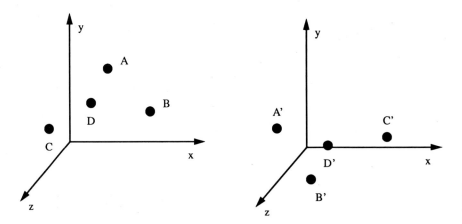

Figure 5.29. Four-point rigid body motion solution: using homogeneous coordinates solve for rotation and translation:

$$
\begin{bmatrix}
x_A \; y_A \; z_A \; = \; 1 \\
x_B \; y_B \; z_B \; = \; 1 \\
x_C \; y_C \; z_C \; = \; 1 \\
x_D \; y_D \; z_D \; = \; 1
\end{bmatrix}
\times
\begin{bmatrix}
M
\end{bmatrix}
=
\begin{bmatrix}
x_{A'} \; y_{A'} \; z_{A'} \; = \; 1 \\
x_{B'} \; y_{B'} \; z_{B'} \; = \; 1 \\
x_{C'} \; y_{C'} \; z_{C'} \; = \; 1 \\
x_{D'} \; y_{D'} \; z_{D'} \; = \; 1
\end{bmatrix}
$$

will be a best-fit solution across the entire 3-D image space. The best-fit solution improves markedly with additional markers, but each marker requires additional patient preparation time, and the correspondence between markers also requires more time for the image expert.

The physical limitations of markers can be sidestepped by using internal landmarks in the images, but this has its own set of practical limitations. Many common landmarks are poorly specified, ambiguous, or simply too large to be used as point markers. In addition, it requires greater expertise to identify anatomic landmarks than to identify corresponding external markers.

Surface-matching algorithms have shown promise for complete automation of multimodal 3-D image registration. Surface matching is based on identification of object surfaces (not necessarily those of interest) common among all multimodal images to be registered. Complete anatomic image surfaces can be used for best-fit matching, but their use presents a number of computational challenges.

The number of points in a complete surface precludes the use of correspondence information to estimate the registration error. An expected matching geometry can be imposed on the surfaces, such as the "head and hat" algorithm,[28,29] where the registration error is calculated from the linear distance between the surfaces along rays from the base surface centroid. Another approach is to base the registration error on the minimum Euclidean distance from the match surface to the base surface. Even computationally efficient estimations of the Euclidean distance[31] have a strong global minimum at the best-fit match point.

To find the ideal transformation for 3-D images, the images must be normalized to the same size. If the voxel dimensions are not known, then this normalization factor must be determined as part of the transformation process. The application of the transformation to one image will often involve interpolation of data values. Generally, trilinear interpolation will give a satisfactory result. Nonlinear graylevel interpolation or shape-based interpolation may be desired if the original image has a large interslice distance.

A promising approach to 3-D image registration using surfaces is based on Chamfer matching.[31-33] The implementation[10] of this method in ANALYZE™ is combined with a straightforward measure of registration cost applicable to arbitrarily complex multidimensional surfaces, and uses a multiscale/multiple starting point search strategy to significantly increase the probability of efficiently locating the global minimum without manual intervention. Although current results of this algorithm are very promising, and extensive simulation and phantom-based evaluation have been carried out,[10] it needs comprehensive validation on clinical images (as do most current multimodality coregistration algorithms). The questions as to which surfaces to use with which imaging modalities and which anatomic regions are best for automated matching must also be addressed and answered.

5.3.1 Chamfer Matching

In the Chamfer matching method, two (or more) volume images are selected to be registered—one image as the "base image" and the other image as the "match image," in ANALYZE™ nomenclature. The match image will subsequently be transformed to align with the base image and resectioned relative to it. Object contours are extracted from both base and match images by using semiautomatic image segmentation algorithms available in ANALYZE™ (see preceding sections of this chapter). The contours from the base images are stacked together to form 3-D base surfaces. If the base image voxel is noncubic, then shape-based surface interpolation[34,35] is applied to interpolate intermediate contours between every consecutive pair of actual contours. A limited number of points are uniformly sampled from the match contour data set, and only these points are used for the registration, i.e., for the cost calculation and minimization process.

Chamfer matching is accomplished by performing a distance transformation that converts a binary surface image into a graylevel image in which all voxels have a value corresponding to the distance to the nearest surface voxel. Because the surface is extracted from a digital image and represented by a discrete image form, calculation of exact Euclidean distances is not necessary. A good integer approximation of Euclidean distance can be computed using the Chamfer 3/4/5 algorithm.[31] In the initial distance image, each surface voxel is set to zero and nonsurface voxels are set to infinity. The distance image is modified with two sequential passes. The forward pass moves over the volume left to right, top to bottom, and front to back. The backward pass moves in exactly the opposite way.

5.3.2 Cost Function Formulation

The distance transformation is applied only to the base surface. Match surface points are geometrically transformed (e.g., translated and/or rotated) as the algorithm searches through 6-D parameter space. At each point in parameter space, the cost function is derived from the root mean square average (r.m.s) of the voxel values in the distance image which correspond to each of the transformed match points:

$$\frac{1}{3}\left(\frac{1}{n}\sum_{m=1}^{n} d^2{}_{i_m,j_m,k_m}\right)^{1/2} \tag{5.3}$$

where (i_m, j_m, k_m) are the coordinates of the mth sample point after geometric transformation, and n is the number of points sampled from the match surface. The root-mean-square average is divided by 3 to compensate for the unit distance 3 in the Chamfer 3/4/5 distance transformation.[31]

5.3.3 Robust Matching

Chamfer matching assumes that the best registration is achieved at the point where the cost function reaches the global minimum. This assumption is true only if:

1. There is only one global minimum point in the cost function;
2. The match surface is not severely distorted relative to the base surface; and
3. Every sampled match surface point has a corresponding point existing on the base surface.

Assumption (1) is satisfied for most medical images that have no rotational symmetry, i.e., there exists only one true matching position. Assumption (2) must be satisfied in order for the assumption of rigid body motion to be true. If it is not satisfied, then a more complicated algorithm, like elastic matching),[36] should be used (although the rigid body transformation can be used as a first-order approximation). Assumption (3) will be satisfied if the images are acquired so that the base volume contains the match volume, and if there is no noise or distortion to add an extra component to the match volume.

The match surface points can be described as either real match points, which have corresponding points on the base surface, or as outliers, which have no such corresponding points. Outliers include noise, extra components, and distorted match points. The total cost is then the sum of costs caused by real match points and outliers. The contribution to the cost from real match points will yield the global minimum at the true registration point, but the cost contributed by outliers may result in a global minimum at a different point. In other words, the presence of outliers may cause a shift in the global registration point. Ideally, one would eliminate all outliers from the match surface to avoid this shift, but automatic recognition of these outliers is difficult and manual editing requires conceptualization of complex spatial transformations (except in the simplest of cases). If a threshold is set for the maximum cost contribution from outliers, then the component cost for outliers is held constant near the true registration point. It may be assumed that for correct registration, the true match points are near the base surface, and most of the outliers are farther away. Therefore, a threshold term (t) can be introduced into the cost function as follows:

$$\frac{1}{3}\left(\frac{1}{n}\sum_{m=1}^{n}\min(t^2, d^2_{i_m,j_m,k_m})\right)^{1/2} \qquad t = \text{threshold} \qquad (5.4)$$

Match surface points having a distance value greater than the threshold will be considered outliers and set to a constant. The value is chosen such that it is large enough to tolerate small degrees of noise, distortion, and transformation error associated with the true matching surface, but small enough to threshold outliers.

A simple 2-D contour image may be used for illustration, as shown in Figure 5.30 (see color figure 20). The base contour and the match contour are depicted as a_1 and a_2, respectively. The respective distance images are b_1 and b_2 (without thresholding), and c_1 and c_2 (with thresholding). The thresholding operation results in a sharper and narrower dip around the true registration point and introduces more local minima around the global minimum (c_3), making it harder to find. However, as the threshold increases, the shallow local minima around the global minimum tend to be smoothed out, and the dip around the global minimum gets wider but stays near the true registration point. As the algorithm searches around the global minimum,

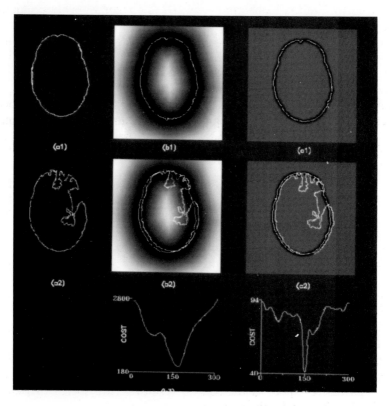

Figure 5.30. When matching difficult surfaces, greater robustness can be achieved by thresholding the Chamfer distance function. In this example a match contour (center row) with regions not present on the base contour (top row) is displaced by 150 pixels in x. Matching with an unthresholded Chamfer distance function locates an error minimum at approximately 160 pixels displacement (bottom row), because the high error associated with the nonmatching parts biases the low error of the matching region. By thresholding the Chamfer distance function (right column), the bias is removed, and the error minimum is found at the correct 150 pixels displacement. See color figure 20.

the cost caused by outliers is held nearly constant and the cost of the real match surface points is minimized.

Instead of applying one threshold directly, a multilevel threshold approach is used, starting with a higher threshold and gradually reducing it while iterating through multiscale space. Currently, the threshold for the highest resolution level (t_0) is empirically decided, and the thresholds for the lower levels are determined by multiplying t_0 by the square root of the scale factor for that resolution level. Using a straight downhill search method, the minimization begins at each level with the result from the previous level as an initial search point. A multithreshold approach decreases the number of local minima to some extent but does not entirely eliminate the problem, even when outliers do not exist. A systematic search of parameter space is guaranteed to find the global minimum but is computationally prohibitive. Even less exhaustive search methods, such as simulated annealing,[37] are not practical. The ANALYZE™ approach is to use multiple starting points, searching downhill towards a local minima for each point. The minimum among these minima is considered to be global. The interval between starting points should be small enough to find the global minimum.

A multiresolution approach is also used to speed the registration process. Borgefors[32] combines this technique with the Chamfer matching to match two-dimensional contours. Matching begins at the lowest resolution level and the result is used to guide higher-level computation. At the highest level, only fine adjustment is needed.

The distance transformation (with thresholding) is performed at each resolution level of the base surface image. The lower-resolution images should preserve rough shape information about the original surface so that the matching result at lower resolutions can guide the matching process at successively higher resolutions. For most medical images, the initial image can be reduced to as small as 20×20 pixels.[2] At low resolution, the size of the image and therefore the size of the search space is reduced substantially, and fewer starting points are needed. At each level, all the resulting local minima are sorted, and the average cost of the smallest 10% of the starting points is calculated. Starting points whose cost is smaller than twice this average are used at the next resolution level. Therefore, most of the starting points are rejected at low resolution levels, and only a small portion are used at the highest resolution levels. Finally, the local minima associated with each point in parameter space at the highest resolution are sorted to yield the global minimum used for the registration transformation.

A priori knowledge about image orientation and position can be effectively used by specifying a search range for the parameter space that will be centered on a "best initial guess" (e.g., the centroid or approximate orientation). The starting search points are uniformly distributed within this search range. The whole process can be implemented iteratively by repeating the matching process with the previous result as the best initial guess at the next iteration. The search space is substantially reduced at the following iteration so that it may be implemented with a smaller grid interval for a finer search result. The iterative process may be terminated when the difference between transformations from two consecutive iterations is less than a prespecified threshold. This threshold is usually determined empirically.

The combination of multithreshold and multiresolution approaches implemented with a multilevel distance transformation makes the algorithm efficient and robust. It has been demonstrated to rapidly converge in a large number and variety of test cases.[10] Computation time may be decreased further by approximating the distance value using the value of the corresponding voxel at a lower-resolution distance image. Since a threshold is already applied to the distance image, the cost function reverts to the same as Equation 5.3.

For illustration, the algorithm is applied to a 3-D set of T1- and T2-weighted MR images, as shown in Figure 5.31. Several slices through the original T1 volume (top row) and registered T2 volume (bottom row) are selected for display. The fused (integrated) images for each respective slice

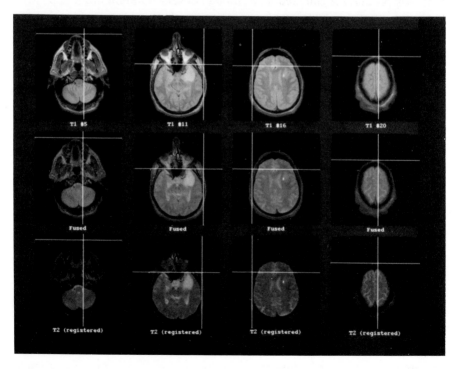

Figure 5.31. These T1 and T2 volumetric MR images of the head have been coregistered by surface matching using the skin surfaces from both scans. Four sections at different levels in the head of the original T1 (top), registered T2 (bottom), and fused (center) images are shown with linked cursors. The correspondence of features in the images at multiple levels indicates the excellent global quality of the match.

are shown in the center row. Since a surface-matching best-fit solution is a compromise of errors distributed over a fairly large surface, it is very likely to lie near a best-fit solution for the entire 3-D image space, as shown in Figure 5.31.

Many problems plague global minimum search algorithms, including avoiding local minima and sensitivity to surface noise. Nonetheless, proper application of multiscale search and noise thresholding techniques can yield rapid automated image registration, even though anatomic surfaces generally have many local minima. Additional immunity to noisy surfaces can be provided by thresholding the error function. This causes the error due to widely divergent regions of the surface to be limited, so as not to unduly influence the correctly matching surface components.

Surface matching, as compared to point or landmark matching, also provides a natural solution to matching images that only partly overlap with each other. This is frequently the case when one imaging modality will provide only a partial scan of the anatomy relative to a more complete scan by another imaging modality. If the partial "match" surfaces are sufficiently large and properly segmented, even though in very different orientation from the more complete "base" surface, a robust surface-matching algorithm can accurately register the two data sets.

As mentioned, this registration algorithm has been fully implemented in ANALYZE™. ANALYZE™ contains many useful tools complementary to the image registration and fusion process. These include highly automated 3-D segmentation routines for preparing surfaces for registration, and powerful display algorithms, including fast volume rendering, for visual confirmation of registration accuracy.

5.3.4 Examples of 3-D Registration on Patient Data

The ANALYZE™ algorithm has been applied to several sets of multimodality volume image data from clinical patient studies. In these cases, the ground truth transformation among two image data sets is not known, and the registration accuracy can only be visually confirmed. Using appropriate color-wash superposition displays and accurate linked cursors, pixel-to-pixel correspondence can be objectively evaluated.

An MR head image of dimension $256 \times 256 \times 123$ with voxel size 0.98 $\times$ 0.98 $\times$ 1.5 mm^3, and a PET brain image from the same patient, dimensions $128 \times 128 \times 15$ and voxel size $2.0 \times 2.0 \times 6.5$ mm^3, were selected for registration, as shown in Figure 5.32. Note the significant differences in orientation (sagittal for the MR, transverse for the PET) between the two acquired data sets. This presents no difficulty for the registration process, as long as appropriate corresponding surfaces can be obtained. The brain was segmented from both images and used as the common object for registration. The MRI brain was used for the base surface and the PET brain was used for the match surface. The threshold was set to 2.0% of the match

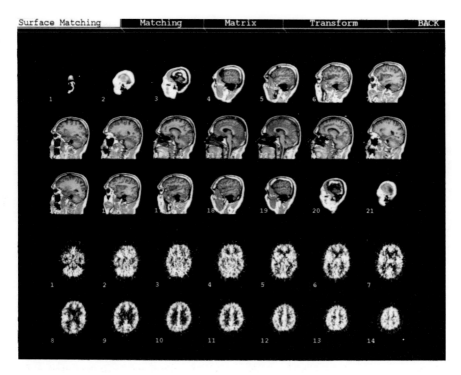

Figure 5.32. Upper three rows show original MR head images. Lower two rows show original PET images of same head, which have been enlarged (2×) for display purposes only. Note significantly different orientation and scale of scans. Yet robust surface matching can register these two data sets.

surface dimension for the highest level of resolution. In this case, the PET brain surface was completely contained within the MRI brain surface. The results demonstrate good registration (within one or two pixels) and can be displayed in different ways. In Figure 5.33 (see color figure 21) representative transverse images are shown for the original PET (upper left) and registered MRI (lower right); the MRI slice was resectioned to the PET slice orientation. The two slices are shown fused by color wash (upper right). The computed transformation matrix and global matching error are also shown (lower left). Figure 5.34 (see color figure 22) shows fused sections throughout the entire 3-D volume in the sagittal orientation (PET slices resectioned to MRI slices). These images show the limited extent of the PET scan.

In another patient, an MR head image of dimensions $256 \times 256 \times 124$ with voxel size $0.781 \times 0.781 \times 1.2$ mm³, and a SPECT brain image from the same patient, dimensions $64 \times 64 \times 15$ and voxel size $2.0 \times 2.0 \times 6.5$ mm³, were selected for registration. The brain was segmented from both images and used as the common object for registration. The patient was scanned with special markers attached to the skin surface, which can be

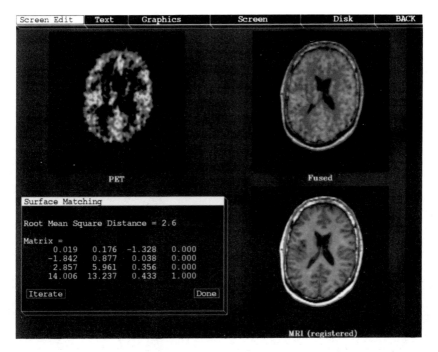

Figure 5.33. A selected slice from MRI and PET volume data demonstrating coregistration. Upper left is an original transverse PET slice from volume and lower right is a corresponding registered MRI slice, resectioned by computed transformation matrix shown at lower left. Fused images are shown at upper right. See color figure 21.

seen in both MR and SPECT images, so that the results are displayed in two and three dimensions, as shown in Figures 5.35 to 5.37 (see color figures 23 to 25). All external markers and internal anatomic landmarks are in good registration.

In one final example, an MR head image of dimensions $256 \times 256 \times 26$ with voxel size $0.938 \times 0.938 \times 3.0$ mm^3 and a CT head image from the same patient, dimensions $512 \times 512 \times 10$ and voxel size $0.674 \times 0.674 \times 3.0$ mm^3, were selected for registration. The skin surface was segmented from both images and used in the matching process. The patient was scanned in a stereotaxic head frame with markers visible in both MR and CT images. Although the markers were not used in the registration process, registration accuracy can be evaluated visually by observing the alignment of the markers, using a linked cursor, as shown in Figure 5.38. These prominent anatomic landmarks appear to be in good registration.

It is difficult to test registration accuracy without "ground truth" information. The average r.m.s. distance between the base and match surfaces may not accurately reflect the quality of registration because the measured

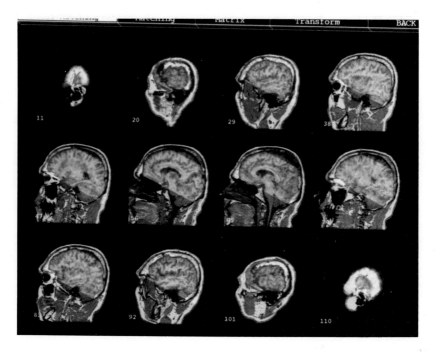

Figure 5.34. PET volume data transformed to match MRI volume data. Multiple slices from 3-D MRI and registered PET image are superimposed using color diffusion ("colorwash") technique to illustrate registration accuracy. See color figure 22.

cost contains contributions from misregistration, noise, and/or distortion of contours. Even in the case of simple misalignment, the exact transformation between base and match surfaces must be known to usefully measure registration accuracy. In the ANALYZE™ matching algorithm, the point-to-point correspondence between the match surface points and the base surface points is not known, and the minimal distance surface point on the base surface is used as the corresponding point for the match surface point. Therefore, the cost function value does not measure true registration accuracy. For example, one pixel misregistration in the x-axis direction may yield a different cost value than one pixel misregistration in the y-direction. To validate the ANALYZE™ algorithm using simulation studies, match images were generated by transforming the base image with a set of *known* parameters, and then the algorithm was used to register the match surface with the base surface. From the applied transformation, true registration accuracy could be calculated.[10] A disadvantage of this approach is that the simulated data may differ in some critical way from real data.

Registration accuracy depends on the algorithm's ability to find the global minimum and the faithfulness with which the global minimum represents accurate registration. The characteristics of the cost function, such as the

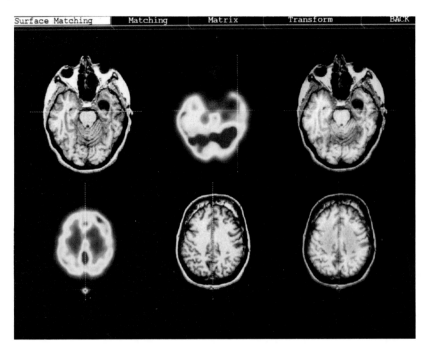

Figure 5.35. Sections of MRI and SPECT volume scan used as base and match images (top row); and a different section matching MRI to SPECT (bottom row). Registered, resectioned image is in center; fused images are at right. See color figure 23.

local minimum property and the concave property, are very complex and depend on the shape of the two surfaces being matched. There is simply no straightforward way of characterizing such a cost function. Generally, for the base object, having more surfaces of different slopes in different orientations can help in detecting subtle misregistration. Outliers from the match surface introduced by the imaging process or by contour segmentation may influence a shift of the global minimum point away from the point of true registration. Threshold values must be carefully chosen to eliminate their effect on the cost function. Noise that affects points close to the surface cannot be simply discriminated by a single distance threshold. However, the noise effect will largely be averaged out by using a sufficiently large number of points in the matching process.

Computation time scales with the number of sampled points from the match surface used and with the size of the search space and number of starting search points. For a volume image of $256 \times 256 \times 256$ elements (16 megabytes), an elapsed time of approximately 3 minutes is typically required to find an optimal transformation on a modern desktop workstation.[10] User interaction or monitoring of the matching process is usually not needed.

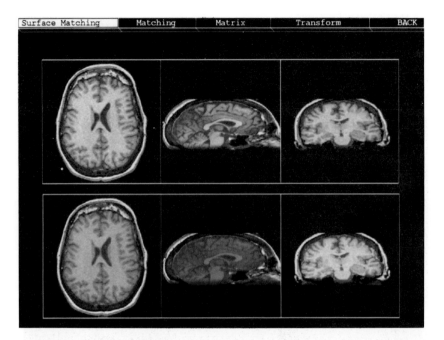

Figure 5.36. Three orthogonal section views of registered and fused MR and SPECT images. Segmented SPECT image with markers is superimposed on MRI. Markers are in good registration in all three orthogonal planes. See color figure 24.

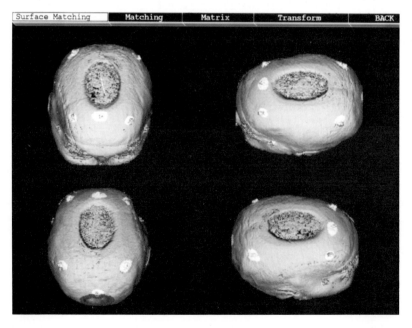

Figure 5.37. Four views of MRI head surface with superimposed overlapping markers from registered SPECT image. Registered MRI markers are visible beneath SPECT markers. Markers are in good registration on displayed surface. See color figure 25.

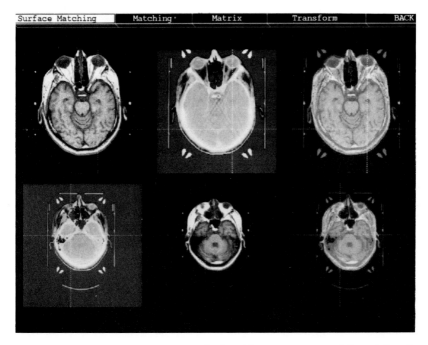

Figure 5.38. Registration of MRI and CT head images; top row, left to right, shows MRI base image, corresponding registered CT match image, and fused image of MRI and CT using color diffusion technique, respectively. Presence of stereotaxic frame markers and use of linked cursors allow visual confirmation of accuracy of registration. Both bone from CT and brain from MRI are visible in fused image. Bottom row shows different slice level, using CT as base image and MRI as match image.

The registration results for the patient data are very promising. Examination by qualified experts (radiologists) suggests that all obvious landmarks are in good registration with visually confirmable accuracy. Determining a statistically significant value for the registration accuracy in such studies is nearly impossible, however, without extensive applications to a large number of data sets. However, the registration accuracy depends on statistical characteristics, such as spatial sampling, noise level and type, percent of surface overlap, and complexity of surface features. Ongoing validation of the algorithm will take these factors into consideration.

5.4 References

1. Pizer, S. M., Cullip, T. J., Fredericksen, R. E. "Toward interactive object definition in 3D scalar images." In: Höhne, K. H., Fuchs, H., Pizer, S. M. (Eds.) *3D Imaging in Medicine, Algorithms, Systems, Applications.* NATO ASI Series, Series F: Computer and Systems Sciences, Vol. 60, Springer-Verlag, Berlin, Heidelberg, 1990.

2. Kübler, O., Gerig, G. "Segmentation and analysis of multidimensional data-sets in medicine." In: Höhne, K. H., Fuchs, H., Pizer, S. M. (Eds.) *3D Imaging in Medicine, Algorithms, Systems, Applications*. NATO ASI Series, Series F: Computer and Systems Sciences, Vol. 60, Springer-Verlag, Berlin, Heidelberg, 1990.

3. Griffin, L. D., Colchester, A. C. F., Robinson, G. P. "Scale and segmentation of grey-level images using maximum gradient paths." In: Colchester, A. C. F., Hawkes, D. J. (Eds.) *Information Processing in Medical Imaging. 12th International Conference, IPMI '91*, Wye, United Kingdom, Proceedings, No. 511, Springer-Verlag, July 1991.

4. ter Haar Romeny, B. M. Florack, L. M. J., Koenderink, J. J., Viergever, M. A. "Scale-space: its natural operators and differential invariants." In: Colchester, A. C. F., Hawkes, D. J. (Eds.) *Information Processing in Medical Imaging. 12th International Conference, IPMI '91*, Wye, United Kingdom, Proceedings, No. 511, Springer-Verlag, July 1991.

5. Merickel, M. B., Jackson, T., Carman, C., Brookeman, J. R., Ayers, C. R. "A multispectral pattern recognition system for noninvasive evaluation of atherosclerosis utilizing MRI." In: Höhne, K. H., Fuchs, H., Pizer, S. M. (Eds.) *3D Imaging in Medicine, Algorithms, Systems, Applications*. NATO ASI Series, Series F: Computer and Systems Sciences, Vol. 60, Springer-Verlag, Berlin, Heidelberg, 1990.

6. Höhne, K. H., Hanson, W. A. "Interactive 3D-segmentation of MRI and CT volumes using morphological operations." *J. Comput. Assist. Tomogr.*, 10, 41–53, 1990.

7. Collins, D. L., Peters, T. M., Dai, W., Evans, A. "Model-based segmentation of individual brain structures from MRI data." In: Robb, R. A. (Ed.) *Proceedings of Visualization in Biomedical Computing 1992. SPIE*, Vol. 1808, Chapel Hill, NC, October 13–16, 1992.

8. Pelizzari, C. A., Tan, K. K., Levin, D. N., Chen, G. T. Y., Balter, J. "Interactive 3-D patient-image registration." In: Colchester, A. C. F., Hawkes, D. J. (Eds.) *Information Processing in Medical Imaging. 12th International Conference, IPMI '91*, Wye, United Kingdom, Proceedings, No. 511, Springer-Verlag, July 1991.

9. van den Elsen, P. A., Maintz, J. B., Pol, E. D., Viergever, M. A. "Image fusion using geometrical features." In: Robb, R. A. (Ed.) *Proceedings of Visualization in Biomedical Computing 1992. SPIE*, Vol. 1808, Chapel Hill, NC, October 13–16, 1992.

10. Jiang, H., Robb, R. A., Holton, K. S. "New approach to 3-D registration of multimodality medical images by surface matching." In: Robb, R. A. (Ed.) *Proceedings of Visualization in Biomedical Computing 1992. SPIE*, Vol. 1808, Chapel Hill, NC, October 13–16, 1992.

11. Evans, A. C., Beil, C., Marrett, S., Thompson, C. J., Hakim, A. "Anatomical-functional correlation using an adjustable MRI-based region of interest atlas with position emission tomography." *J. Cereb. Blood Flow Metabol.*, 8, 513–529, 1988.

12. Hawkes, D. J., Hill, D. L. G., Lehmann, E. D., Robinson, G. P., Maisey, M. N., Colchester, A. C. F. "Preliminary work on the interpretation of SPECT images with the aid of registered MRI images and an MR derived neuro-anatomical atlas." In: Höhne, K. H., Fuchs, H., Pizer, S. M. (Eds.) *3D Imaging in Medicine, Algorithms, Systems, Applications*. NATO ASI Series, Series F: Computer and Systems Sciences, Vol. 60, pp. 241–252, Springer-Verlag, Berlin, Heidelberg, 1990.

13. Colchester, A. C. F., Hawkes, D. J. (Eds.) *Information Processing in Medical Imaging. 12th International Conference, IPMI '91*, Wye, United Kingdom, Proceedings, No. 511, Springer-Verlag, July 1991.

14. Robb, R. A. (Ed.) *Proceedings of Visualization in Biomedical Computing 1992. SPIE,* Vol. 1808, Chapel Hill, NC, October 13–16, 1992.

15. Barrett, H. H., Gmitro, A. F. (Eds.) *Information Processing in Medical Imaging. 13th International Conference, IPMI '93,* Flagstaff, AZ, No. 687, Springer-Verlag, June 1993.

16. Foley, J. D., Van Dam, A., Feiner, S., Hughs, J. *Computer Graphics: Principles and Practice.* 2nd Ed. Addison-Wesley Publishing Co., Reading, MA, 1990.

17. Robb, R. A., Camp, J. J. "A paradigm for using multispectral images in evaluating tumor response to treatment." *XIIIth International Conference on Information Processing in Medical Imaging,* Northern Arizona University, Flagstaff, AZ, June 14–18, 1993.

18. Llacer, J., Veklerov, E. "The maximum likelihood estimator method of image reconstruction: its fundamental characteristics and their origin." In: de Graaf, C. N., Viergever, M. A. (Eds.) *Proceedings of the 10th International Conference on Information Processing in Medical Imaging.* Plenum Press, New York, 1988.

19. Specht, D. F. "Probabilistic neural networks for classification, mapping, or associative memory." In: Rumelhart, D. E., McClelland, J. L. (Eds.) *Proceedings of the IEEE International Conference on Neural Networks,* San Diego, CA, July 1988, pp. 525–532.

20. Specht, D. F. "Probabilistic neural networks." *Neural Networks,* 3, 109–118, 1990.

21. Serra, J. *Image Analysis and Mathematical Morphology.* Academic Press, London, 1982.

22. Haralick, R. M. Sternberg, S. R., Zhuang, X. "Image analysis using mathematical morphology." *IEEE Trans. Pattern Anal. Machine Intell.,* Vol. PAMI-9, 1987, pp. 532–550.

23. Merickel, M., McCarthy, M. "Registration of contours for 3-D reconstruction." *IEEE Annual Conference of the Engineering in Medicine and Biology Society,* 1984, pp. 616–620.

24. Fleming, J. S. "A technique for motion correction in dynamic scintigraphy." *Eur. J. Nucl. Med.,* 9, 397–402, 1989.

25. Boesecke, R., Bruckner, T., Gabriele, E. "Landmark based correlation of medical images." *Phys. Med. Biol.,* 35, 121–126, 1990.

26. Abu-Mostafa, Y. S., Psaltis, D. "Recognitive aspects of moments invariants." *IEEE Trans. Pattern Anal. Machine Intell.,* PAMI-6, 1984, pp. 698–706.

27. Faber, T. L., Stokely, E. M. "Orientation of 3-D structures in medical images." *IEEE Trans. Pattern Anal. Machine Intell.,* PAMI-10, September 1988, pp. 626–633.

28. Pelizzari, C. A., Chen, G. T. Y. "Registration of multiple diagnostic imaging scans using surface fitting." *Proc. 9th ICCR,* 1987, pp. 437–440.

29. Pelizzari, C. A., Chen, G. T. Y. "Accurate three-dimensional registration of CT, PET, and/or MR images of the brain." *J. Comput. Assist. Tomogr.,* 13, 20–26, 1989.

30. Goldstein, H. *Classical Mechanics.* 2nd Ed. Addison-Wesley, Reading, MA, 1970, pp. 93–142.

31. Borgefors, G. "Distance transformations in arbitrary dimensions." *Comput. Vision Graphics, Image Proc.,* 27, 321–345, 1984.

32. Borgefors, G. "Hierarchical Chamfer matching: A parametric edge matching algorithm." *IEEE Trans. Pattern Anal. Machine Intell.,* 10, 849–865, 1988.

33. Barrow, H. G., Tenenbaum, J. M., Bolles, R. C., Wolf, H. C. "Parametric correspondence and Chamfer matching: Two new techniques for image matching." *Proc. 5th Int. Joint Conf. Artificial Intell.*, 1977, pp. 659–663.

34. Raya, S. P., Udupa, J. K. "Shape-based interpolation of multidimensional objects." *IEEE Trans. Med. Imag.* TMI-9, 1990, pp. 32–42.

35. Herman, G. T., Bucholtz, C. A., Zheng, J. "Shape-based interpolation using modified cubic splines." *Annual International Conference of the IEEE Engineering in Medicine and Biology Society,* Vol. 13, No. 1, 1991.

36. Bajcsy, R., Broit, C. "Matching of deformed images." *IEEE Proc. 6th Int. Conf. on Pattern Recognition,* 1982, pp. 351–353.

37. Kirkpatric, S. "Optimization by simulated annealing." *Science,* 220, 671–680, 1983.

6

Image Measurement
and Meaning

What is observable is only a sign of the physical fact ... The problem of observation is all but eclipsed by the problem of meaning.
Suzanne K. Langer, *Philosophy in a New Key*

6.1 Introduction

In addition to the power of images for visualization and intuitive comprehension of complex physical relationships,[1-3] digital images are inherently measurable—and measurements provide insights, understanding, and meaning. However, the usefulness of image measurements depends on the accuracy and reproducibility of the measurements, which in turn are dependent upon image type, fidelity, and "realness," and on the method or algorithm used for measurement.

Images have many different attributes that may be measured reflecting the properties and features of the imaged object(s). One attribute which is relatively straightforward to measure is simply the spatial extent (length, area, volume) of imaged objects. This type of measurement might be used to calculate the surface area of skin needed in plastic surgery, to estimate the change in volume of brain tumors in response to radiation therapy treatment, or to determine the size and shape of prosthetics to be implanted in reconstructive surgery (all examples of applications in Chapter 7).

More complex measures of imaged objects, such as shape,[2,3] moments,[4,5] fractal signature,[6,7] average boundary energy,[4] etc., hold promise for automated image segmentation and understanding. These could facilitate improved or new diagnostic procedures. Measures of image grayscale statistics within selected object regions are also useful. Examples of their use include and form the basis for estimates of blood volume and blood flow from dynamic CT contrast scans,[8] quantization of regional brain metabolism using functional imaging modalities PET and SPECT,[9] and brain function mapping from MRI neurofunctional studies.[10]

Because the explicit segmentation of a region of interest in 3-D medical images has so many valuable uses (only one of which is visual verification of anatomy), measurements are most commonly made after manual or automated segmentation of an image or group of images into specific sets of substructures and/or features. However, there are also powerful statistical sampling techniques that can be used as an alternative to explicit segmentation. In many cases, accurate automated segmentation is not possible due to insufficient image quality, and the time required for careful manual segmentation is prohibitive. In such cases, statistical approaches often offer higher accuracy and reproducibility in measurements.

ANALYZE™ features both simple and complex, both deterministic and stochastic methods and tools for measuring the attributes of 3-D biomedical images. Several of these are demonstrated in this chapter. The errors important in measurements and their effect on understanding the "meaning of the numbers" will also be discussed.

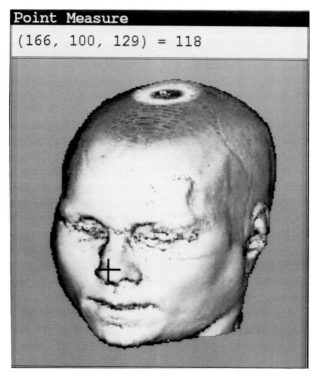

Figure 6.1. 3-D pixel coordinates and corresponding values are easily determined interactively by selecting a pixel on a 3-D image.

6.2 Region of Interest Measurements

The most basic measurements in medical images are simply computing 3-D coordinate locations. These might be made interactively by scanning through a stack of sections to find a certain structure, and then pointing to a feature on that structure in the desired section. More intuitively, it can be obtained by pointing to any location on a 3-D image, as shown in Figure 6.1. (The voxel value can be displayed at that point, as well.) Alternatively, 3-D points and planes can be obtained by selecting an exact or approximate location on a surface in a 3-D volume rendering of the object and seeing the orthogonal sections related to (intersecting) the selected point, as shown in Figure 6.2. Another useful measure is to identify all image pixels having the same value, either in a specific region, or for the entire image, as shown in

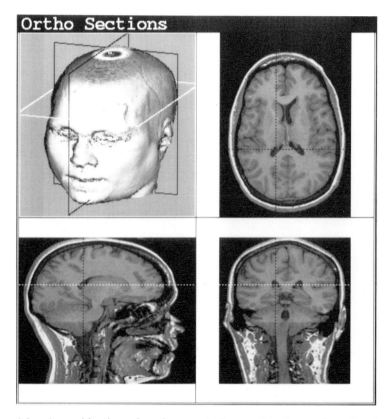

Figure 6.2. A combination of surface renderings and orthogonal section images makes locating structures intuitive and straightforward. The user may point to a voxel on the rendered surface or to a pixel on one of the orthogonal sections, and the 3-D coordinates and grayscale value of the chosen voxel or pixel are updated continuously.

Figure 6.3. Measurement of "line profiles" reveal the changing progression of image grayscale values along any traced line, as illustrated in Figure 6.4. Both straight and curvilinear traces can be profiled, providing both local distance and intensity information.

Linear and curvilinear distances may also be calculated in the 3-D coordinate system of the volume image. Euclidean distances between coordinates selected on different 2-D slices must often be calculated manually. But Euclidean and curvilinear distances between points on a 3-D volume rendering of a surface can be easily calculated automatically. The surface pixels lying in the "shadow" of the 2-D projection of a line traced on the surface from a selected viewpoint constitute samples on a curve in 3-D space, as shown in Figure 6.5. The length of the curved line is estimated by counting the scaled Euclidean distance between projected surface pixel centers along the curve. For the case of square 2-D pixels, only unit pixel and $\sqrt{2}$ pixel steps are possible in summing distance along the traces. For the 3-D cubic voxel case, unit voxel, $\sqrt{2}$ unit voxel, and $\sqrt{3}$ unit voxel steps are possible.

Figure 6.6 shows an example of various types of regions that may be specified and positioned on an image for measurement. The regions may be labeled for identification, annotation, and reproduction. When measurements are made, these labels can be recorded with the measurements, for preserving the association between the numbers and the region from which

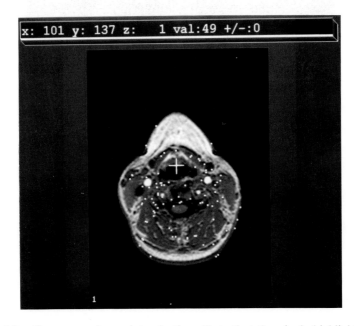

Figure 6.3.   Common value point selection. Note that the pixels highlighted have the same grayscale value as the selected pixel.

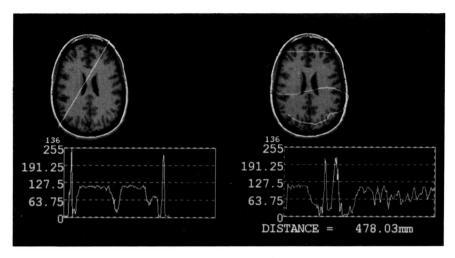

Figure 6.4. Straight and curved line profiles. Profiles reflect progression of pixel values along path of line.

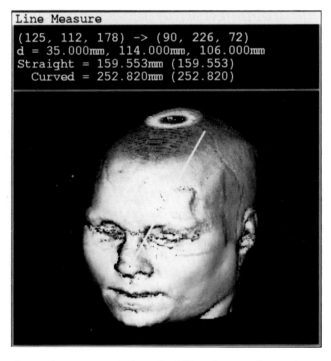

Figure 6.5. Two points on a rendering of a 3-D surface can be used to measure 2-D and 3-D straight and curvilinear distances.

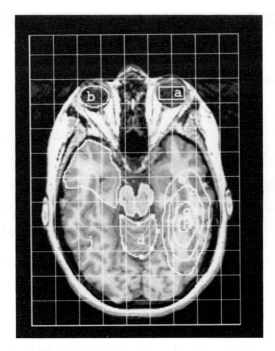

Figure 6.6. Various types of regions defined and positioned on an image for measurement.

they came. The labeled regions in Figure 6.6 have the following shapes: a) rectangle, b) ellipse, c) manual trace, d) spline with control points, e–h) divided traces where the user supplies an inside and outside trace and the computer calculates the specified number of interior dividing traces, i) an auto trace which is the border of a region defined by a user supplied seed point and a threshold range, and j) a grid region. Each of these regions can be individually sampled, measured in a variety of ways, and recorded for subsequent analyses.

The use of coregistered data from different imaging modalities often makes region definition and measurement more precise. For example, to measure the functional activity within a specific anatomic region of the brain, MR images are often used to precisely define the desired region(s), but the actual measurements are made on the same regions in coregistered PET data. Figure 6.7 (see color figure 26) shows such an anatomic region defined on an MRI properly positioned on the corresponding registered PET image.

Regional areas in 2-D images may be measured two different ways, as illustrated in Figure 6.8. The most straightforward way is simply to count all pixels included in the region and scale (multiply) the result by the known

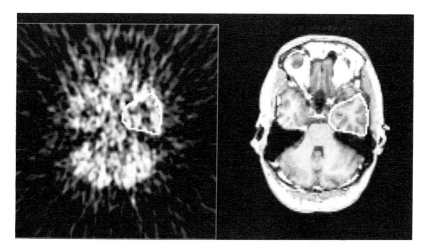

Figure 6.7. Defined regions of interest for measurement of coregistered data sets (MRI and PET). The desired anatomic region is specified in the high-resolution MRI, and the functional measurement made in the corresponding regions in the PET image. See color figure 26.

area of a pixel. However, this approach assumes that the border lies exactly along the edges of the boundary pixels in the region, and that the region was segmented to contain all pixels known to be entirely part of the object. Under these conditions, pixel counting gives highly reproducible results, although they are likely to consistently overestimate the area and perimeter of the actual object.

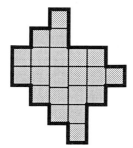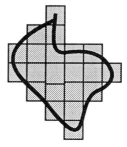

Figure 6.8. On the left, the object boundary is assumed to lie along the pixel borders. Both the area and the perimeter of small objects may be estimated using this method, although it generally overestimates them both. On the right, the boundary pixel coordinates lie on an analytic curve which is the true boundary (curves of varying complexity may be used). This method is more accurate for the measurement of the area and perimeter of large objects, but will tend to slightly underestimate them both.

On the other hand, if the image region was segmented to contain all pixels thought to be even partially in the object of interest, area may be more accurately estimated by considering the region boundary as a curve connecting the centers of the edge pixels, and calculating the area bounded by that curve. Simple line-segment boundaries provide useful estimates, but the detailed boundary formed by analytical curves is more accurate when knowledge about the anatomy and imaging modality used can be included in the definition of the curve. It may slightly underestimate the actual perimeter and area of the object.

In addition to the area and perimeter of a 2-D region of a 2-D image, various shape-descriptive measurements can be made. The minimum enclosing rectangle (MER), its attitude and aspect ratio, give some indication of the orientation and compactness of a region. The ratio of the area of the region to the area of the MER, known as the rectangular fit factor (RFF), indicates how well the region fills its MER, while measurements such as circularity ($C = P^2/A$) indicate how efficiently the shape encloses space.[3]

In many applications, the measurement of interest may be the statistical distribution of grayscale values within the region. This is the basis, for example, of the measurement of blood flow and perfusion from changes in dye concentration, of average metabolism rate in PET or other functional brain images, and of comparative exposure in autoradiograms. The maximum, minimum, mean, and standard deviation are the most commonly derived statistical measures. The grayscale histogram of an image region contains the entire statistical distribution. The properly scaled sum of all pixel values in the region of interest (or the summation over the region's histogram) is known as the integrated optical density (IOD).[4] If the image is thresholded, the sum of pixel values above the threshold in the region is known as the brighteness area product (BAP). The BAP is useful for estimating the amount of high-contrast material in a region, such as radiopaque dye injected into the bloodstream.[8]

Measuring the distribution of grayscale values within a region (rather than the mass and shape properties of the region itself) for common geometric shapes can be very useful. Figure 6.9 illustrates that circular, elliptical, or rectilinear subregions of a homogeneous image region give very similar statistical measures. Subcompartment measures are often desired in biological perfusion and diffusion studies. Figure 6.10 illustrates the use of "pie-wedge" dividers defined by equally spaced radial lines extending to anatomic boundaries to measure differential diffusion around the wall of the heart.

Regions of interest can be selected manually on each image or extruded through a defined number of successive sectional images in a volume to facilitate measurements in 3-D. Such a series of adjacent 2-D regions forms a 3-D volume of interest (VOI). Figure 6.11 shows a VOI defined for a brain tumor on a series of MR images of the head.

Extending the analysis and measurement of regions from 2-D to 3-D exposes a paradox: tomographic sections contain unambiguous information

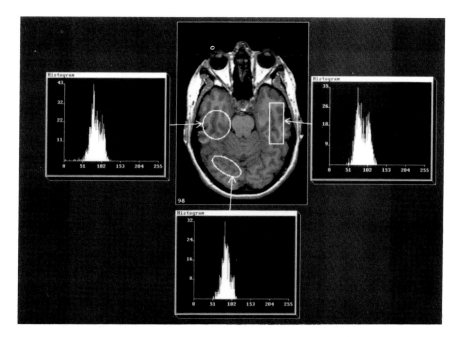

Figure 6.9. The use of geometric regions in image measurement. Note that the mean and standard deviation of the grayscale are nearly identical in the various-shaped regions.

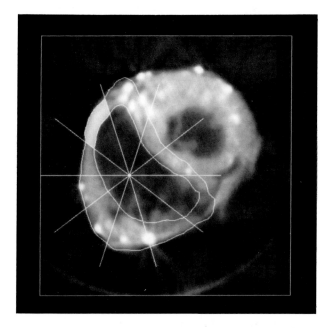

Figure 6.10. A radial divider bounded by the anatomic outline of the heart is used to measure differential transmoval perfusion in the myocardium. The brightness area product (BAP) can be calculated for each individual region to measure the amount of radiopaque dye in the local tissue compartments.

215

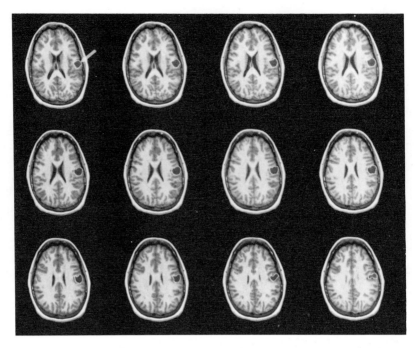

Figure 6.11.   Definition of volume of interest (VOI) for measuring tumor (arrow) in MRI scan.

about the interior of objects in a basically unintuitive and difficult-to-analyze form, whereas 3-D renderings of objects are intuitively natural, familiar forms, which contain no direct information about their interiors. Thus, while there is usefulness in tools that allow regions to be defined intuitively from 3-D renderings, a section-by-section review is often necessary to critically analyze the information interior to a region. Conversely, there is significant

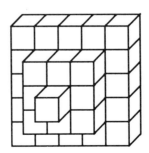

Figure 6.12.   This solid object contains 35 voxels; 34 of them lie on the surface, with a total of 86 exposed voxel faces.

utility in tools that allow section-by-section specification of region bound-aries, but 3-D rendering allows intuitive verification of the correct 3-D shape and full extent of the region. Therefore, both of these capabilities need to be maintained to facilitate efficient analysis of 3-D biomedical images.

The volume of 3-D solid regions is easily estimated by voxel counting; the precision of the measurement is inversely proportional to the number of voxels in the object. The surface area of a 3-D region presents more resis-tance to straightforward voxel-based estimation. If the image voxels are iso-tropic in dimension, the count of surface voxels (i.e., all object voxels hav-ing at least one nonobject neighbor) scaled by the squared voxel dimension may be a good estimate of surface area for large (several thousands of vox-els) objects. However, this generally produces an underestimation of the true surface area. Counting exposed voxel faces, as illustrated in Figure 6.12, produces a better estimate of surface area for small objects, but usually overestimates the true surface area. These two approaches are equivalent to the perimeter estimates described previously, and once again, greater accu-racy can be achieved by fitting a low-energy analytical boundary to the sur-face voxel coordinates and calculating the area mathematically.

6.3 Stereological Measurement Techniques

Another useful approach to measurement of object properties in 3-D images bypasses the interactive and presegmentation processes required by conven-tional region of interest (ROI) techniques. This approach makes estimations of area, volume, surface area, etc. through stereological techniques.[11] This process involves the simple and fast method of segmenting an object by counting the number of intersections a randomly oriented and positioned grid makes with the object being measured. Such approaches are based on the Cavalieri Principle,[12] which states that the volume of an object can be estimated by cutting the object into N equally spaced sections, finding the area of the object on each section, and appropriately weighting the sum of all such section areas. The estimate of the volume may be given by

$$V_{est} = T * (A_1 + A_2 + \ldots A_n)$$
(6.1)

where T is the thickness of each object slice.

The error in using this type of measuring scheme is based on how the measured area changes from slice to slice. An approximate coefficient of error (CE = SE/mean) for Equation 6.1 is

$$CE \simeq \left(\sum_{i=1}^{n} A_i \right)^{-1} * \left[\frac{1}{12} \left(3 \sum_{i=1}^{n} A_i^2 + \sum_{i=1}^{n-2} A_i A_{i+2} - 4 \sum_{i=1}^{n-1} A_i A_{i+1} \right) \right]^{\frac{1}{2}}$$
(6.2)

Clearly, voxel counting is one variant of this approach, in which the sub-divisions of the objects are the voxels themselves, and an explicit voxel-by-voxel segmentation of the object is required. Another approach involves the placement of a systematic grid of points over each section and counting the number of intersections between the points and the object. The spacing of the points determines the area contributed by each point that intersects the object. In this approach, fewer border decisions are needed, as many of the points will be either clearly on or off the object of interest. Also, the counting of the intersections has proven to be quicker than tracing the border of an object. Using this method

$$V_{\text{est}} = T * A_p * (P_1 + P_2 + \ldots P_n)$$ (6.3)

where A_p is the area associated with each point and P_n is the number of intersections counted on slice n. The error for this measurement can be broken into two parts, the error due to sectioning (Equation 6.2) and the error due to point counting. The error due to point counting is related to the ratio of the mean boundary length ($\bar{B}$) and the mean area of a section ($\bar{A}$):

$$\tilde{C}E^2 = 0.0724 \cdot \frac{\bar{B}}{\sqrt{\bar{A}}} \cdot \frac{\sqrt{n}}{\left(\sum_{i=1}^{n} P_i\right)^{\frac{3}{2}}}$$ (6.4)

Figure 6.13 shows a randomly positioned and rotated stereology grid superimposed on an image. Grid points that intersect the object can be easily

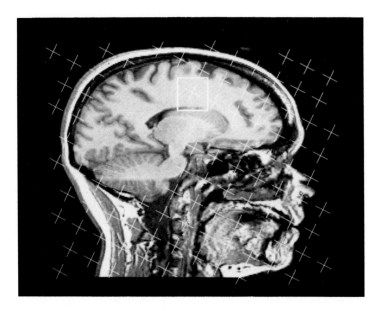

Figure 6.13. Randomly rotated and positioned grid for stereologic measurement of volume. A rectangular cursor collects points for statistical measure as it is passed over grid points.

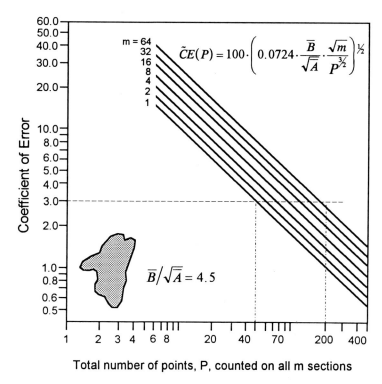

Figure 6.14.   Nomogram illustrates error contributions in point counting for defined shapes. Coefficient of error up to 3% is generally acceptable for useful measures.

collected by interactively positioning the square cursor over them. The question arises, "How many points need to be collected in order to obtain statistically significant, useful measurements?" Figure 6.14 shows a nomogram that plots the CE of the point-counting method against the total points sampled. For determining the volume of an organ from a group of subjects, it has been shown that 50–150 points per organ are usually sufficient to determine the volume[11,13] Using this number of points provides a 5% to 10% level of precision for a wide variety of shapes. Therefore, relatively accurate volume measurements can be made quickly using this method. The stereological grid technique also can be used to approximate the surface area of an object. This is accomplished by determination of the number of parallel grid lines which intersect with the border of the object.

6.4 Measurement in the Frequency Domain

Certain types of image features (such as patterns) are best measured in the frequency domain. Figure 6.15 (see color figure 27) illustrates an application

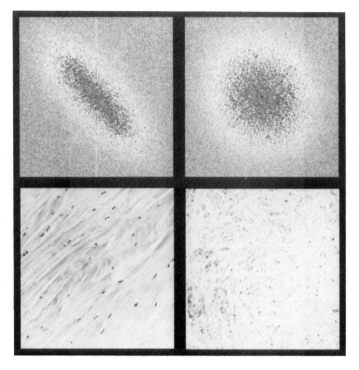

Figure 6.15. Fourier transform (color-scaled magnitude only) of anisotropic (left) and isotropic (right) photomicrographs of collagen show a clear Fourier feature related to the direction of anisotropy. See color figure 27.

of Fourier techniques to the analysis of photomicrographs of collagen. Collagen is an elastic connective tissue which often exhibits a directional pattern or texture under the microscope. Although the automated detection of subtle texture is often very difficult in the original image, the Fourier transform of anisotropic samples shows clearly the presence and direction of the texture. The summation of the Fourier spectrum in radial wedges further reduces the analysis to a vector that can be easily searched for the presence and direction of anisotropic texture.

6.5 Meaning

Measurement is both the process and the purpose of imaging. Meaning is the purpose of measurement. In its canonical form, an image is simply an array of samples (measurements) of the spatial distribution of some physical and/or functional property of an object or set of objects. However, understanding of the object and its properties cannot be completely gained by only observing these canonical data. Human knowledge of biology is founded on notions of anatomy and physiology, which are further based upon geometry and texture, and can only be augmented directly by measurements expressed in such terms.[1-3]

As a simple example, a set of adjacent CT sections of the entire head might be used to calculate the cranial volume of the skull. Notions such as "volume" and "the space inside the cranium" are basic models of the desired measurement, and measurements are necessary in this form if one is to make objective use of the image information. Neither "volume" nor "the space inside the cranium" is directly measured by the imaging device, only the distribution of radiopacity in space. Nonetheless, the required measure can be extracted from the image because the structures of interest are differentiated by their radiopacity.

In this case, the skull can be rather easily separated from soft tissue by its CT number. But there remain fundamental differences between "the skull" of a patient in the physical world and "the skull" as it appears in a 3-D medical image. A real-world skull is an object having an exact and unambiguous boundary. There is no part of space that can be conceptualized as "partially" skull: we consider all points in space to be either part of the skull or not part of the skull. The "skull" in an image, however, is represented by a statistical probability density function. Somewhere between voxels representing bone with 100% certainty and voxels representing non-bone with 100% certainty there are voxels that can only be described as being "partially" or "probably" bone with varying degrees of certainty (or perhaps uncertainty is a better term). This is the first philosophical impediment to deriving fully accurate and precise measurements from images: physical objects have definite boundaries and exact volumes, whereas images of objects have probabilistic borders from which discrete boundary estimates must be determined in order to calculate an approximate volume. Even intricate measurement schemes that attempt to increase the precision of volume measurement by collecting subvoxel contributions from "partial" skull voxels must specify precisely which voxels are allowed to make such a contribution to the volume calculation. Image finiteness and noise limit such precision, leading to uncertainty in measures made on them.

As another example, radiopaque dyes or microspheres may be used to quantify blood perfusion in myocardial tissue. With such techniques, it is possible to measure the dynamic global distribution of blood perfusion during the heartbeat from a sequence of high-speed multiplanar CT scans. The difficulty is that measurements are to be made of objects as they move (e.g., the perfusion in the cardiac muscle fiber decreases as it contracts, and increases as it relaxes). The inherent function of the imaging device is to sample space as objects move through it. The "perceived" perfusion in any voxel may be influenced by a piece of the myocardium ejecting blood, a less perfused piece of myocardium moving into the voxel space, or the myocardium moving partially out of any given voxel—a condition not sensed by the imaging device. All these contribute to uncertainty in the measure.

As a final example, it is common to use high-resolution images, such as obtained from MRI, in conjunction with low-resolution functional images, such as obtained from SPECT or PET, of the brain to measure the metabolism of specific brain structures under various conditions, such as aging, psychological disorders, drug effects, etc. The functional images can be calibrated such that voxel values are scaled exactly to uptake rates of specific isotopes or chemicals, but the complete extent of certain brain structures cannot be readily identified from the functional images alone (particularly if there is a partial functional deficit, a condition often to be expected in such studies). The high-resolution images are used (after coregistration with the functional images) to identify structures of interest, and the regions so defined are then reflected into the functional image data for measurement. However, a philosophical conundrum occurs: the low-resolution PET images not only have larger voxels than the region-defining MR images (as illustrated in Figure 6.7), but the image is blurred such that all of the uptake which occurs in a voxel-sized piece of tissue does not end up in a single voxel, but is partially added into neighboring voxels, resulting in uncertainty.

These examples illustrate both the blessing and the bane of modern digital/electronic medical imaging. The advantage is the significant potential for obtaining meaning from measurements of the numbers constituting the images. If these numbers are robust, then accurate, reproducible, quantitative assessments of anatomy and function of organs and tissues and cells of the body can be made for more sensitive and specific assessment of human disease—including improved accuracy in diagnosis of disease and enhanced effective clinical treatment with assured and reproducible positive outcome. The continually improving resolution, precision, and consistency of modern imaging systems to faithfully capture digital representations of anatomy and function underscore the hope for achieving this potential. Somewhat paradoxically, this same improvement in capabilities suggests the principal limitations of quantitative imaging. Imaging systems and imaging methodologies, as advanced as they are, are still imperfect and finite, and in the infinite perspective, digital images are coarse samples of real-world objects and their properties. Therefore, mensuration on images must be carefully done, accounting for a variety of linear and nonlinear, systematic and random sources of error. Resulting calculations become approximations, rather than exact measurements, hopefully always with error bounds to assist in characterizing the relative value of the measures.

Notwithstanding these imperfections, approximations, and errors, digital imaging has rapidly evolved toward its promise as a quantitative science: the "meaning" of structure and function in health and disease is unfolding as many *useful* measures, both absolute and relative, are now possible using

3-D biomedical imaging. The addition of the third dimension in imaging, especially when isotropic 3-D sampling is provided, has significantly extended the number, type, and value of quantitative, objective measurements helpful in characterizing and assessing form and function and in diagnosing and treating disease and pathology, both in biology and in medicine.

6.6 References

1. Olson, Ð. R., Bialystok, E. *Spatial Cognition*. Lawrence Erlbaum Associates, Hillsdale, NJ, 1983.

2. Uttal, W. R. (Ed.) *Visual Form Detection in 3-Dimensional Space*. Lawrence Erlbaum Associates, Hillsdale, NJ, 1983.

3. Koenderink, J. J. *Solid Shape*. MIT Press, Cambridge, MA, 1990.

4. Castleman, K. R. *Digital Image Processing*. A. Oppenheim (Ed.) Prentice-Hall, Englewood Cliffs, NJ, 1979.

5. Jain, A. K. *Fundamentals of Digital Image Processing*. Prentice-Hall, Englewood Cliffs, NJ, 1989.

6. Peleg, S., Naor, J., Hartley, R., Avnir, D. "Multiple resolution texture analysis and classification." *IEEE* PAMI-6 (4):518–532, 1984.

7. Pentland, A. "Fractal based descriptions of natural scenes." *IEEE* PAMI-6 (6):661–674, 1984.

8. Ritman, E. L., Robb, R. A., Wood, E. H. "Synchronous volumetric imaging for noninvasive vivisection of cardiovascular and respiratory dynamics: evolution and current perspectives." In: Brandenburg, R. O., Fuster, V., Giuliani, E. R., McGoon, D. C. (Eds.) *Cardiology—Fundamentals and Practice*. Year Book Medical Publishers, Chicago, 1987, Chapter 63, pp. 1968–1984.

9. Robb, R. A. *Three-Dimensional Biomedical Imaging. Vol. I & II*. CRC Press, Boca Raton, FL, 1985.

10. Jack, C. R., Thompson, R. M., Butts, R. K., et al. "Sensory motor cortex: correlation or presurgical mapping with functional MR imaging and invasive cortical mapping." *Radiology,* 190, 85–92, 1994.

11. Pache, J. C., Roberts, N., Zimmerman, A., Vock, P., Cruz-Orive, L. M. "Vertical LM sectioning and parallel CT scanning designs for stereology: application to human lung." *J. Microsc.,* 170, 3–24, 1993.

12. Cavalieri, B., 1635, Geometria Indivisibilibus Continuorum. Typis Clementis Ferronij, Bononiae. Reprinted 1966 as Geometria degli Indivisibili. Unione Tipografico-Editrice Torinese, Torino.

13. Michel, R. P., Cruz-Orive, L. M. "Application of the Cavalieri Principle and vertical sections method to lung: estimation of volume and pleural surface area. *J. Microsc.,* 150, 117–136, 1988.

7

Practical Applications

Tell me and I will forget, show me and I will remember, involve me and I will understand.

Old Chinese Proverb

7.1 Introduction

3-D biomedical imaging has matured sufficiently to be used in a variety of important clinical and advanced biological applications. These applications attest to the current effectiveness and future promise of 3-D imaging for solving certain problems better than "traditional" techniques, and for addressing other problems that have long resisted any solution at all. They represent achievement of the goal to move from science to practice, to refine laboratory methods into hospital procedures, to transfer the bench to the bedside.

The applications included in this chapter are meant to be exemplary, not exclusive. They illustrate the use of display, editing, and measurement of 3-D biomedical images for identifying, isolating, modifying, simulating, and quantifying data in support of specific clinical and/or scientific goals. All applications are illustrated using ANALYZE™, but several other software systems can provide similar, if not as comprehensive, capabilities. ANALYZE™ has been used extensively for faithful simulation, realistic rehearsal, and effective planning of medical treatment procedures, especially surgery. It provides direct support for incorporating 3-D visualization and virtual reality technology into the operating room. It has been used for both functional and structural analyses of cells, receptors, organs, and organ systems. Additionally it has been used for computer-aided education to teach anatomy using actual 3-D volume images of all regions of the body.

7.2 Neurofunctional Imaging and Neurosurgery Planning

Neuroimaging of brain structure and function presents complex visualization and analysis tasks for which many techniques and solutions are currently being developed[1,2] Visualization and measurement of structure–function relationships in the brain are fundamental to the understanding of specific cause-and-effect processes in both health and disease. Several invasive techniques are currently used to establish the relationship between abnormal function and specific neuroanatomical structures, including surgical placement of subdural electrode strips for both stimulating and measuring evoked central nervous system responses. 3-D image acquisition, processing, and visualization techniques which provide noninvasive correlation of the functional characteristics of the brain with its anatomic structure have the advantages of reducing patient risk, discomfort, and morbidity while providing acurate in vivo detection of function undisturbed by the invasive procedures.

Neurofunctional imaging of the brain frequently requires the integration of multimodality or multiscan image data for precise localization of structures and functions. Structural definition of the brain can be accomplished with X-ray CT and MR imaging, but neither alone can capture all of the structural definition of the brain and surrounding structures, particularly when specific devices are implanted or applied to the head. Together (correlated) they can provide 3-D image volumes for full 3-D localization of brain structures with certain constraints on spatial resolution and extent of 3-D coverage. Functional imaging of the brain has been primarily done using nuclear medicine techniques, including SPECT and PET imaging, using specific radioisotopes selected to measure cerebral blood volume (CBV), cerebral blood flow (CBF), and regional metabolism. The relatively poor spatial resolution of these devices significantly restricts accurate localization of function within specific structures, resulting in useful but limited measurement of global function within the context of the entire image. Recent advances[3–5] in neurofunctional imaging with MRI have provided noninvasive techniques for imaging the functional characteristics of the brain, usually as the result of an evoked response to a stimulus. The areas of evoked functional activity can be localized by obtaining additional MRI data for the 3-D structure of the brain, again requiring an integration of these image sets prior to visualization.

With functional MRI (fMRI) techniques, the functional information is gathered using blood oxygen level-dependent (BOLD) criteria.[6–7] Nuclear medicine imaging studies have demonstrated a local change in physiological activity in selected areas of the cortex associated with certain stimulation techniques.[8] Similarly, functional MRI is based on the local increase in cerebral perfusion required to deliver oxygen to regions of the cortex activated by certain stimuli. The oxygen delivery exceeds the metabolic need of the activated area, resulting in an increase in tissue perfusion and a net decrease

in the concentration of deoxyhemoglobin. Oxygenated hemoglobin is dia-
magnetic, whereas deoxyhemoglobin is paramagnetic, and this paramagnetic
property of deoxyhemoglobin creates local field inhomogeneities that reduce
the signal intensity on T2- or T2*-weighted MR images.[7] With the net overall
decrease in the concentration of deoxyhemoglobin in the activated region of
cortex, a net signal increase in the MR field occurs, resulting in an image
reflecting the functional area in the brain activated by the stimulus. These
techniques can be applied with conventional medium-field (1.5 T) clinical
scanners.[3,4]

Figure 7.1 illustrates an exemplary neurofunctional MRI process, indicating the steps used to integrate a functional activity image with an anatomic reference image. The study was performed[4] using an unmodified clinical MR scanner with a standard quadrature head coil, and processing all
images with ANALYZE™. The functional images were acquired during
photic stimulation using a flashing red light at a frequency of 8 Hz to stimulate the visual cortex. The functional image (bottom left) was acquired

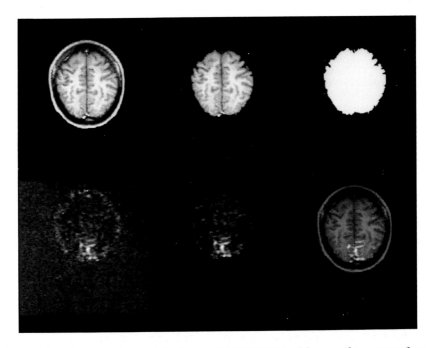

Figure 7.1. Segmentation and fusion in ANALYZE™ of images from neurofunctional MRI (fMRI) (lower row) and a T1-weighted spatial localization image (upper
row). The final integrated image (lower right) demonstrates the capability to visualize
functional information in the occipital cortex with the structural context for spatial
localization (Data courtesy of Drs. Richard Thompson and Clifford Jack, Mayo
Foundation.)

along an oblique plane through the calcarine cortex using an SPGR (spoiled gradient recalled echo) sequence with pulse sequence parameters optimized for functional signal activation.[4] The oblique plane was determined using a standard T1-weighted localization image (upper left) which was saved for integration with the functional image. Sequences of six "off" images (without photic stimulation) followed by six "on" images (with photic stimulation) were repeated twice, for a total of 24 images in the study. The first two images of each sequence were eliminated, as regional analysis of the time sequence showed these images to be at a signal level indicating a transition between the "off" and "on" states. The resulting eight "off" images were averaged to provide a baseline image, and the eight "on" images were similarly averaged to provide a single image of the activated state. These averaged images were then subtracted, providing the functional response image shown in the lower left of Figure 7.1.

The functional images were acquired within a short time following the selection of the oblique plane with the T1-weighted image, and the volunteer's head was structurally supported in the coil, so the two images were assured to be spatially registered, subject only to physiological motion in the head. The structure of the brain in the T1-weighted image was segmented (top center) using a region-growing technique. This image was used as a binary mask (top right) applied to (multiplied) the functional subtraction image (lower left) to specifically define the portion of the functional image corresponding to the brain (lower center image). A threshold was then applied to the segmented functional image to isolate the functional activity, and a grayscale map was applied. This functional image was then overlaid on the original T1-weighted image using grayscale compositing, resulting in the final integrated image shown in the lower right of Figure 7.1. This image provides direct 2-D visualization of the functional activity evoked by the photic stimulus localized with anatomic detail in the occipital cortex of the brain.

Figure 7.2 (see color figure 28) depicts visualization and analysis of neurofunctional activity in full 3-D context using ANALYZE™. The patient has a left frontoparietal lesion in the left sensory motor cortex which caused partial motor seizures of the right side of the face and hand.[5] This is depicted as the green structure in the volume-rendered image in the lower left panel of Figure 7.2. A 3-D SPGR sequence was used to image the structural anatomy of the entire brain, from which the renderings of the cortical surface and tumor were created using an object map for each structure. The brain was automatically segmented from the MRI volume image using 3-D mathematical morphology operations. Subdural electrodes were placed on the cortical surface in the vicinty of the left motor cortex and surrounding the tumor, followed by cortical stimulation studies to identify functionally essential cortex in the region of the tumor. A 3-D CT scan was done through this region to image the stainless steel electrode positions. The CT and 3-D MRI volume images were coregistered using surface matching on the corti-

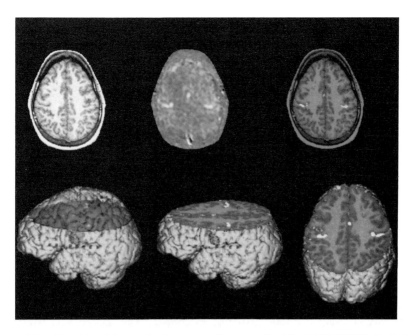

Figure 7.2. Functional images (upper row) integrated with ANALYZE™ depicting function in the motor cortex can be further visualized in full 3-D context (lower row), showing the location of the function (orange) in comparison to full 3-D brain anatomy (white) and tumor pathology (green). (Data courtesy of Dr. Clifford Jack, Mayo Foundation.) See color figure 28.

cal surface of the brain extracted from the two modalities. The electrodes were then segmented from the correlated CT and added into the volume-rendering object map, allowing direct visualization of the electrode positions (from CT) on the cortical surface of the brain (from MRI), as shown in red in the lower left image. The patient was then imaged using the neurofunctional techniques just described, using bilateral finger-to-thumb opposition and contraction and relaxation of the lip and lower face muscles as the evoked response stimulus (head and face muscle tightening were symptoms of the tumor-induced seizures). A T1-weighted oblique image was determined so as to section through the left sensory motor cortex (upper left), and the resultant neurofunctional evoked response (upper middle) and integrated structural and functional image (upper right) showing bilateral activation of the sensory motor cortex were computed. This activity can be observed adjacent to the tumor in this image (upper right), with the tumor visible immediately above the area of activation on the right side of the image (patient's left). The functional image plane was matched to the 3-D volume image, and an object indicating the position of this plane was added to the object map, as shown by the blue structure in the rendering (lower left).

Finally, the area of functional activity above a selected threshold was added to the object map, allowing the functional activation area to be rendered with all other structures, as depicted by the orange regions in the lower panel of images. The rendering in the lower left of Figure 7.2 uses 24-bit transparency to visualize the extent of the plane, tumor, and functional regions within the entire cortical surface of the brain. The renderings in the lower middle and lower right depict the areas of functional activation by clipping the volume at the location of the functional acquisition plane, revealing the T1-weighted image of the brain tissue and the precise location of the evoked response function.

Such direct visualization of the multimodal components of structure and function provides an anatomic link between the areas of functional activation and both normal tissue and pathology. Such displays provide important insights in planning optimal surgical resection of the tumor while preserving normal critical tissues where damage would possibly lead to postoperative neurologic deficit.

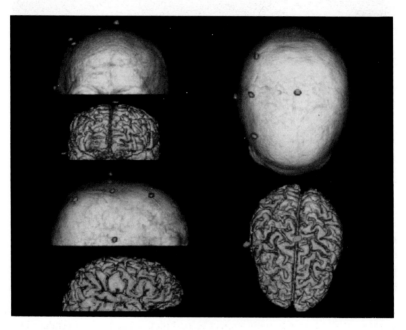

Figure 7.3. These volume renderings of 3-D acquired MRI data used for neurosurgical planning depict the soft tissue and brain structure of an epilepsy patient. The green structures visualized on the skin surface are capsules used as markers of EEG electrode positions indicating the electrical focus of the seizure activity (center marker). These can be projected from the skin surface to map the seizure focus to a specific gyrus in the brain parenchyma prior to surgery to aid the surgeon in optimally resecting the offending tissue. (Data courtesy of Drs. Frank Sharbrough and Clifford Jack, Mayo Foundation.) See color figure 29.

Computer-assisted surgery planning methods have been applied in neurosurgery and skull base surgery for several years, primarily through the use of stereotaxic systems for intraoperative 3-D localization of structures.[9] These techniques require accurate segmentation and visualization of multimodality image data of the head, including external soft tissue, skull, brain tissues, cerebrospinal fluid, eyes, paranasal sinuses, and musculature. Often external reference frames and markers or internally applied devices must also be imaged and localized within the context of the 3-D anatomic volume image. Neurosurgery planning in stereotaxic systems[10] depends on mapping the patient coordinate space provided by the reference frame into that of the acquired images. This mapping is established from points in the image corresponding to the frame in order to support intraoperative navigation of instruments during the surgical procedure. This is currently done with display of 2-D section data from the acquired volume image, often using only the anisotropic data and displaying the orthogonal sections.

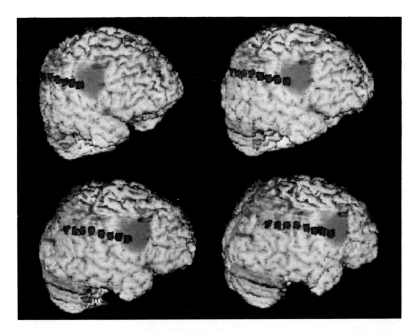

Figure 7.4. Composite renderings of CT and MRI data can be used to localize subdurally implanted electrodes with respect to pathology. The brain is rendered from a 3-D SPGR MRI volume image, demonstrating a large tumor (dark region). After MR imaging, subdural electrodes placed on the cortical surface of the brain are imaged with CT and used with evoked response studies to identify viable tissue surrounding the tumor. Proper visualization of electrode position is critical to analyzing these electrical potentials in relation to pathology and surgical decisions. This is directly facilitated by coregistering and visualizing the electrodes (black dots) from the CT in conjunction with the cortical brain surface from the MRI. (Data courtesy of Drs. Frank Sharbrough and Clifford Jack, Mayo Foundation.)

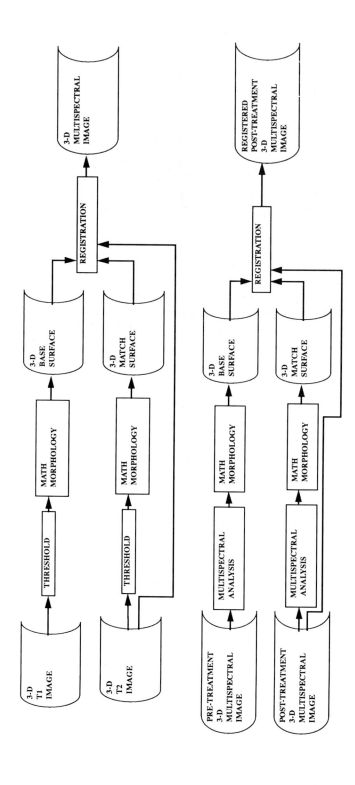

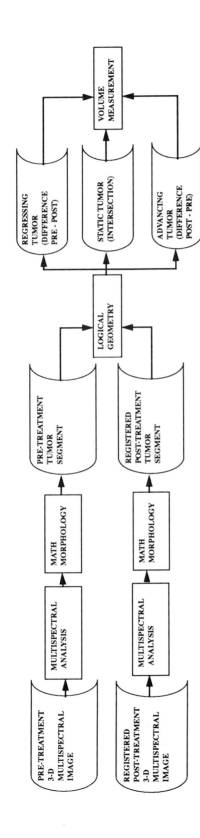

Figure 7.5. A paradigm for quantifying tumor response to treatment. The method of tumor segmentation relies on morphological and multispectral analysis of MR images. The individual spectral components (e.g., T1 and T2) must first be coregistered into a 3-D multi-spectral image (top row). The pre- and posttreatment multispectral images are then aligned and tumor segmentation is accomplished by multispectral classification followed by morphological processing to produce the pre- and posttreatment tumor volumes (center row). Since the tumor segments are in physical registration, the parts of the original tumor that have been destroyed, that are static, and that represent new growth can be determined (bottom row).

3-D visualization techniques using multimodality data can significantly augment such neurosurgical simulations. Markers placed on the patient's head provide a reference between the coordinate space of the patient and that of the volume image, but these markers may also serve to identify specific locations of functional activity acquired by other means. For example, Figure 7.3 (see color figure 29) depicts 3-D visualizations created with ANALYZE™ from a 3-D acquired MRI SPGR sequence of a patient with epilepsy. The patient's epileptic activity is not directly attributable to pathology, so the anatomic origin or focus of the seizure activity is unknown. However, the electrical activity causing the seizure can be localized using standard electroencephalography (EEG) techniques by placing multiple electrodes on the head and identifying the one associated with the strongest electrical activity, either during seizure or during evoked response testing to mimic seizure-like brain function. Once this primary electrode has been determined, it is marked with a small capsule (vitamin E), and other markers are placed on the scalp approximately orthogonal to this marker. When scanned with MRI, the capsules provide a high signal that can be easily segmented and separately rendered (green structures) along with other anatomic features, like the soft tissue of the head. To localize the portion of the brain causing the seizure focus activity, these markers can be triangulated for projection onto the cortical surface of the brain. Since the MRI volume image permits direct visualization of the cortical surface of the brain, the projected marker positions can be accurately localized on the surface of the brain. This localizes the portion of the brain causing the seizure activity prior to surgery, providing valuable information in guiding the neurosurgeon in planning resection of the focus of epileptic activity.[11]

When pathology is present, identification of vital tissue surrounding the pathology is critical in planning an optimal surgical approach that minimizes risk to such tissue. Subdurally implanted electrodes are often used either to measure the electrical activity of the brain tissue surrounding the pathology (e.g., tumor) or to stimulate a response through electrical activation of the electrodes. Thus, functional correlates to the tissue in a region of each electrode are determined, which is important to establish the location and extent of the pathology prior to surgery. Visualization allows the direct detection of the position of the electrodes in the region of the pathology, as shown in Figure 7.4. A 3-D SPGR MRI volume image is acquired to visualize the cortical surface of the brain, including a tumor (dark structure). After placement of the subdural electrodes, CT scanning can image the position of the electrodes relative to the brain anatomy, and with spatial coregistration of the CT and MRI volume images, the electrodes can be assigned as a specific object and rendered (shown as dots in Figure 7.4) with the surface of the brain from MRI. This type of visualization utilizes multimodality information to provide an integrated vision of function and structure necessary for effective preoperative neurosurgical planning.

7.3 Tumor Response to Treatment

Figure 7.5 is a diagram depicting a new paradigm for evaluating the response to treatment of tumors using 3-D imaging. The basic principle in the paradigm is to produce a volumetrically accurate representation of the pre- and posttreatment tumor in a coregistered framework by segmenting it from the 3-D image data using a combination of multispectral analysis and morphological processing.[12] This approach is potentially much more robust and clinically reproducible than traditional edge-strength methods and has been incorporated into ANALYZE™.

Figure 7.6 (see color figure 30) illustrates the step of multispectral analysis. Both the T1- and T2-weighted MRI data contain information that can be used to identify the tumor region, but the combined T1/T2 signature of tumor voxels is sufficiently unique to allow automated extraction of the entire tumor region. Some isolated misclassified voxels are included, however.

Figure 7.7 illustrates how shape information (in this case the compactness of the tumor) can be used to remove extraneous voxels. The figure illustrates

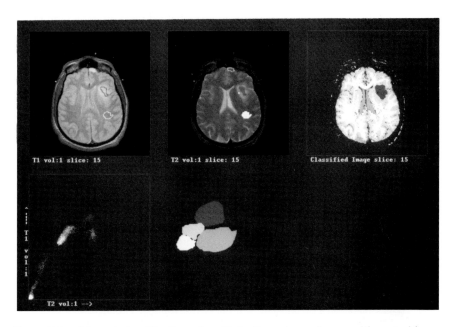

Figure 7.6. Manual classification of multiple tissue types from multispectral image data. The "clusters" of voxels having unique T1 and T2 values allow straightforward segmentation of the spatially complex regions of the images including white and gray matter (blue and yellow), cerebral spinal fluid (green), and tumor (red). The segmentation has identified all of the most likely tumor voxels as well as some obviously extraneous voxels with similar tissue characteristics. See color figure 30.

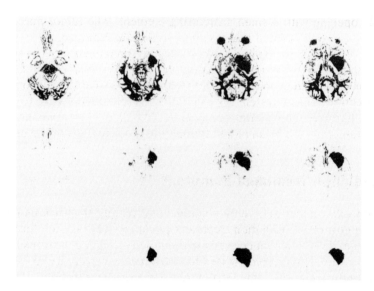

Figure 7.7. Morphological processing (in this case opening with a 3 × 3 square) makes use of knowledge about the shape of the tumor (e.g. "large," "compact") to remove extraneous voxels. Top row shows classified regions on several different slices; center and bottom rows show iterations to segment/isolate tumor.

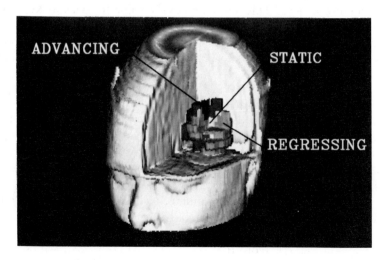

Figure 7.8. Since the tumor segments are in physical registration, determination can be made of which parts of the original tumor are regressing, which remain static, and whether or not new tumor regions are advancing (refer also to Figure 7.5). See color figure 31.

a simple opening with a small structuring element. The tumor mass is unchanged, but small isolated misclassified voxels are removed.

Figure 7.8 (see color figure 31) illustrates the final analysis. The parts of the original tumor that have been destroyed, the parts that remain, and new regions of tumor can be identified and measured. This paradigm should lead to an effective clinical system for evaluating the effectiveness of treatment regimens like radiation therapy or chemical "bullets" for reducing or destroying tumors in the brain and potentially in other regions of the body.

7.4 Radiation Treatment Planning

Radiation kills cancer cells only slightly more readily than it kills healthy cells. The goal of 3-D radiation treatment planning (RTP) is therefore to deliver a lethal dose to all cancer cells without delivering a dangerous dose to healthy tissue.[13] This is complicated by the extreme sensitivity to radiation exhibited by certain anatomic structures, for example the brain stem and optic nerve.

Since radiation therapy treatment can consist of a number of beams from any direction, each having its own unique profile and dosage level, there potentially exist several satisfactory treatment plans for any given patient. However, finding an optimal or near-optimal plan is difficult due to the essentially infinite search space. Historically, the solution space has been restricted to opposed pairs of beams having identical profiles located in the image scanning planes.[14] This restriction of the solution space makes finding a satisfactory clinical treatment plan feasible, but it is highly likely that more optimal plans are possible outside of this severely restricted solution space. 3-D multimodality imaging offers significant promise for developing effective RTP approaches and systems[15,16,17] for routine clinical use.

The relaxation of current RTP constraints in search of more optimal plans requires tools[18] for the facile display and analysis of the complex distributions of radiation dosage[19] associated with unrestricted loci and profiles of treatment beams. Figure 7.9 (see color figure 32) shows one tool for exploring a 3-D treatment plan. The dose distribution arising from a 7-beam conformal nonplanar treatment plan has been applied as a color wash over a 3-D image of the patient's head rendered in ANALYZE™ from MRI data. Each color represents an "isodose volume," with orange representing dose levels between 90% and 100% of prescribed dose, yellow representing 70% to 90%, etc. The red region represents dosage in excess of the prescribed dose (i.e., "kill" level). Note that the same 3-D color distribution is displayed on both the rendered image of the skin surface and the individual 2-D orthogonal sections.

Figure 7.10 illustrates the same dose–volume as computed for Figure 7.9 (see color figure 33), but color mapped on surfaces of selected important structures inside the head. The tumor itself is principally enclosed within the

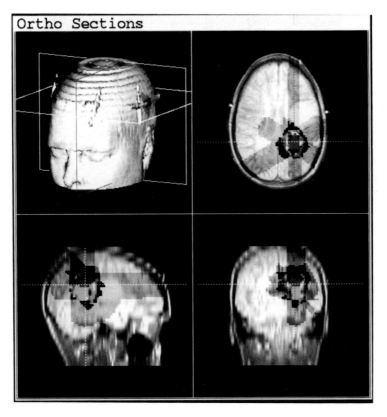

Figure 7.9. The dose distribution of a 7-beam non-coplanar radiation treatment therapy plan is shown as a color wash in the 3-D image volume rendered with ANA-LYZE™. Intersecting orthogonal planes may be displayed by picking a point of intersection on the skin surface or by pointing to the intersection point on any displayed section. See color figure 32.

90% isodose surface, and only a small region of 30–50% dose is affecting the brain stem.

Figure 7.11 (see color figure 34) is a stereo transparency rendering of the entire dose distribution. Note that the shapes perceived in the image are isodose surfaces, rather than the surfaces of target objects. Such visualizations provide significant potential for optimizing 3-D RTP in conforming to the mutually inseparable goals of destroying tumors while preserving normal tissue.[20]

7.5 Craniofacial Surgery Simulation and Planning

Craniofacial surgery involves surgery of the facial and cranial skeleton and soft tissues, often done in conjunction with plastic surgical techniques to

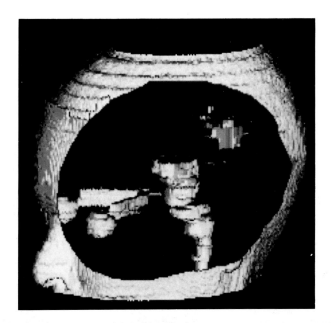

Figure 7.10. The same dose distribution of Figure 7.9 is shown on the surface of the tumor and on critical structures inside the head. Although most of the tumor volume is enclosed within the 90–100% prescribed dose region (orange), a small "tendril" of the tumor has escaped high dosage. One beam also brushes the brain stem, delivering only 30–50% prescribed dose (blue). See color figure 33.

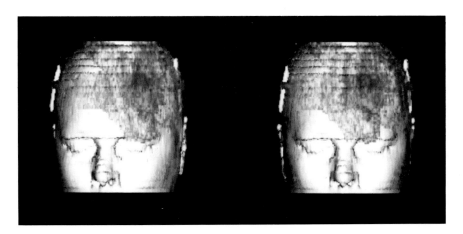

Figure 7.11. The same dose distribution of Figures 7.9 and 7.10 is shown as a stereo pair transparency. Rotational sequences of this type of rendering give a strong intuitive impression of the location and shape of the high-dose region, and thereby of the "goodness of fit" of the plan to simultaneous goals of tumor ablation and healthy tissue preservation. See color figure 34.

correct congenital deformities, or for the treatment of deformities caused by trauma, resection of tumors, infections, and other acquired conditions.[21] These same techniques are often applied to other bony and soft tissue structures in the body. Surgical treatment of these cases requires both quantitative and qualitative knowledge of the anatomy, preferably prior to the actual surgical procedure. Currently, preoperative information is most commonly acquired using X-ray CT scanning for the bony structures,[22] with MRI used for imaging the internal musculature. Assessment of postoperative results is often qualitative, consisting primarily of comparison of pre- and postoperative photographs. Visualization and quantitative analysis of postoperative CT and MRI scans allow accurate, objective assessment of the results of the surgery, permitting evaluation of such uncontrollable factors as growth in children, resorption of bone grafts, and the tendency of moved segments of bone to return to their original positions. Quantitative assessment of the results of the computer-aided surgery provides statistical data for the analysis of results, quality assurance, and the establishment of normative values necessary to facilitate analysis of pathological conditions.[23]

Although the data presented by the scanners themselves are useful, the information obtained is significantly increased by direct visualization of the full 3-D context of the structures involved in the surgery,[24] which also facilitates accurate measurement of structures of interest. The risk of complications in craniofacial and plastic surgery has been shown in several studies to be directly related to the duration of the operation. Precise presurgical planning minimizes the duration of the surgical procedure, thus minimizing the risks. With interactive computer planning and simulation of the surgical procedure, it is possible to prepare an accurate preoperative plan, minimizing the need to spend time designing complex operative plans with the patient already under anesthesia and often with the intracranial contents exposed.

Figure 7.12 (see color figure 35) demonstrates the use of 3-D surface-rendering techniques in the planning and quantitative analysis of craniofacial surgery.[25] Image data acquired using conventional X-ray CT provide the base volume image from which the bone can directly be rendered via thresholding to the voxel values corresponding to the dense bone (high values in CT). The rendering in the upper left demonstrates the utility of direct 3-D visualization of these structures for the assessment of defects, here the result of an old facial fracture. One approach to the surgical correction of such a defect is to use the undamaged contralateral structures, which can be segmented directly from the 3-D rendering and mirror imaged for placement in the damaged side (upper middle). This artificial structure can be further refined using cutting tools in the 3-D rendering that act only upon the new object created by segmentation and mirroring of the contralateral structures. Such tailored objects can then be used for simulation of direct implantation, as shown in the upper right, lower left, and middle renderings. Upon creating the final shape and dimension of the implantable structures, accurate size and dimension measurements can be estimated from the structures (lower

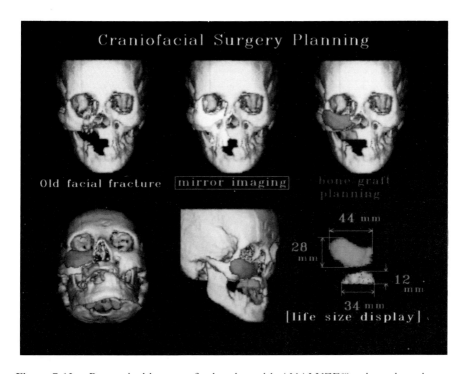

Figure 7.12. Presurgical bone graft planning with ANALYZE™ using mirror imaging (top row) and subsequent editing of the graft prostheses (top right, bottom left, and center), including accurate quantitative assessment of prosthesis size and shape (bottom right). See color figure 35.

right) and their contours can be extracted for use in devices (e.g., milling machines) that can create the prosthetics for implantation.[26]

7.6 Orthognathic Surgery

Patients undergoing orthognathic surgery can be scanned both pre- and post-operatively to evaluate displacement of the temporomandibular joint (TMJ) with 3-D imaging. Orthognathic procedures involve repositioning of portions of the skull or mandible to improve the meshing of the teeth. One rather common procedure is bilateral split-ramus osteotomy, an operation in which the mandible is separated at two points so that the chin may be repositioned (usually forward). Some patients exhibit postoperative symptoms associated with displacement of the TMJ. Measurements of TMJ displacements immediately after surgery are useful to determine if the measured movements fall within acceptable limits of the theoretical geometry for normal function.[27,28]

MR images can be used to analyze the procedure and to minimize patient risk (by comparison with using X-ray CT). However, since both the surfaces used for registration and those used for analysis are bony, the MR images are difficult to segment, since in MR images bony structures give rise to no signal. Only a small set of coronal sections in the TMJ region are scanned. Although a customized, removable head restraint can be used for each patient, pre- to postoperative manual registration is not reliable. Using selected traces of the temporal fossae, the pre- and postoperative images can be successfully registered to a common reference frame using 3-D registration techniques in ANALYZE™. Figure 7.13 illustrates coregistered MRI scans of pre- and postoperative MR images of the TMJ. Figure 7.14 (see color figure 36) illustrates a phantom study undertaken to validate the TMJ analysis method. A dry skull including mandible was scanned by X-ray CT. A spacer was then inserted between the mandible and the temporal fossa on one side only and the skull was rescanned. The upper part of the skull surface was then extracted from each image and used to coregister the two scans. In

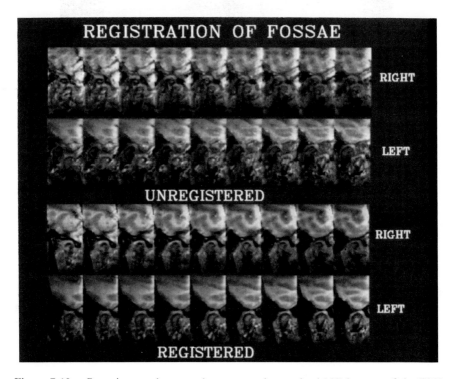

Figure 7.13. Superimposed pre- and postoperative sagittal MR images of the TMJ. In the top two rows, the two sets of images are not in proper spatial registration, and the resulting combined images are undecipherable. In the bottom row, the 3-D images have been coregistered using ANALYZE™ and the superimposed images clearly show the TMJ structures.

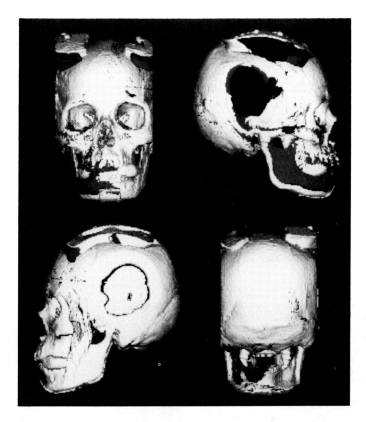

Figure 7.14. Two sets of 3-D CT scans of a dry skull were used to evaluate 3-D image effectiveness of analysis in orthognathic surgery. The first scan (red volume) was made with the mandible in its normal position. The second scan (white volume) had spacers placed between the temporal condyles and fossae. The right spacer was larger than the left, resulting in rotation and shifting of the mandible to the left. After coregistration, the two 3-D images are accurately fused into one skull, but the two jaws are in different positions, as expected. See color figure 36.

Figure 7.14, the two scans are displayed simultaneously, the first in white and the second in red. The figure clearly shows the registration of the upper part of the skull and the displacement of the mandible by the spacer. Such validation has led to confident applications of 3-D imaging for postoperative evaluations of TMJ operations.

7.7 Orthopedic Surgery

Imaging in support of orthopedic visualization and surgical planning has traditionally been done using standard radiographic techniques. Plain films have been the primary modality of choice when imaging the bone and joints in the body, and they remain a common imaging technique for diagnostic purposes in orthopedics. However, these traditional X-ray-based techniques are not able to sufficiently image the soft tissue components of the orthopedic structures of interest, and the superposition of structures in 3-D when projected onto 2-D plain films severely limits the usefulness of any one viewpoint in providing accurate diagnostic and therapeutic information. Often it is necessary to reposition the patient and record multiple radiographs from different views. X-ray CT imaging has provided the basis for advanced imaging techniques for the bone and joints, allowing full 3-D volume images to be acquired and used by the orthopedic surgeon. This is useful in a variety of orthopedic applications, including trauma evaluation, congenital defects, and degenerative diseases.[29]

Orthopedic visualization can take advantage of many of the inherent features for manipulation and measurement in digital imaging[30] of 3-D volume imaging for the investigation of the skeletal structures in the body. Creation

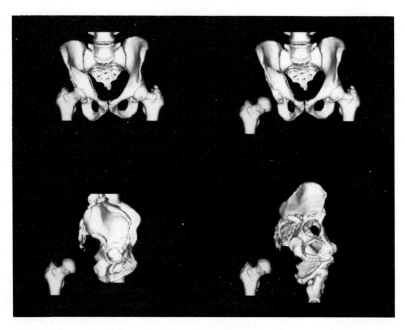

Figure 7.15. Volumetric X-ray CT of skeletal structures provides image information for direct visualization of various structures in orthopedic applications, including visual inspection of trauma damage. These images rendered via ANALYZE™ are from 3-D X-ray CT data of the hip of a trauma patient with a large intraacetabular fracture. This fracture cannot be visualized from the initial AP rendering (upper left), but by segmenting the head of the femur and translating it away from the hip (upper right), the hip can be rotated independently (lower left) to visualize clearly the fracture (lower right). (Data courtesy of Dr. David Lewallen, Mayo Foundation.)

of orthogonal and oblique multiplanar reformatted images permits the orthopedic surgeon to visualize the structure in full context, rather than only
in the plane of acquisition, and results in the ability to create images necessary for direct quantitative analysis. 3-D rendering techniques are easily applied to the visualization of bone from X-ray CT volume images, as shown
in Figure 7.15. From CT data, the bone can be segmented using simple
thresholding and directly rendered, as shown in this rendering of the pelvis
and partial femurs. These renderings are from a patient with an intraacetabular fracture. The fracture cannot be visualized directly from the initial an-
terior-posterior (AP) rendering (upper left), and may not be well appreciated
in conventional plain films or by reviewing a standard set of transaxial CT
sections through this region. Using multiple object segmentation and rendering techniques in ANALYZE™, the head of the femur can be defined
as a separate object and manipulated independently from the pelvis. By
translating the femur away from the hip (upper right) and rotating the hip

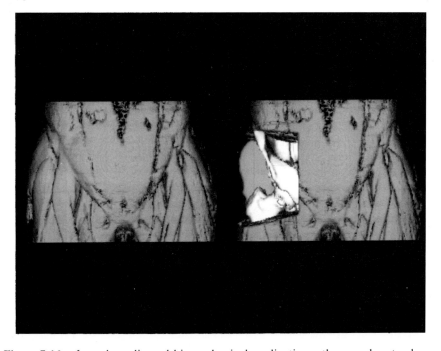

Figure 7.16. In orthopedic and biomechanical applications, the muscles, tendons,
and ligaments are often as important as the bone. From X-ray CT data, these soft
tissue structures can be segmented with ANALYZE™ and rendered in their natural
relationships to the bone (left). Sections of the overlapping musculature can be cut
away to reveal the underlying hip bone, providing direct visualization of the relationships between these structures (right). (Data courtesy of Dr. David Lewallen, Mayo
Foundation.) See color figure 37.

(lower left), a direct view into the acetabulum can be obtained (lower right), providing a view of the fracture to the surgeon otherwise impossible to obtain.

In orthopedic applications, it is frequently necessary to understand the soft tissue structures surrounding the skeletal structure of interest. In many biomechanical and prosthesis design studies,[31] the muscles, tendons, and ligaments are as important as the bone. Soft tissue structures can be segmented from the same X-ray CT data used to image the bone, or image information from other modalities more appropriate for imaging the soft tissue, like MRI, can be correlated with the CT to provide an integrated visualization of soft and hard tissues. Figure 7.16 (see color figure 37) demonstrates a visualization of combined bone and soft tissue where the soft tissue structures have been segmented from the CT data used to image the hip. These soft tissues are rendered on top of the underlying skeletal structures, with cutaway sections allowing for correlated visualization of the bone and soft tissue.

7.8 Physeal Bar (Bone Growth Plate) Resection

The physis is a disk of living tissue that separates the shaft from the joint processes at both ends of the long bones in children and young adolescents. It is from this disk that all growth of the bone shaft and joint surfaces progresses. At maturity, the physis fuses and becomes mineralized bone. Trauma or disease can cause the physis to prematurely and partially fuse, leaving a sector of the bone unable to grow. The normal growth in the surrounding regions causes the bone to deform. If the fused region is relatively small, and if sufficient growth remains in the remaining physis, the fusion can be broken and removed, and normal growth will correct the deformation. The clinical indicators for success are the relative size of the fused region and the precision of the surgical procedure.[32]

The physis can be adequately imaged by MRI. The growth tissue is detectable as a faint signal in the zero-signal bone region. It is so faint, however, that it is not evident in the thin sections needed for accurate measurement, and the often-used thicker sections present wide variations in signal strength that may indicate differences in tissue viability, thickness, geometric artifacts, or partial-volume effects of image acquisition. Automated segmentation of these images is highly prone to the detection of "pseudobars" and to misestimation of physeal areas. Currently, the most useful estimates of true physeal shape and area are those manually extracted by a radiologist familiar with the anatomy, physiology, and image characteristics.

Measuring areas of the bar by orthogonal projection has large potential errors because of the highly conical shape a partially fused physis can acquire. But perhaps even more important than improved quantification of pa-

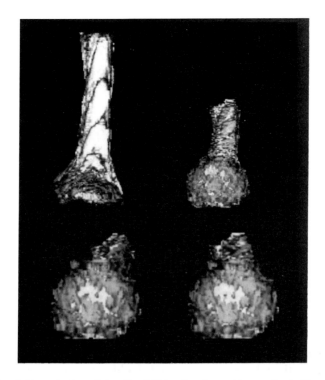

Figure 7.17.   3-D rendering of the distal tibia of a physeal bar patient. Top row shows two views of shaft. Bottom row is stereo pair of shaft end. The bone is made transparent to expose the physeal plate (orange) and interior bar (white). These images are cross-fused (i.e., the left eye image is on the right and vice versa), so a 3-D image of the physis and bar can be seen by crossing the eyes. See color figure 38.

thology from the images is the usefulness of the rendered images in helping the surgeon determine a precise and effective surgery.

Figure 7.17 (see color figure 38) shows 3-D renderings from MRI scans of the distal tibia of a young physeal bar patient. The physis is shown in place by rendering the bone transparently. The top two images show the tibial shaft and the bottom two images are a stereo pair of the distal articulating surface of the tibial shaft. Note the conical appearance of the physis due to continued growth of the bone around the central bar. Such 3-D renderings have facilitated improved surgical plans (i.e., more precise delivery of surgery and correction of problem) in several patients at the Mayo Clinic.

7.9 Cardiac Imaging

Imaging the heart is a challenge both for imaging technology and for visualization and analysis because of the high rate of motion and complex interdependent cardiac structures, including muscle, blood vessels, and valves. Imaging systems must acquire images with sufficiently high temporal resolution to capture the heart in near stop action (i.e., within a few milliseconds) in order to visualize the structure clearly. For dynamic studies, such scans must be repeatable at different points in the cardiac cycle, most commonly accomplished by gating the acquisition to the electrocardiogram for several points in the ECG. For 3-D structural visualization and analysis, this must be done through the entire axial extent of the heart in order to capture all structural components.[33] All together, these aspects of cardiac imaging present an enormous problem to acquisition technology to capture the true structural to functional relationships of this complex, dynamic organ.

Several scanning technologies today can accomplish parts of this task, that is, acquiring high temporal resolution images without gating, but at the expense of full 3-D coverage (e.g., fast CT), or full 3-D coverage at the sacrifice of temporal resolution using gating (e.g., MRI). X-ray CT imaging, such as with the fast CT scanners, can image cardiac structure, often with the use of blood pool contrast agents to visualize the chamber anatomy, coronary arteries, and vessels connected to the heart. With image acquisition gated over several cardiac cycles, both CT and MRI modalities[34,35] can acquire time sequence images throughout the cardiac cycle with good structural detail, but spontaneous physiological events are averaged out. Nuclear medicine imaging systems can obtain information about heart function through the use of specific radiopharmaceuticals using gating to specific points in the cardiac cycle, although at low spatial resolution.[36] Such information includes myocardial perfusion and blood pool imaging. Ultrasound can acquire real-time cardiac imagery for evaluation of function, including valve structure and movement, and with recent linear array technologies, multiple axial slices can be acquired for 3-D time sequence visualization and analysis.[37]

To obtain synchronous volumetric images of the heart, a unique scanner called the Dynamic Spatial Reconstructor (DSR) was developed at the Mayo Foundation in the late 1970s.[38] The DSR uses X-ray CT principles with multiple X-ray sources to achieve high-speed, repetitive imaging capability. Volume images isotropically sampled with approximately 1 mm^3 voxels can be acquired in $1/100$ sec, with repetitive volumetric acquisitions every $1/60$ sec, producing a unique 4-D data set with high temporal and spatial resolution. This imaging system has been applied to many aspects of cardiac imaging.[33,39] Figure 7.18 (see color figure 39) depicts four views of an intact heart scanned with the DSR within which the myocardium (pink), ventricular and atrial chambers (blue), and coronary arteries (red) can be visualized. With the injection of iodinated contrast media into the vasculature, the coronary arteries were segmented with simple thresholding, as was the chamber anatomy. Each component has been assigned to an object map, given different colors, and rendered using 24-bit transparency to visualize the structural dimensions and geometric relationships of these cardiac components. These

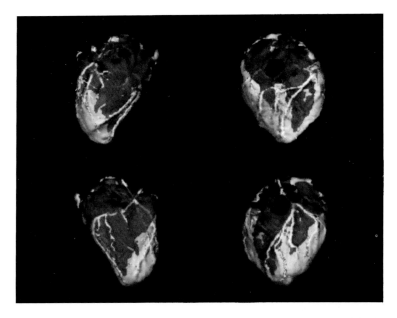

Figure 7.18. Transparent 3-D rendering of an intact heart scanned with the DSR showing the myocardium (pink), chambers (blue), and coronary arteries (red) from four different views. See color figure 39.

are static volume images taken from a single time point in the DSR scanning sequence.

The stop-action volumetric images illustrated in Figure 7.18 can be acquired throughout the cardiac cycle without gating, producing instant-to-instant volume images as shown in Figure 7.19 (see color figure 40). These rendered images depict the left ventricular (red) and right ventricular (blue) chambers of the heart at 15 time points throughout the cardiac cycle. Each chamber has been segmented separately using thresholding and region growing, with the chambers in the original volume images enhanced with iodinated contrast material. In order to render an image of the chambers where both are filled with dye, the left ventricular filling phase and right ventricular filling phase have been separately segmented and added together to achieve a time sequence display of the structure and function of both chambers. The renderings begin at end diastole (upper left) and continue left to right, top to bottom, through end systole (lower left), returning back to near end diastole (lower right). The "hole" seen in the left ventricular chamber is the invagination of the papillary muscle from the surrounding myocardium during the contraction. Although such 4-D data sets are unique to the DSR, modern fast X-ray CT and 3-D real-time ultrasound are beginning to produce data for similar comprehensive structure–function studies of the heart.

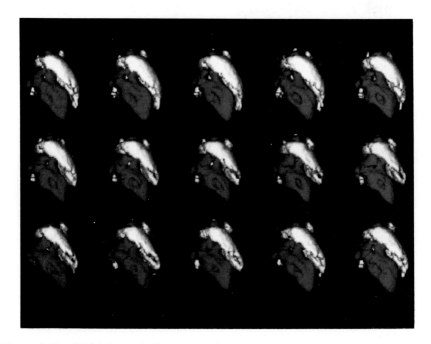

Figure 7.19. Multiple renderings throughout the cardiac cycle of an intact heart scanned by the DSR depicting the left ventricular chamber (red) and right ventricular chamber (blue) from end diastole (upper left) through systole (lower left) and back to diastole (lower right). See color figure 40.

When a pacing impulse reaches the heart, it is distributed around the organ by a network of nerve fibers. The precise pattern in which nerve-initiated muscle contractions spread through and about the myocardium keeps the heart synchronously and efficiently contracting and relaxing to eject and receive blood in meeting the circulatory demands of the body. Any interruptions or alterations in the pattern of these nerve conductances are accompanied by changes in the mechanical sequence of the heartbeat, with potentially severe consequences. Studies to correlate and couple myocardial electrophysiology with myocardial mechanics therefore have important implications for characterizing cardiac behavior and performance and for signaling danger when anomalies in this coupling occur.

Figure 7.20 (top) (see color figure 41) is a 3-D volume rendering of a fast CT scan of a heart which has been correlated with and colorized by the activation times recorded from 52 electrodes placed around the surface of the epicardium. The red colors signal early activation sites near the beginning of the heartbeat, and the blue colors signal late myocardial activity near the end of the heartbeat.

Figure 7.21 (see color figure 42) illustrates the effect of the drug quinidine on the pattern of nerve activation. The effect of quinidine is to slow the heart

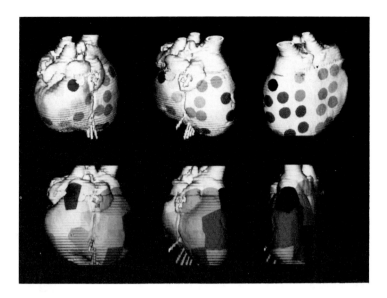

Figure 7.20. Heart surface colorized by evoked response activation delay. Each spot (top row) indicates the position of one of 54 electrodes on the surface of the heart. The color indicates the activation time at the electrode from early (red) to late (blue) in the heartbeat. The entire surface of the heart is colorized (bottom row) by interpolating an activation time for each point on the heart surface from the nearest two electrodes. See color figure 41.

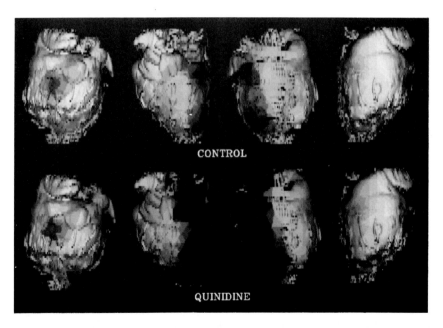

CONTROL

QUINIDINE

Figure 7.21. 3-D volume renderings of fast CT scan of a heart colorized with activation time as recorded by 54 electrodes placed around the heart surface. The upper images represent a normal heartbeat, while the lower images represent a heartbeat after the administration of an anti-arrhythmic drug, which slows the heartbeat. See color figure 42.

251

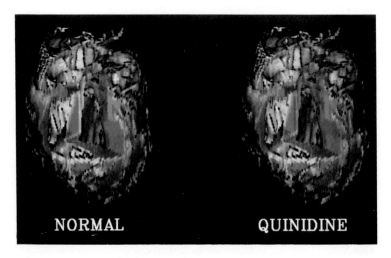

Figure 7.22.   A cutaway view of the same data shown in Figure 7.21, showing the activation delay pattern on the interior surfaces of the heart. A "wedge" is placed in the center of the 3-D rendering to reveal the myocardial transmural activation patterns. See color figure 43.

rate. This is illustrated by the extended color range on the heart after drug administration by comparison to the control state. However, the pattern (activation sequence) has not been altered. Figure 7.22 (see color figure 43) shows a cutaway "wedge" view which illustrates the activation pattern transmurally, extending from the epicardium to the endocardial wall. With the advent of 4-D imaging systems and minimally invasive electrophysiologic monitoring devices, coupling of myocardial polarization sequences to myocardial contractility using such visualization mappings will become an important clinical technique in diagnosis and treatment of heart disease.

7.10 Lung Transplant Analysis

Differential lung volume can be measured by periodic 3-D CT imaging of single-lung transplant patients over time. A transplanted lung usually does not fill with air to the same extent as the original lung, and although this condition generally improves within a few months of surgery, timely and accurate evaluation of transplant lung performance within a few months of surgery is critical to determination of outcome.

Lungs can be readily segmented from 3-D fast CT images using global thresholding. But errors due to partial volume effect and reduced ratios of air to mass of tissue by comparison to the original lung (i.e., higher CT numbers) need to be taken into account. To obtain accurate measurements, the

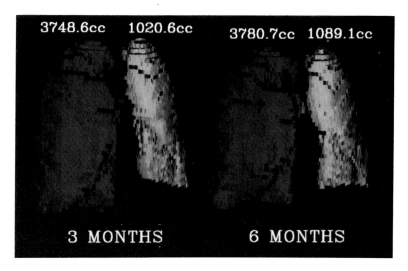

3748.6cc   1020.6cc   3780.7cc   1089.1cc

3 MONTHS   6 MONTHS

Figure 7.23. A volume rendering of the lung surfaces of a single-lung transplant patient 3 months (left) and 6 months (right) postsurgery. The transplanted left lung is noticeably smaller than the native right lung in both images, but volume measurement shows a 10% increase in transplant lung volume in 3 months, a favorable outcome. See color figure 44.

images must often be segmented more carefully than by simple thresholding, such as by morphologic processing.

Figure 7.23 (see color figure 44) illustrates a comparison of lung volume measurements using 3-D CT scans taken 3 and 6 months after the transplant surgery. The desired improvement in lung volume is evident (10% increase for transplant lung, 1% increase for normal lung).

7.11 Prostate Cancer Evaluation

The likelihood of benign or malignant prostate growth approaches certainty as men age past 50.[40] Accurate diagnosis (particularly differentiating malignant from benign tumors) is difficult, and the severity of malignant prostate cancer leads to a significant amount of benign prostatic disease being treated surgically. Since the complications of prostate surgery (notably impotence and incontinence) can be psychologically devastating, any improvement in diagnostic ability leading to fewer unnecessary surgeries, or any improvement in surgical planning leading to fewer complications, would have a significant impact on health care. MRI has been used as a screening procedure, but the current final arbiter of malignant tumor diagnosis is digital palpitation. However, the use of MRI as a diagnostic and surgical planning tool for this disease has excellent promise.[40]

One of the most commonly performed surgical procedures in major hospitals is radical retropubic prostatectomy for treatment of prostate cancer. One of the most confounding factors and causes of morbidity in radical prostatectomy is the difficulty of visualizing the highly variable individual pelvic anatomy of each patient. For clinically localized cancer confined to the prostate gland, the treatment of choice is surgery. Radical retropubic prostatectomy offers the best chance for permanent cure. However, radical retropubic prostatectomies are not without significant morbidity. Up to 50% of patients become impotent following surgery because of injury or sacrifice of the neurovascular bundle traveling next to the prostate gland. Second, because the prostate gland is intimately involved with the external urinary sphincter, radical retropubic prostatectomy can damage the sphincter, resulting in temporary or permanent urinary incontinence.

With new advances in MRI techniques, high-resolution, 3-D volume MRI can be obtained of the prostate gland. With these data, 3-D reconstructed images of the bladder, prostate gland, external urinary sphincter, neurovascular bundle, and associated musculature can be segmented and displayed with programs like ANALYZE™, as shown in Figures 7.24 and 7.25 (see color figures 45 and 46). The ability to three-dimensionally render an image of the prostate gland as it relates to surrounding organs and structures may aid the surgeon in protecting adjacent vital structures and preventing significant morbidity, such as impotence, following surgery.

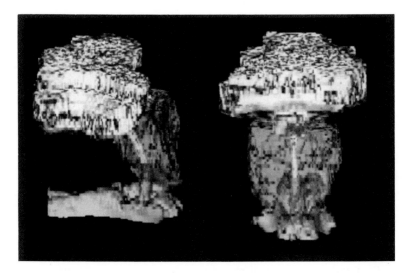

Figure 7.24. Transparent volume rendering of the urinary anatomy from 3-D MRI scan of pelvis. Segmented structures shown are bladder and urethra (yellow), prostate gland (green), external urinary sphincter (pink), and erectile support bodies (blue). Note that the external sphincter is fully visible through the transparent structures that would otherwise obscure it. See color figure 45.

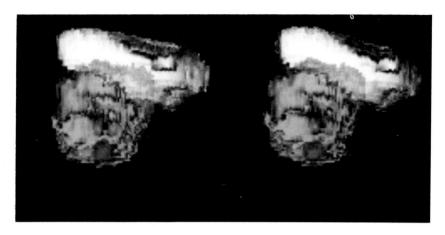

Figure 7.25.   Stereo pair (cross-fusion) of transparent rendering of the bladder (yellow), prostate (green), and external urinary sphincter (red). Radical prostatectomy patients suffer temporary or permanent urinary incontinence due to damage to the external sphincter. This type of imagery may help surgeons visualize each patient's unique anatomic configuration and reduce such morbidity. See color figure 46.

Figure 7.26 shows a representative sagittal and transverse MRI from a pelvic scan of normal anatomy. The bladder is an easily identifiable bright region. The internal urinary sphincter is likewise a visually identifiable but inhomogeneous region. The prostate has a clearly defined border, providing adequate features for manual segmentation, but is highly inhomogeneous in grayscale, rendering conventional automated segmentation impossible.

It has been shown[41] that deformable models may be used to automatically segment the prostate. Deformable models are based upon the statistical analysis of shape measurements of normal and pathological prostates determined by manual segmentation. The segmented prostates are statistically analyzed both to determine an "average" prostate shape and to quantify the typical variation of prostate shape in such a way as to define the envelope of "shape space" in which all variations of prostates are contained. If, for example, four shape measures are applied to the segmented prostates, the region of this 4-D measurement domain in which all sampled prostates occur defines the "shape region" for the sampled prostates.

To use the deformable model to segment the prostate from a new image, the "average" prostate shape is inserted into the image at the "average" location, and the average shape is rotated, scaled, and translated repeatedly in search of the best match with edges (i.e., strong gradients) in the 3-D grayscale image. Once the best fit has been found, those regions of the average shape which do not lie directly on edges in the grayscale image are "warped" to the nearest edge. The resulting shape is then analyzed to determine whether or not it lies in the region of shape space which is "accept-

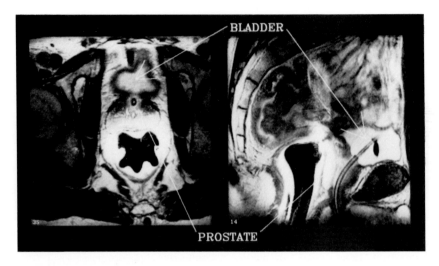

Figure 7.26. Representative transverse (left) and sagittal (right) MR images from a pelvic scan. The bladder is a fairly uniform region with sharp boundaries, and is easily segmented automatically. The prostate is inhomogeneous throughout its extent, but still shows sharp boundaries which allow it to be segmented manually or by more sophisticated automated methods.

able" for a prostate. If it is, the deformable model will accurately segment the prostate from the image. If the resulting warped shape is not an acceptable prostate shape, the warping is corrected to bring the model within acceptable parameters, and the process is repeated. The sequence of rigid motion matching, warping, and shape analysis is repeated until the model converges to an acceptable boundary or some maximum number of iterations suggests failure.

The deformable model is a very sophisticated image processing technique that depends on a large sample of normal and pathological images, and on the selection of powerful and appropriate shape measures. There is significant evidence[41] that this technique will perform well for many different areas of human anatomy (the external urinary sphincter is another good candidate) if the model is carefully constructed for the particular organ to be identified.

Therefore, the greatest obstacle to routine presurgical 3-D visualization of urologic anatomy is the difficulty in segmenting (i.e., separating a region from the surrounding image) the structures of interest. Only the bladder can be easily segmented using straightforward methods; the most crucial structures in Figure 7.26 were manually outlined in each section. Manual segmentation is so time- and expertise-intensive as to preclude routine clinical application of 3-D imagery. However, a number of sophisticated new schemes (such as deformable models, as just described) hold excellent promise for the automated segmentation of these structures. The possibility now exists for completely automated segmentation of 3-D pelvic imagery from standard MRI protocols. The promise is that providing such presurgical imagery will positively affect clinical outcome.

Optimal 3-D imaging of MRI volume data sets for accurate study of the 3-D relationships of the prostate gland and adjacent organs, such as the bladder, external urinary sphincter, and neurovascular structures, should aid the surgeon in reducing the significant morbidity following prostate cancer surgery, including impotence or urinary incontinence.

7.12 Glaucoma Studies

The trabecular tissue of the eye is a sponge-like, fluid-laden tissue that forms an annular ring around the cornea at the point where the sclera and iris meet. It is a main focus of study into the basic mechanisms underlying the clinical progression of glaucoma.[42] The tissue consists primarily of fluid-filled voids surrounded by beams (trabeculae) of connected tissue. Cell nuclei are distributed sparsely (but not randomly) throughout the tissue, while cell cytoplasm extends in tendrils along the trabeculae and on the interior surface of the larger fluid spaces. The trabecular tissue regulates the flow of aqueous

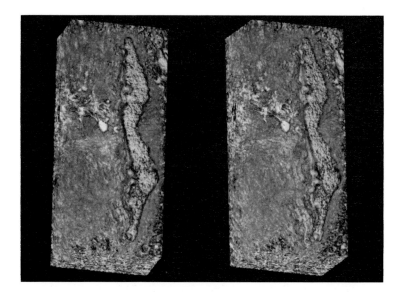

Figure 7.27. Stereo pair transparent rendering of a block of trabecular tissue reconstructed from microphotographs of 1-μm tissue sections. The green object is Schlemm's canal, a major drainage path for aqueous humor in the eye. The blue regions are aqueous humor in the spongy tissue coming from the anterior chamber of the eye. Pink material is solid tissue, either cytoplasm, cell nuclei, or collagen. See color figure 47.

humor out of the eye and back into the venous blood system. Analysis of
2-D sections has not yielded the sought-for understanding of flow change,
but reconstruction of the complex 3-D topology of this tissue may lend important insights.

Figure 7.27 (see color figure 47) is a stereo-pair rendering of a block of
trabecular tissue in which both the solid tissue and the fluid space have been
rendered transparently. The images shown are rendered from a series of digitized photomicrographs of 64 1-μm fixed sections of trabecular tissue. The
large interior object is Schlemm's canal, the primary drainage route for the
aqueous humor. One apparently independently connected "system" of fluid
spaces has been given slightly higher opacity than the remaining fluid
spaces, which seem to have no lateral connections into this isolated system.

Figure 7.28 (see color figure 48) is an opaque rendering of the same block
of tissue showing Schlemm's canal as an open space. The large "bumps" on
the surface of Schlemm's canal are cell nuclei. The orientation and appearance of this rendering were chosen to mimic an artist's rendering of the tissue.[42] Such studies are precursors to breakthroughs in determining the cause
of glaucoma and to developing 3-D imaging techniques for early detection of

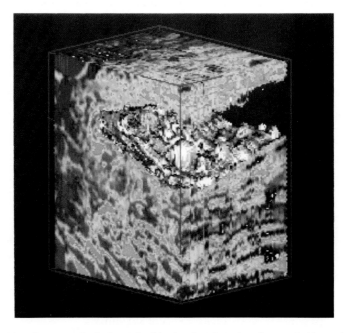

Figure 7.28. Opaque rendering of a block of trabecular tissue. Schlemm's canal is
shown as a cavernous space. The "bumps" in the floor of the canal are cell nuclei.
See color figure 48.

(or even screening for) the disease, as well as providing strategies for optimal microsurgical or medical treatment.

7.13 Corneal Modeling

Keratorefractive surgery refers to several procedures that surgically alter the corneal surface for the purpose of correcting vision. Radial keratotomy (rk) is one such procedure in which fairly deep radial incisions are made at intervals around the cornea to effectively "relax" the curvature of the eye and move the focal plane of a myopic eye back onto the retina.[43]

Some patients who have undergone this surgery report visual aberrations, including loss of contrast/night vision, ghost images, and disconcerting glare or flare, while testing 20/20 in a well-lit clinical setting.[43–45] It is believed that these aberrations are due to the irregular corneal surface resulting from the surgical procedure, but it is only in the last few years that technology has been available to noninvasively measure corneal topography and definitively evaluate this hypothesis.

The vision channel is composed of 3-D anatomy that captures 3-D signals (scenes), yet the measurement system is restricted in its ability to faithfully sample the full dimensionality of the signal (not unlike other optical systems). Hence modeling plays an important role in evaluation of the human visual system and its components. But for realistic modeling of the vision channel, one needs reasonable input data.

The digital keratoscope[46] measures the shape of the cornea by analyzing the position of light sources on a photograph of the cornea. Since the geometry of the camera, cornea, and light sources is fixed, the position of the reflections directly indicates local corneal curvature. Unfortunately, corneal topography measurements do not directly conform to our models of vision, which are based on optical science, i.e., it is impossible to gain any useful insight from directly viewing maps of the varying topography of the cornea. Normal corneas can certainly be identified by their regularity, but there is no easily identified feature that separates satisfied from unsatisfied rk patients.

By modeling[47,48] the refraction of light at this irregular surface, as shown in Figure 7.29, a transformation is made between the topography measurement space and the measurement space of optical systems. Rays of light from a point source are refracted at the measured points and collected in a focal plane. The 2-D image of the point source thus created is the point-spread function (psf) of the optical system and is analogous to the impulse response of an electronic signal-processing system.

The psf provides many possibilities for further analysis of the cornea. Figure 7.30 (see color figure 49) shows the Fourier transform of a normal corneal psf on the left and of an unsatisfied rk patient on the right. The

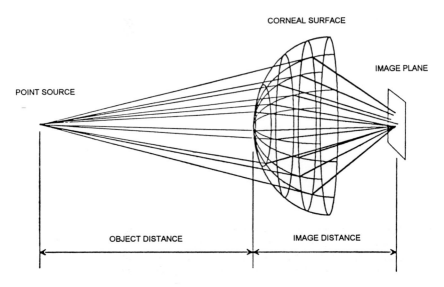

Figure 7.29. Model of an irregular corneal surface. When rays of light refracted at measured points on the model are accumulated into an image plane, they produce a point-spread function (psf), which analytically characterizes the optical performance of the cornea.

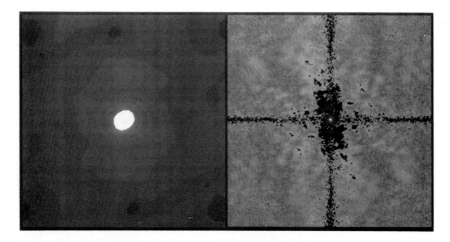

Figure 7.30. Color-coded Fourier transform of the psf of a normal cornea (left) and of an irregular cornea (right) of a patient after radical keratotomy. The violet color represents the first order of magnitude of attenuation in the modulation transfer function. Dark blue, light blue, and green represent the second, third, and fourth orders, respectively. See color figure 49.

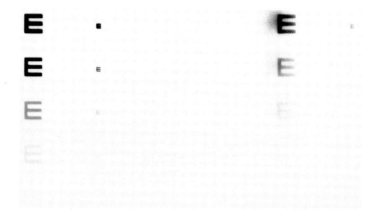

Figure 7.31. Using the model, a contrast test chart can be generated, simulating what the subject actually sees. The left and right charts correspond to the normal and surgically modified corneas, respectively, shown in Figure 7.30. Note that both contrast and acuity are severely reduced in the irregular cornea.

normal transform stays essentially in the first order of magnitude in spatial frequency attenuation (the violet color) and is very symmetrical, whereas the rk transform falls rapidly into the second and third order of magnitude (blue and green) and is highly irregular.

By convolving the modeled psf with an image of a contrast test chart, the loss of contrast/night vision reported by the patient can be simulated as shown in Figure 7.31 (again compared to the normal cornea on the left). The importance of this part of vision is further illustrated in Figure 7.32, which shows the result of convolving the two psfs with a night driving scene. Such 3-D image modeling techniques are leading the way to vastly improved care of the eye in both ophthalmologic and optometric practice.

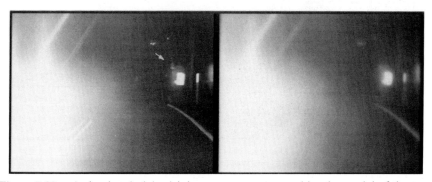

Figure 7.32. A simulated night driving scene as processed by the model of the two corneas in Figure 7.30. Note the darkly dressed jogger (arrow on left image), and the increased glare which obliterates this silhouette in the surgical cornea (right).

7.14 Special Surgical Procedures

3-D imaging can be used for special or unusual procedures that without 3-D visualization might not be possible. For example, ANALYZE™ has been used to plan the successful separation of two sets of conjoined twins, as illustrated in Figures 7.33 and 7.34 (see color figures 50 and 51). Volume rendering and the interactive tools associated with realistic 3-D visualization, manipulation, and measurements in ANALYZE™ were used to plan these sensitive and challenging operations. In Figure 7.33, full-body fast CT scans (upper left) reveal the joined sternum, abdomen, and liver of the first set of conjoined twins. 3-D renderings (upper right) can be viewed and dissected from any orientation to accurately evaluate anatomic spatial relationships. Special "cutting tools" (lower left) can be used to interactively determine the optimal bisection to minimize the size of the surgical opening. After

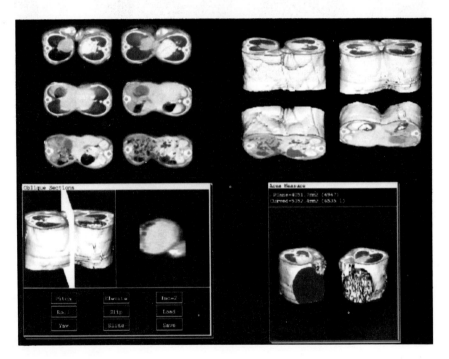

Figure 7.33. Full-body fast CT scans reveal several cross sections through connected body trunks of infant conjoined twins (top left). ANALYZE™ volume rendering of these CT scans can be rotated, tilted, etc. to visualize and study the connected bodies in 3-D (top right). Using a planar dissection tool (bottom left) the optimal approach to bisecting the bodies can be planned, directed at minimizing the surgical opening. The simulated bisection can then be used to accurately measure the area of the surgical openings (bottom right) to determine the amount of skin graft required to close the actual openings. (Data courtesy of Dr. Uldis Bite, Mayo Foundation.) See color figure 50.

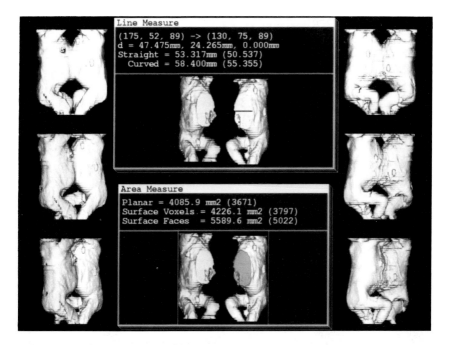

Figure 7.34. Another set of conjoined twins processed almost identically to those in Figure 7.33. Shown are simulated 3-D renderings of connected bodies, simulated bisection and segmentation, and measurement of area of surgical openings for calculation of skin graft. (Data courtesy of Dr. Uldis Bite, Mayo Foundation.) See color figure 51.

simulating the bisection, the surgical openings can be accurately measured (lower right) to estimate the quantity of skin and grafting material required to cover the openings. An almost identical procedure was repeated for the second set of twins (Figure 7.34). Such operations are concrete and compelling examples of the three major components of biomedical visualization needed to support sophisticated surgery planning: realistic display, interactive manipulations (editing), and quantitative measurement. The successful results are prototypical of the growing evidence that 3-D visualization and analysis of medical images have bridged the gap from science to practice—from the computer laboratory to the operating room—heralding a new era in surgery.

7.15 Microscopy Imaging

Application of 3-D visualization and analysis techniques to the field of microscopy has grown significantly in recent years.[49] These techniques have been successfully applied in light and electron microscopy, but the advent of confocal microscopy has led to the rapid growth of 3-D visualization of microscopic structures. Light microscope images digitized directly from the microscope can provide a 3-D volume image by incrementally adjusting the focal plane, usually followed by image processing to deconvolve the image, removing the blurred out-of-focus structures. Similarly, electron microscopy will generate multiple planes by controlling the plane of focus, with further processing necessary for selective focal plane reconstruction. Confocal microscopy, however, uses laser energy with precise optical control to selectively image specific sections within the microscopic structure. Multiple image planes can be selected, providing direct volume image acquisition without the need to remove signal from structures outside of the plane of interest. Often these images are acquired using specific fluorescent dyes to selectively image a particular component of the structure being examined.

Visualization techniques have been used to examine the morphology and function of neurons from selected ganglia in the mammalian peripheral autonomic nervous system.[50] To understand neuron physiology, information about a neuron's shape and dimensions is needed to integrate and localize multiple synaptic inputs. The number and location of selective neurotransmitter receptor sites provides valuable information about the potential response of a neuron to a specific neurotransmitter. These properties of the neuron have been successfully imaged and visualized using ANALYZE™ volume rendering, as in Figure 7.35 (see color figure 52). Laser scanning confocal microscopy was used to acquire images of a neuron from a wholemount preparation of the inferior mesenteric ganglion from a guinea pig. The single neuron was filled with the fluorescent dye Lucifer Yellow, which fluoresces with yellow-wavelength laser light. The ganglion was bathed in a solution containing antibodies against the neurotransmitter vasoactive intestinal polypeptide (VIP), a neuropeptide that functions as an inhibitory transmitter to vascular and nonvascular smooth muscle and as an excitatory transmitter to glandular epithelial cells. The antibodies were conjugated with the photofluor Cy-5, a red dye that fluoresces with red wavelength laser light. The ganglion and solution were then scanned twice with confocal microscopy, once with yellow-wavelength laser followed by a scan with red-wavelength laser, forming two volume images containing the structure of the single neuron and the location of the neurotransmitter VIP, respectively.

The neuron was segmented from the first volume image using simple thresholding with region growing. A binary mask was created from the segmented neuron for application to the VIP volume image. The VIP volume image was processed using 3-D morphological processing to segment out only connected collections of fluorescent dye larger than a prescribed number of voxels using connected component techniques to remove background noise. The binary mask for the neuron was then used to mask and segment only those voxels which constituted the body of the neuron, followed by application of the mask to the VIP volume image to open a hole in which the

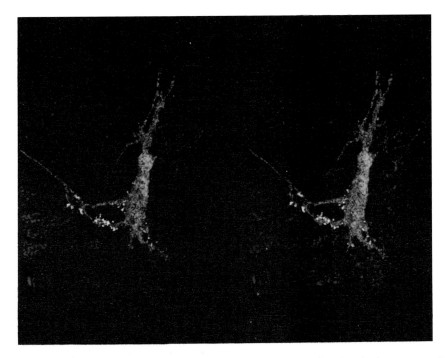

Figure 7.35. Multiple object stereo volume rendering from confocal microscopy of a neuron (yellow) from the inferior mesenteric ganglion bathed in a solution containing labeled VIP neurotransmitter (light blue), demonstrating receptor sites for VIP along the dendrites and somal body of the neuron (red). (Data courtesy of Dr. Joe Szurszewski, Mayo Foundation.) See color figure 52.

neuron voxels were inserted. This resulted in a combined image volume containing the desired structures from the two different fluorescent confocal scans. Objects were created in an object map for this volume corresponding to the neuron, shown in yellow in Figure 7.35, and the surrounding VIP shown in light blue. The volume renderings of these structures were computed as a stereo pair. 3-D region growing within the volume-rendered image was then performed by selecting the body of the neuron and finding any VIP connected to the neuronal body. The connected VIP was then assigned to an independent object and rendered with a red color. Therefore, the resulting renderings shown in Figure 7.35 show both the form of the neuron and indications of its function, demonstrating the location of putative synaptic regions for VIP along the dendrites and somal body of this neuron.

Figure 7.36 (see color figure 53) shows another example of multifluorescent confocal imaging and the resultant 3-D visualizations. These stereo pair 3-D renderings are of an amphipod appendage infected with bacteria. The original image series was collected using scanning laser fluorescent micros-

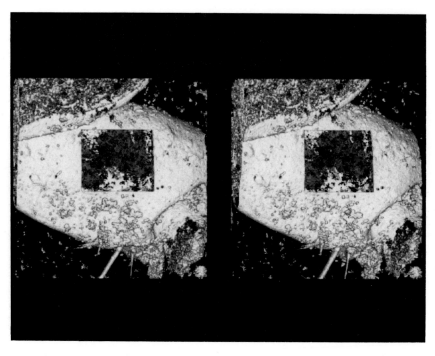

Figure 7.36. Multiple object stereo volume rendering from confocal microscopy of an amphipod appendage (white) infected with bacteria (red), with a cutaway view showing the relationship of the bacteria to the internal muscle (brown). (Data courtesy of Drs. Wilma L. Lingle and Dennis J. O'Kane, Mayo Foundation.) See color figure 53.

copy with propidium iodide as a fluorescent label for the bacteria. The exoskeleton and muscle were autofluorescent in the volume image. The bacteria, muscle, and exoskeleton were segmented using thresholding for each structure. The exoskeleton of the amphipod is shown in white, with a selective subregion cut from the exoskeleton without removing the internal musculature shown in brown and the bacteria shown in red. This was accomplished using separate objects for each of these structures, with the cutout subregion selectively applied to only those voxels which were part of the amphipod exoskeleton.

7.16 Anatomy Teaching

ANALYZE™ is also being used as an educational adjunct to surgery, as illustrated in Figure 7.37 (see color figure 54), providing computer-assisted teaching of anatomy to surgical trainees and residents. Interactive computer-aided teaching sessions on workstations or videodisc can be developed using

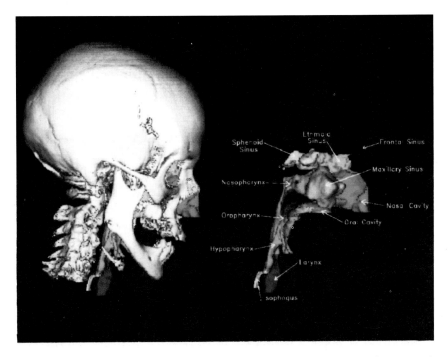

Figure 7.37. ANALYZE™ segmentation and volume rendering techniques can be used for the anatomic education of surgeons and physicians. For example, from cadaveric X-ray CT data of the head, the paranasal sinuses and other air spaces in the head can be segmented and rendered intact in the skull for localization to familiar anatomy (left), or without the skull to visualize internal spaces unobscured (right). Each sinus and air space can be assigned a different color and examined individually or in relation to the other spaces or structures, with labels identifying each component. (Data courtesy of Dr. Stephen Carmichael, Mayo Foundation.) See color figure 54.

extensive screen editing tools and sequence scripting. Static and dynamic displays produced using real 3-D imagery provide significant advantages over conceptual illustrations of anatomy, being closer to the real thing. Such 3-D presentations, when supported with realistic displays, faithful editing techniques, and accurate measuring tools as described in previous chapters, may replace or at least importantly augment anatomy teaching as traditionally accomplished using cadaver dissection. For those who might scoff at such a notion, arguing that such visualization experiences cannot provide the tactile learning associated with such "morbid" experience, the specter of virtual reality looms in answer on the horizon.[51] Virtual reality systems of the near future will feature sensory input and feedback, including visual, auditory, olfactory, and tactile, as well as realistic dynamic 3-D displays. The "virtual cadaver" is just around the corner. Educational systems using high-resolution 3-D imaging and virtual reality, augmented with natural language user query and system response functions, will constitute powerful and important uses of these techniques in the twenty-first century.

7.17 References

1. Thatcher, R. W., Hallett, M., Zeffiero, T., John, E. R., Huerta, M. (Eds.) *Functional Neuroimaging: Technical Foundations*. Academic Press, San Diego, CA, 1984.

2. Robb, R. A. "Visualization methods for analysis of multimodality images." In: Thatcher, R. W., Hallett, M., Zeffiero, T., John, E. R., Huerta, M. (Eds.) *Functional Neuroimaging: Technical Foundations*. Academic Press, San Diego, CA, 1984.

3. Connelly, A., Jackson, G. D., Frackowiak, R. S. J., et al. "High-resolution functional mapping of activated human primary cortex using a clinical magnetic resonance imaging system." *Radiology*, 188, 125–130, 1993.

4. Thompson, R. M., Jack, C. R., Butts, R. K., Hanson, D. P., et al. "Imaging of cerebral activation at 1.5T: optimizing a technique for conventional hardware." *Radiology*, 190, 873–877, 1994.

5. Jack, C. R., Thompson, R. M., Butts, R. K., et al. "Sensory motor cortex: correlation or presurgical mapping with functional MR imaging and invasive cortical mapping." *Radiology*, 190, 85–92, 1994.

6. Thulborn, K. R., Waterton, J. C., Matthews, P. M., et al. "Oxygenation dependence of the transverse relaxation time of water protons in whole blood at high field." *Biochem. Biophys. Acta*, 714, 265–270, 1982.

7. Ogawa, S., Lee, T. M., Kay, A. R., et al. "Brain magnetic resonance imaging with contrast dependent on blood oxygenation." *Proc. Natl. Acad. Sci. USA*, 87, 9868–9872, 1990.

8. Fox, P. T., Raichle, M. R. "Focal physiological uncoupling of cerebral blood flow and oxidative metabolism during somatosensory stimulation in human subjects." *Proc. Natl. Acad. Sci. USA*, 83, 1140–1144, 1986.

9. Robb, R. A. "Interactive and quantitative analysis of biomedical images." In: Kelly, P. J., Kall, B. A. (Eds.) *Computers in Stereotactic Neurosurgery*. Blackwell Scientific Publications, Cambridge, MA, 1992, Chapter 2, pp. 17–32.

10. Kelly, P. J., Kall, B. A. (Eds.) *Computers in Stereotactic Neurosurgery*. Blackwell Scientific Publications, Cambridge, MA, 1992.

11. Cascino, G. D., Jack, C. R., Parisi, J. E., Sharbrough, F. W., Hirschorn, K. A., Meyer, F. B., Marsh, W. R., O'Brien, P. C. "MRI-based volume studies in temporal lobe epilepsy: pathological correlations." *Ann. Neurol.*, 30, 31–36, 1991.

12. Robb, R. A., Camp, J. J. "A paradigm for using multispectral images in evaluating tumor response to treatment." *XIIIth International Conference on Information Processing in Medical Imaging Conference*, Northern Arizona University, June 14–18, 1993.

13. Mohan, R., Barest, G., Brewster, L. J., Chui, C. S., Kutcher, G. J., Laughlin, J. S., Fuks, Z. "A comprehensive three-dimensional radiation treatment planning system." *Int. J. Rad. Oncol. Biol. Phys.*, 15, 481–495, 1988.

14. Goitein, M. "Limitations of two-dimensional treatment planning programs." *Med. Phys.*, 9, 580–587, 1982.

15. Fraas, B. A., McShan, D. L., Diaz, R. F., Ten Haken, R. K., Aisen, A., Gebarski, S., Glazer, G., Licter, A. S. "Integration of Magnetic Resonance Imaging into Radiation Therapy Treatment Planning. I. Technical Considerations." *Int. J. Rad. Biol. Phys.*, 13, 1897–1908, 1987.

16. Kessler, M. D., Pitluck, S., Petti, P., Castro, J. R. "Integration of multimodality imaging data for radiotherapy treatment planning." *Int. J. Rad. Biol. Phys.*, 21, 1653–1667, 1991.

17. Sherouse, G. W., Bourland, J. D., Reynolds, K., McMurry, H. L., Mitchell, T. P., Chaney, E. L. "Virtual simulation in the clinical setting: Some practical considerations." *Int. J. Rad. Oncol. Biol. Phys.*, 19, 1059–1065, 1990.

18. "Radiotherapy Treatment Planning Tools Collaborative Working Group, Technical Report" 91-2, Purdy, J., Chaney, E., Kalet, PIs, NCI contract numbers N01-CM097564, 97565, 97566.

19. Drzymala, R. E., Mohan, R., Brewster, L., Chu, J., Goitein, M., Harms, W., Urie, M. "Dose-volume histograms." *Int. J. Rad. Biol. Phys.*, 21, 71–78, 1991.

20. Bourland, J. D., Camp, J. J., Robb, R. A. "Volume rendering: application in static field conformal radiosurgery." In: Robb, R. A. (Ed.) *Proceedings of Visualization in Biomedical Computing 1992.* SPIE, Vol. 1808, Chapel Hill, NC, October 13–16, 1992.

21. Vannier, M. W., Marsh, J. L., Warren, J. O. "Three-dimensional CT reconstruction images for craniofacial surgical planning and evaluation." *Radiology*, 150, 179–184, 1984.

22. Bite, U., Jackson, I. T. "The use of three-dimensional CT scanning in planning head and neck reconstruction." *Plastic Surgical Forum, Vol. VIII.* Annual meeting of the American Society of Plastic and Reconstructive Surgeons, Kansas City, MO, 1985.

23. Vannier, M. W., Yates, R. E., Whitestone, J. "Electric imaging of the human body." In: Robb, R. A. (Ed.) *Proceedings of Visualization in Biomedical Computing 1992.* SPIE, Vol. 1808, Chapel Hill, NC, October 13–16, 1992.

24. Kikinis, R., Cline, H. E., Altobelli, D., Halle, M. W., Lorensen, W. E., Jolesz, F. A. "Interactive visualization and manipulation of 3-D reconstructions for the planning of surgical procedures." In: Robb, R. A. (Ed.) *Proceedings of Visualization in Biomedical Computing 1992.* SPIE, Vol. 1808, Chapel Hill, NC, October 13–16, 1992.

25. Fukuta, K., Jackson, I. T., McEwan, C. N., Meland, N. B. "Three-dimensional imaging in craniofacial surgery: a review of the role of mirror image production." *Eur. J. Plastic Surg.*, 13, 209–217, 1990.

26. Marsh, J. L., Vannier, M. W., Bresina, S. J., Hemmer, K. M. "Applications of computer graphics in craniofacial surgery." *Clin. Plastic Surg.*, 13, 441, 1986.

27. Bell, W. H. (Ed.) *Modern Practice in Orthognathic and Reconstructive Surgery.* Saunders, Philadelphia, 1992.

28. Katzberg, R. W. "Temporomandibular joint imaging." *Radiology*, 170, 297–307, 1989.

29. Fishman, E. K., Ney, D. R., Magid, D. "Three-dimensional imaging: clinical applications in orthopedics." In: Höhne, K. H., Fuchs, H., Pizer, S. M. (Eds.) *3D-Imaging in Medicine: Algorithms, Systems, Applications.* Vol. 60 of NATO ASI Series F, pp. 425–440, Springer-Verlag, Berlin, 1990.

30. *Digital Imaging in Orthopaedic Surgery: A Dialogue Between Physicians and Engineers.* Interactive Symposium, St. Petersburg, FL, 1990.

31. Chao, E. Y. S., Ivins, J. C. (Eds.) *The Design and Application of Tumor Prostheses for Bone and Joint Reconstruction.* Thieme-Stratton, New York, 1983.

32. Peterson, H. A. "Partial growth plate arrest and its treatment." *J. Pediat. Orthoped.,* 4, 246–258, 1984.

33. Ritman, E. L., Robb, R. A., Wood, E. H. "Synchronous volumetric imaging for non-invasive vivisection of cardiovascular and respiratory dynamics: evolution and current perspectives." In: Brandenburg, R. O., Fuster, V., Giuliani, E. R., McGoon, D. C. *Cardiology—Fundamentals and Practice.* Year Book Medical Publishers, Chicago, 1987, Chapter 63, pp. 1968–1984.

34. Breen, J. F., Sheedy, P. F., Schwartz, R. S., Stanson, A. W., Kaufmann, R. B., Moll, P. P., Rumberger, J. A. "Coronary artery calcification detected with ultrafast CT as an indication of coronary artery disease." *Cardiac Radiol.,* 185, 435–439, 1992.

35. Higgins, C. B., Caputo, G. R. "Acquired heart disease." In: Hricak, H., Helms, C. (Eds.) *Magnetic Resonance Imaging of the Body.* 2nd Ed. Raven Press, New York, 1992.

36. Cooke, C. D., Garcia, E. V., Folks, R. D., Peifer, J. W. "Three-dimensional visualization of cardiac single-photon-emission computed-tomography studies." In: Robb, R. A. (Ed.) *Proceedings of Visualization in Biomedical Computing 1992.* SPIE, Vol. 1808, Chapel Hill, NC, October 13–16, 1992.

37. Belohlavek, M., Foley, D. A., Gerber, T. C., Kinter, T. M., Greenleaf, J. F., Seward, J. B. "Three- and four-dimensional cardiovascular ultrasound imaging: A new era for echocardiography." *Mayo Clinic Proc.,* 68, 221–240, 1993.

38. Robb, R. A., Hoffman, E. A., Sinak, L. J., Harris, L. D., Ritman, E. L. "High-speed three-dimensional x-ray computed tomography: The Dynamic Spatial Reconstructor." *Proc. IEEE,* 71, 308–319, 1983.

39. Ritman, E. L., Robb, R. A., Harris, L. *Imaging Physiological Functions.* Praeger Scientific, New York, 1985.

40. Quinn, S. F., Franzini, D. A., Demlow, T. A., Rosencrantz, D. R., Kim, J., Hanna, R. M., Szumowski, J. "MR imaging of prostate cancer with an endorectal surface coil technique: correlation with whole-mount specimens." *Radiology,* 190, 323–327, 1994.

41. Cootes, T. F., Hill, A., Taylor, C. J., Haslam, J. "The use of active shape models for locating structures in medical images." *Proceedings of the 13th Annual Conference on Information Processing in Medical Imaging,* Flagstaff, AZ, June 1993, pp. 33–47.

42. Alvarado, J. A., Murphy, C. G. "Outflow obstruction in pigmentary and primary open angle glaucoma." *Arch. Ophthalmol.,* 110, 1769–1778, 1992.

43. Maguire, L. J., Bourne, W. M. "Corneal topography of transverse keratotomies for astigmatism after penetrating keratoplasty." *Am. J. Ophthalmol.,* 107, 323, 1989.

44. McDonnell, P. J., McClusky, D. J., Garbus, J. J. "Corneal topography and fluctuating visual acuity after radial keratotomy." *Ophthalmology,* 96, 665, 1989.

45. Wyzinski, P., O'Dell, L. "Subjective and objective findings after radial keratotomy." *Ophthalmology,* 96, 1608, 1989.

46. Gormley, D. J., Gersten, M., Koplin, R. S., Lubkin, V. "Corneal modeling." *Cornea,* 7, 30, 1988.

47. Camp, J. J., Maguire, L. J., Cameron, B. M., Robb, R. A. "A computer model for the evaluation of the effect of corneal topography on optical performance." *Am. J. Ophthalmol.,* 109, 379–386, 1990.

48. Camp, J. J., Maguire, L. J., Robb, R. A. "An efficient ray tracing algorithm for modeling visual performance from corneal topography." *Proceedings of the First Conference on Visualization in Biomedical Computing*, Atlanta, GA, May 22–25, 1990.

49. Kriete, A. (Ed.) *Visualization in Biomedical Microscopies*. VCH Publishers, Germany, 1992.

50. Miller, S. M., Schmalz, P., Ermilov, L., et al. "Three-dimensional structure of neurons from peripheral autonomic ganglia using confocal microscope images." *Proceedings of Visualization in Biomedical Computing 1992, SPIE*, Vol. 1808, 640–650.

51. Robb, R. A. "Surgery simulation and virtual reality workshop." In: *Proceedings of Virtual Reality Meets Medicine II*, San Diego, CA, 1994.

8

Summary and Prognostications

We shall not cease from exploration, and the end of all our exploring, will be to arrive where we started, and know the place for the first time.

T. S. Eliot

8.1 Overview of Current Approaches and Systems

The advances in medical imaging capabilities since 1970 have been developed, applied, and accepted at a volume and pace unprecedented in medical history. Computer and digital radiographic technology and techniques have significantly expanded the possibilities for accurate, quantitative, and noninvasive visualization and measurement of intracorporeal morphology and function. These advances have provided a variety of new diagnostic methodologies for clinical evaluation of health and disease. 3-D imaging is emerging as the method of choice in many clinical examinations, replacing some previously routine procedures, and significantly complementing others. The continuing evolution of 3-D imaging promises even greater capabilities for accurate noninvasive clinical diagnoses and treatment, as well as for quantitative biological investigations and scientific exploration, targeted at ever increasing our understanding of the human condition and how to improve it.

3-D imaging modalities based on a variety of energy sources, including X-ray, radionuclide emissions, ultrasound, and nuclear magnetic resonance have demonstrated significant practical clinical utility. The variety of disease processes and abnormalities affecting all regions of the human body are so numerous and different that each imaging modality possesses some attribute(s) that makes it uniquely helpful in providing the desired understanding or discrimination of the disease or abnormality, and therefore no single method has prevailed to the complete exclusion of others. The advantages and limitations of each modality are primarily associated with the specific

273

implementation of the basic governing physical and mathematical principles involved, and with the particular medical or biological applications sought. However, in the most general sense, the methodologies are complementary, together providing a powerful new armamentarium of clinical diagnostic and biomedical research capabilities which has advanced and will continue to significantly advance the practice of medicine and the frontiers of biological understanding.

Table 8.1 provides a brief summary of the major attributes of some imaging modalities discussed in this book, as well as an indication of certain desirable and apparently achievable future advances. Table 8.1 is not intended to provide direct categorical comparisons among the different imaging methods, since such comparisons cannot be valid unless an equitable accommodation is made of the variety of factors that influence and change the imaging characteristics of each modality. In particular, the resolution values given in Table 8.1 are intended to be representative of those achievable under practical operating conditions, but these may vary considerably from system to system, even of the same modality type. There are always trade-offs in the performance and application of imaging systems, so that maximum resolution in the spatial, contrast (sensitivity), and time dimensions is generally not simultaneously achievable. For example, longer scan times may improve spatial and contrast resolution if there is no object movement during the scan. Conversely, short scan times may give better-quality images of moving objects. Also noteworthy about Table 8.1 is that harmful biological effects do not generally occur at the diagnostic dose levels employed in medical imaging. Therefore, Table 8.1 indicates only the possible effects of excessive doses, or perhaps accumulative doses, of the energies used in the various imaging methods.

The ability to extract objective and quantitatively accurate information from 3-D biomedical images has struggled to keep pace with the ability to produce the images themselves. This is somewhat of a paradox, since on the one hand the new 3-D imaging capabilities promise significant potential for providing greater specificity and sensitivity (i.e., precise objective discrimination and accurate quantitative measurement of body tissue characteristics and function) in clinical diagnostic and basic investigative imaging procedures than ever before possible, but on the other hand, the momentous advances in computer and associated electronic imaging technology which have made these 3-D imaging capabilities possible have only recently been developed for full exploitation of these capabilities. The long-sought horizon has been reached—that of efficient capabilities to extract and analyze the intrinsic and relevant information contained in multidimensional image data, that is, the true morphologic, pathologic, biologic, physiologic, and/or metabolic "meaning" of the numbers produced by 3-D imaging modalities.

Powerful new microcomputer-based systems and software packages have been integrated into networks that permit many simultaneous detailed investigations and evaluation of 3-D and 4-D (dynamic 3-D) biomedical im-

Table 8.1. Comparison of Some Attributes of Different 3-D Imaging Modalities

	Spatial Resolution (mm)	Contrast Sensitivity (%)	Scan Time (sec)	Measured Parameters	Biological Effects	Medical Applications	Principal Limitations	Future Improvements
Digital Radiography	~ 0.1	~ 5 (attenuation relative to H₂O)	.03	X-ray absorption, contrast distribution	Ionization of cells	Bone abnormalities, vascular problems, artherosclerosis, cardiac flows	Structure superposition (not 3-D), contrast sensitivity	Quantitative i.v. angiography
CT	~ 0.5	~ 0.5 (attenuation relative to H₂O)	2	X-ray attenuation, electron density, average atomic number	Ionization of cells	Central nervous system disorders, spinal cord problems, abdominal masses and infections, soft tissue tumors	Scan time, beam hardening, soft tissue sensitivity	High-speed, full 3-D scans (60/sec, 200 simultaneous, adjacent 0.5-mm sections)
MRI	~ 1	~ 0.1 (T₂ spin-lattice relaxation)	200	Nuclide relaxations and concentrations, proton density	Electrophysiologic disturbances	Degenerative brain disease, neoplasms, infections, ischemia, edematous conditions	Scan time, number of ubiquitous naturally occurring magnetic nuclides	Improved spatial resolution, faster scans, functional imaging
SPECT	~ 5	~ 5 (counts relative to radioactivity)	300	Gamma source distribution and magnitude, radionuclide concentration	Ionization of cells	Bone cancer, liver and gallbladder disease, brain lesions, myocardial infarction	Scan time, body attenuation, spatial resolution, radioisotopes	Faster scans, improved sensitivity
PET	~ 5	~ 3 (Counts relative to radioactivity)	30	Gamma source distribution and magnitude, radionuclide concentration	Ionization of cells	Metabolic processes, brain glucose activity, brain tumors, myocardial ischemia	Scan time, body attenuation, number of radiosotopes (cyclotron required), spatial resolution	Improved efficiency, time-of-flight accuracy
Ultrasound	~ 1	~ 0.00001 (fractional acoustic velocity)	100	Acoustic velocity, impedance, attenuation, and frequency shift	Thermal heating, cavitation	Obstetrics, breast cancer, testicular cancer, cardiac function	Scan time, ray bending (refraction and diffraction), spatial resolution	Faster scans, ray tracing methods

ages. Modern computer networks are "intelligent" managers for efficient allocation of resources and ready access to all the information available in large 3-D image databases, facilitating rapid display, manipulation, and measurement of those data. Advanced imaging software provides important capabilities for visualizing, editing, and quantitatively analyzing both structural and functional information and their relationships in various organs of the body. Although the overall power of the networked approach comes from the synergistic integration and utilization of a variety of computational components, the architecture also fosters development of advanced image processing software which is transportable to stand-alone workstations.

Integrated systems (computers and software) for the analysis of 2-D, 3-D, and 4-D (and beyond) images are available in both the commercial and research markets. As yet, no system has appeared that has entirely satisfied the needs of both biomedical research and clinical applications. The reason for this may be that the focuses of the two areas have been different. The medical imaging systems and hence the commercial image analysis workstations have been largely targeted at the practice of radiology, where it may be sufficient to simply visualize structures within the body. This philosophy has spawned the development of the so-called PACS (picture archiving and communications system), which aims to duplicate the capabilities of a film-based radiology department but without the use of film. This limited focus has diluted enthusiasm for generalized use of such systems, particularly in view of the high cost required to achieve the desired performance. Emerging systems are now available that are aimed at medical specialties uniquely or in conjunction with radiology. For example, several companies sell workstations or services that are designed for surgery planning. A variety of image analysis workstations have been developed for a range of research applications. These systems vary widely in their goals and capabilities. Some of the systems have been designed to handle volume images from a variety of sources and so could find application in a variety of medical circumstances.

8.2 New Concepts

The effective extraction of accurate quantitative information from 3-D and 4-D images requires new conceptual approaches and methodologies in image processing. Multidimensional image analysis is largely an exploratory process, directed at understanding better the nature of the object imaged. There are essentially three major tasks associated with any analysis of biomedical imagery: 1) display, 2) editing, and 3) measurement. These tasks are inter-related, often overlapping, and coexist in a rather classical channel of feedback, feed-forward information passing. The capabilities of a multidimensional image analysis system should be fine-tuned to effectively facilitate these tasks and to provide adroit exploration of all relationships (i.e., structural and functional) existing within the data.

The traditional sequential approach to interactive image analysis is illustrated in Panel A of Figure 8.1. The general purpose of such analysis is to optimize the parameters of some "image transformation," Ti, so that the observer (who applies his own mental transform) can "understand" the image. The critical element of such a concept in both 2-D and 3-D image processing is interactive feedback, allowing the human operator to control some or all of the transformation parameters.

Panel B in Figure 8.1 includes the image transformation produced by the display. Although computers can "understand" 3-D images as 3-D arrays of numbers, humans cannot usefully understand numerical representations as images. In order to present this numerical information meaningfully to humans, a "display transformation," Td, is introduced into the system. This transformation (which includes both a conceptual and a physical element) may often be as complex as the image transformation, but is in general a better-behaved and better-understood function. Nonetheless, if this transformation is to be as useful as possible, the operator must have control of its parameters as well. The observer evaluates what the transformation has accomplished and ascertains if it helps convey or elucidate the information desired. This implies not only that the observer knows what he wants to happen, but that he understands what the transformation actually has done

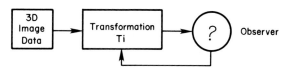

A. Sequential Single Transformation Model

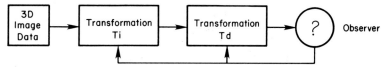

B. Sequential Multiple Transformation Model

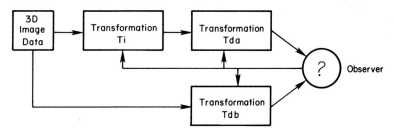

C. Parallel Multiple Transformation Model

Figure 8.1. Three conceptual models for interactive display and analysis of 3-D image data.

to the original data. In the traditional sequential approach applied to a 3-D medical image, this task is analogous to understanding the 3-D structure of an organ by sequentially viewing parallel adjacent slices through the organ, such as is often done in CT imaging. Not only must the observer "know what he wants" (i.e., that these slices together represent an organ with which he is familiar), but he must also mentally reconstruct the separate sectional views of the structure into its complete continuous form.

Panel C of Figure 8.1 introduces the parallel version of interactive image analysis. In this framework, the importance of understanding the transformation, Ti, is explicitly addressed by presenting the operator simultaneous "before and after" views of the image. The difference between the sequential and parallel methods may be compared to the difference between driving an automobile toward a given destination with and without a road map. Not knowing the route results in a random, time-consuming exercise to get from here to there, while using a road map to select the optimal route results in saving of time and reasonable assurance of accuracy in reaching the goal.

The parallel image analysis method includes a divergent case, where Tda and Tdb are conceptually and physically separate. However, conceptually different display methods may be combined on the same physical display device and still fit the model. The central concept is that *3-D image analysis is largely an exploratory task,* and efficient tools for permitting data visualization, processing, reduction, and measurement are critical to the effective performance of this task. The important mechanism associated with this concept is that the observer is allowed to interactively modify the image and be presented "before and after" views of the effects of such modulation.

Turning from conceptual to practical considerations, one must recognize that the large volume of data to be processed in multimodal, multidimensional biomedical image analysis requires simultaneous and efficient management of input/output and computation. This may now be accomplished using distributed processing approaches which are concomitantly *less expensive and more powerful* than large mainframe or supercomputer systems. The significant advances in the microelectronic industry have fostered the distributed processing approach for large-scale computing, and made computers much more useful as tools. Attention to design of system network architecture and utilization of current state-of-the-art microprocessor technology makes this possible. A multidimensional image database can be very large, especially when extended to 4-D (e.g., sets of 3-D images related through time). Therefore, movement of data in the system must take place as efficiently as possible, and data information structures need to be shared between analysis functions to limit the frequency of transfers. This can be done through the use of shared memory segments large enough to hold the entire 3-D image or with software that performs efficient image memory paging. Interactive manipulation of large 3-D images also requires an efficient method for archival image storage and retrieval.

Efficient computation of image transformations is facilitated by maintaining the entire 3-D image in the system memory. Modern computers have large memory banks. Rapid computation and display of the multidimensional data permits highly interactive visual feedback mechanisms to guide the analysis process. The graphics display system needs to be integrally interfaced to the system for high-speed transfers of image data and graphics functions. The display resolution must allow, at a minimum, one image at full size to be displayed, along with some other graphics and text, and ideally should allow for multiple image display at full size, with related graphics and/or text included.

Rapid, multiformat image display and highly interactive graphics are crucial to and should be included in all aspects of multidimensional image analysis. For this reason, the design of the user interface is extremely important to the success of the system.[1] The user interface should be friendly and intuitive and should be supported by a well-designed (ergonomic) station with conveniently arranged display and input device(s). A conceptual approach to designing effective user interfaces[1] for 3-D biomedical imaging applications includes:

1. *Early Focus on Users*. Designers must make direct contact with intended users, to understand the cognitive, behavioral, attitudinal, and anthropometric characteristics and the characteristics of the activities they will perform with the system.
2. *Integrated Design*. All aspects of usability, including the user interface, the help system, training and documentation, etc., should evolve in parallel, rather than be defined sequentially, and should be integrated with each other.
3. *Early and Continual User Testing*. An empirical approach is required, involving observation and measurement of user behavior, careful evaluation of user feedback, insightful solutions to challenges and problems, and strong motivation to make design changes that will increase usability.
4. *Iterative Design*. The system must be continually modified based on the results of behavior functional analysis, user interface, help system, and documentation. The process of implementation, testing, feedback, evaluation, and change should be iteratively applied.

Specifically, the user interface design task should include:

1. Application analysis, involving a determination of the required functions and an analysis of the needs and abilities of the intended users;
2. Dialog design, involving the general design of the virtual world that the system will present to users, including the interaction paradigm, interface metaphors, information presentation framework, and information access, navigation, and transformation methods;
3. Graphic design, involving the specific design of screens, menus, use of color and typeface, and the design of dialogs and interface elements;

4. Iterative user interface prototyping and implementation, involving the implementation of the user interface and function access modules during the dialog design and graphic design phases; and
5. Usability evaluation, including iterative testing and revision.

The rate of evolution and acceptance of 3-D biomedical imaging systems will be increasingly dependent on effective, compliant, and extensible user interfaces. In the near term these will be carefully customized and implemented with user-specific needs and style in mind, but there are exciting prospects for a single universal interface for multiple applications that will greatly facilitate the uniform delivery of health care and sharing of health care resources, resulting in significant savings in health care costs.

8.3 Future Directions

It is perhaps of value to consider where the recent impressive and continuing advances in biomedical imaging capabilities are leading, and how they fit into the overall future picture of diagnostic medicine and associated biological disciplines. Without question, the cutting edge in these disciplines and most other aspects of the biomedical sciences is increasingly in the molecular biochemical and biophysical spheres, and quite certainly the most important advances during the foreseeable future will be in the realms of molecular and genetic engineering.

However, the increases in biomedical investigative power being provided by current imaging modalities to obtain dynamic quantitative images of structural–functional relationships within organs and organ systems by minimally invasive methods will provide the basis for the last frontier of continued important advances in these disciplines, at least in the macroscopic realm. It is a reasonable prediction that further development and exploitation of these techniques will be of continuing importance, but increasingly significant future advances will most probably be at the molecular and submolecular rather than at macroscopic anatomic and functional levels.

Perhaps the most exciting development in this regard will be the ability to image (measure) accurately the spatial distribution and magnitude of any *selected chemical element* or metabolic function in any region of the body. This challenging, but not impossible, extension of the state-of-art in medical imaging might be called "tomochemistry" or "biochemical imaging." Given 1) a selectable and tunable energy source for which the direction of its output beam is accurately known and whose spectral nature could be varied as desired, and 2) an array of miniature detectors surrounding the torso so that the energy emanating from the body induced by the known, fully characterized energy source could be accurately measured, it would be possible to obtain accurate 3-D reconstructions not only of the anatomic structures within the transradiated portions of the torso, but also of the distribution of a variety of selected chemical elements or biologic materials within the tissues of the body under study.

These possibilities for chemical imaging using energies like X-rays or gamma rays may be illustrated by the following general equation for absorption of radiation:

$$S_{jp} = \int I_{ojp}(\lambda) W_p(\lambda) \exp[-iL_{pi\ k}C_{ki}\mu_k(\lambda)]d\lambda$$

in which S_{jp} represents the responses of a particular detector output, p is the index of the ray path for this particular detector, j is the index of the spectral nature of the radiant energy source, i is the index of the geometric elements (e.g., cubic voxels) which ray p traverses within the object, and k is the index of the chemical element in voxel i. I_{ojp} is the intensity of radiation incident on the body, $W_p(\lambda)$ is the efficiency of the detector, L_{pi} is the path length of ray p in voxel i, C_{ki} is the concentration of the kth chemical element in voxel i, and $\mu_k(\lambda)$ is the appropriate coefficient of absorption for the kth chemical element.

This equation indicates that both the spectral content and the amount of radiation incident upon and transmitted by the object must be determined for chemical-element-selective reconstruction. This may be done under properly chosen boundary conditions, in which repeated measurements of S_{jp} are made with various conditions imposed upon I_{ojp}. For example, if I_{ojp} represents a monochromatic photon energy for each value of j, then the corresponding set of integral equations reduces to a set of algebraic equations which may be solved.

Application of this equation, however, requries the use of new types of radiant energy sources and/or energy-selective detectors. Even though the state-of-the-art in radiant energy sources and energy-selective detectors does not permit practical application, both do exist in experimental laboratories. For example, rapid progress is being made in the field of laser X-rays. Furthermore, miniature radiation detectors with adequate energy-discriminating and signal-to-noise characteristics are being developed. Thus, fabrication of a clinically useful 3-D reconstruction machine with both anatomic structural and chemical composition sensing capabilities is possible in the near future. The "ideal" 3-D imaging system would provide *simultaneously* and *rapidly* all of the advantages and eliminate all of the limitations of the different imaging modalities described in this book and other work.[2-8] Although it is difficult to conceive of such a system, certain combinations have already been investigated and used. For example, X-ray CT and emission CT are sometimes used in tandem in radiation treatment therapy planning. MRI and X-ray CT are used in surgical planning. MRI and PET are used in central nervous system studies of disease and behavior.

Major segments of the biological sciences and the practice of medicine are based on study and knowledge of the relationships of anatomic structure to biological function. Traditionally this knowledge has been gained either by influence or by direct surgical vivisection or by postmortem examinations. These types of direct visualization and study of anatomic structure and function of internal organ systems in man have, up to the present, been the preserve of the surgeon and pathologist. The revolutionary capabilities provided by the new 3-D imaging modalities for obtaining similar information noninvasively, nondestructively, and painlessly will provide these data to the internist and surgeon for reproducible examinations of individual patients without disturbing the physiology of the organ system under study or altering its normal integration into the physiology of the body as a whole.

With the expected continuing advances in miniaturization of powerful computing and electronic sensing elements in the solid-state microelectronics industry, the ultimate imaging device may one day resemble the hand-held comprehensive diagnostic instruments used by "Bones" McCoy, the physician on the Star Fleet spaceship Enterprise in the popular science-fiction saga, *Star Trek*. Dr. McCoy simply points the scanning device at the body and the complete anatomic, physiological, biochemical, and metabolic status of the subject is instantaneously determined and displayed.

The extent to which such science-fiction capabilities may ultimately be achieved is speculation, but it is evident that twenty-first-century medicine will represent a culmination of continuing evolutionary progress in multidimensional imaging methods. Well before such "galactic technology" is in place, the medical and scientific communities, and indeed the human race at large, can expect to benefit in improved health care from a continuum of marvelous synergistic advances in imaging technology, particularly 3-D biomedical imaging systems, as well as from new imaging methodologies and paradigms yet to be conceived.

8.4 References

1. Gould, J., Boies, S., Lewis, C. "Making usable, useful, productivity-enhancing computer applications." *Communications of the ACM*, January 1991, pp. 74–85.

2. Robb, R. A. *Three-Dimensional Biomedical Imaging. Vol. I & II*. CRC Press, Boca Raton, FL, 1985.

3. Udupa, J. K., Herman, G. T. *3D Imaging in Medicine*. CRC Press, Boca Raton, FL, 1991.

4. Höhne, K. H., Fuchs, H., Pizer, S. M. *3D Imaging in Medicine, Algorithms, Systems, Applications*. NATO ASI Series, Series F: Computer and Systems Sciences, Vol. 60, Springer-Verlag, Berlin, Heidelberg, 1990.

5. *Proceedings of Visualization in Biomedical Computing 1992*. SPIE, Vol. 1808, Chapel Hill, NC, October 13–16, 1992.

6. Kriete, A. *Visualization in Biomedical Microscopies, 3-D Imaging and Computer Applications*. VCH Publishers, Germany, 1992.

7. Kelly, P. J., Kall, B. A. *Computers in Stereotactic Neurosurgery*. Blackwell Scientific Publications, Boston, MA, 1992.

8. Thatcher, R. W., Hallett, M., Zeffiro, T., John, E. R., Huerta, M. (Eds.) *Functional Neuroimaging: Technical Foundations*. Academic Press, San Diego, CA, 1994.

Index